W9-AUY-118

COMPLEX ADOPTION AND ASSISTED REPRODUCTIVE TECHNOLOGY

SOCIAL WORK PRACTICE WITH CHILDREN AND FAMILIES
Nancy Boyd Webb, *Series Editor*

Complex Adoption and Assisted Reproductive Technology: A Developmental Approach to Clinical Practice
Vivian B. Shapiro
Janet R. Shapiro
Isabel H. Paret

Child Development: A Practitioner's Guide
Douglas Davies

Group Work with Adolescents: Principles and Practice
Andrew Malekoff

Social Work Practice with Children
Nancy Boyd Webb

Complex Adoption and Assisted Reproductive Technology

A Developmental Approach to Clinical Practice

VIVIAN B. SHAPIRO
JANET R. SHAPIRO
ISABEL H. PARET

Foreword by Nancy Boyd Webb

THE GUILFORD PRESS
New York London

A Division of Guilford Publications, Inc.
72 Spring Street, New York, NY 10012
www.guilford.com

Printed in the United States of America

This book is printed on acid-free paper.

Last digit is print number: 9 8 7 6 5 4 3 2 1

Library of Congress Cataloging-in-Publication Data available from the Publisher.

ISBN 1-57230-628-7

About the Authors

Vivian B. Shapiro, PhD, is Emeritus Professor of Social Work, The School of Social Work, The University of Michigan. Dr. Shapiro helped found the Infant Mental Health Association in Michigan, and is in practice in Princeton, New Jersey. Her research and publications have focused on the treatment of children at risk and the use of narrative theory in practice with nontraditional families. Her current clinical work includes treatment of children in international and complex adoption.

Janet R. Shapiro, MSW, PhD, is Assistant Professor and Alexandra Grange Hawkins Lecturer at the Bryn Mawr College Graduate School of Social Work and Social Research. Dr. Shapiro's teaching, clinical work, and research have focused on the translation of developmental theory to practice with special populations of children and families. In particular, her research and clinical work is centered on social and emotional development in infancy and early childhood, with special emphasis on relational development in atypical populations.

Isabel Paret, PhD, is Clinical Associate Professor in the Department of Psychiatry, Robert Wood Johnson Medical School, UMDNJ, and supervises at the Graduate School of Applied Professional Psychology, Rutgers University. Dr. Paret is a member of the executive council of the Association for Child Psychoanalysis, Inc., and a board member of the New Jersey Association for Infant Mental Health. She is in private practice in Princeton, New Jersey, and has published in the clinical literature.

Foreword

As we enter the new millennium, practitioners must be prepared to provide services to an evolving group of children and families with distinctive histories that complicate and challenge their lives. Although the many new ways of forming families—including open adoption, international/transcultural adoption, and kinship care, in addition to a variety of assisted methods of reproduction—help many parents succeed in their efforts to have a child, often parents are unprepared for the complicated aftermath that may accompany these forms of collaborative parenthood. Difficulties in bonding may present problems for both the child and the parents related to parental expectations and fears, differing backgrounds and cultures, and even outside responses to "families of difference."

This book breaks new ground in bringing together the overlapping psychological, sociological, and legal implications associated with various new forms of parentage. Vivian B. Shapiro, Janet R. Shapiro, and Isabel H. Paret have skillfully woven together the complicated issues for children and families who must forge an identity that incorporates the unique circumstances of each child's history. The authors have identified an important new field of social work practice with families and children who need a range of supportive services, including medical, legal, and psychological. Many of these families will require ongoing support as they deal with a growing child whose biological heritage may be unknown or only partly known to them.

I am delighted to have this book as part of Guilford's Social Work Practice with Children and Families series. It successfully employs a developmental/ecological perspective that emphasizes the importance of attachment as the cornerstone of human relationships. Rich clinical examples illustrate the challenge of identity formation, for both the child and the family, raised by the child's and the parents' history and the distinct personal meaning of that history. The question of whether, how much, and when to tell the child about his/her background finds expression through the construction of a personal narrative for the child and the family. Chapter 10, on the use of assisted reproductive technology by single, gay, and lesbian parents, points to the necessity of constructing a narrative for the child about his/her birth history that conforms to the parents' judgment about how much to reveal.

A recurring theme in the book concerns the expanded sense of "family." For example, an in-depth case study in Chapter 4 poignantly deals with the impact of delayed adoption on a child, the prospective adoptive parent, and the child's biological mother. Family therapists will appreciate the multilevel focus on all individuals who contribute, openly or secretly, to a child's conception, birth, and family placement.

This book will serve as a resource for social work education in courses that deal with adoption, and with families and children. It also speaks to the reality of practice needs in the field of adoption and in mental health and medical clinics that deal with couples who are affected by infertility and who wish to utilize assisted reproductive technology. By presenting a range of different forms of parentage, the authors have broadened our understanding and pointed to an important new field of social work practice.

NANCY BOYD WEBB, DSW
Distinguished Professor of Social Work
Fordham University

Preface

This book began as an effort to describe the multiple pathways to family formation represented by new forms of adoption and the increasing use of assisted reproductive technology (ART). As many practitioners who work with children and their families are already aware, family life in the United States has continued to become more diverse and complex. It is within that context that we have explored the meaning of complex adoption and ART for parents, for children, and for our society.

In most societies, the formation of families is both a private and public concern. Complex adoption and ART represent new pathways to family formation and reflect a range of social, psychological, scientific, demographic, and political phenomena. In this book, we have tried to consider these pathways to family formation from individual, familial, and societal perspectives. Thus, we examine not only types of complex adoption and/or ART, but the nature of the family context and structure in which pathways to parenthood are undertaken. This approach has created a matrix of sorts as we look, for example, at the nature of international adoption within both single- and dual-parent families, or the use of ART in either heterosexual or homosexual partnerships. Throughout this volume we focus on the nature of diversity within and across family structures and on the meaning of this complexity for practitioners who work with children and families.

Our own process in the research and writing of this book has led us to the conclusion that the study of complex adoption and ART requires a broad base of knowledge that integrates multiple theoretical perspectives on child development and family life. This book is perhaps most directly addressed to those practitioners who work with children and parents in therapeutic contexts. Many kinds of professionals, however, in a variety of settings have the opportunity to support the competence of parents and children in complex adoption and ART. We hope that this volume provides a framework to help doctors, nurses, teachers, therapists, and child welfare professionals take advantage of everyday opportunities to be sensitive to the unique needs of these children and their parents. We are particularly interested in the ways in which ecological and developmental theory can be applied to various levels of clinical practice and to the delineation of policy regarding complex adoption and ART.

As our understanding of human behavior and development continues to grow in sophistication and nuance, researchers and clinicians are addressing anew basic questions of human development. The role of early experience in development, the capacity to recover from exposure to trauma, the tension between "nature" and "nurture," and the centrality of primary attachment relationships to child development are central themes in developmental research. Each of these is reflected in our exploration of complex adoption and ART, which, by their definition, point to these very questions. We integrate a historical view of developmental theory with emerging research on human behavior to consider the experience of children and families in complex adoption and ART. It is our hope that the study of parents and children in these unique circumstances can be used to inform a more general understanding of the needs of parents and children in our rapidly changing society.

Each of the three authors collaborated on every chapter, except for Chapter 4, which is an adaptation of a previously published paper by Isabel Paret and Vivian Shapiro, and Chapter 11, written by Marsha Levy-Warren. Janet Shapiro is the primary author of Chapters 1, 2, 3, and 12.

We gratefully acknowledge the assistance of Nancy Boyd Webb, Gerald Schamess, and the external reviewers for their critiques and helpful comments. We would also like to thank Rochelle Serwator and Jeannie Tang from the editorial staff at The Guilford Press, as well as the copy editor, Ms. Jacquelyn Coggin. On a personal note, we thank Linda Harrington for her typing of the manuscript, and Peter Paret and Harold Shapiro for reading the material with such thoughtfulness. Janet Shapiro would like to thank her husband, Steven Eisenberg, and her young children, Sophia and Jacob, for their patience, love, and understanding.

Contents

PART I. NEW FAMILY NARRATIVES: AN APPROACH TO PRACTICE

1. A Conceptual Framework for Practice 3

2. Developmental Perspectives and Clinical Issues in Complex Adoption 24

PART II. COMPLEX ADOPTION

3. The Adoption of Children Following Foster Placement 53

4. The Impact of Delayed Adoption: A Case Study 76

5. International Adoption and Family Formation 98

6. Skipped-Generation Kinship Care: Grandparents and Their Grandchildren 125

7. Open Adoption: Family Attachments and Identity Formation 148

PART III. ASSISTED REPRODUCTIVE TECHNOLOGY AND FAMILY FORMATION

8. Social and Scientific Changes in the Formation of Families 173

9. Family Identity and Emerging Psychological Issues 201

10. Single, Gay, and Lesbian Parents: New Family Perspectives 228

PART IV. IMPLICATIONS FOR PRACTICE, TRAINING, AND RESEARCH

11. A Clinical Look at Knowing and Telling: Secrets, Lies, and Disillusionments 251

12. New Forms of Parentage: Summary and Implications for Practice, Training, and Research 276

References 303

Index 323

COMPLEX ADOPTION AND ASSISTED REPRODUCTIVE TECHNOLOGY

I

New Family Narratives: An Approach to Practice

1

A Conceptual Framework for Practice

This book addresses the special and complex set of issues that arises for parents and their children when families are formed through complex adoption and assisted reproductive technology (ART). The emergence of these pathways to parenthood is related to the social, political, demographic, and scientific changes occurring in our society. This book aims to describe the diverse characteristics and needs of families formed through complex adoption and ART. In providing a synthesis of relevant developmental, ecological, ethnographic, and clinical research, it is our hope that this volume can be utilized to inform the work of clinicians and researchers in their efforts to recognize, understand, and respond to the unique needs of these children and families. A deeper understanding of the ways in which complex adoption and ART shape the life experience of children and families has implications not only for more informed clinical practice but also for research, education, and public policy.

We refer to nontraditional forms of adoption as "complex" because they involve significant social and psychological factors that present unique challenges to parents and children. In some complex adoptions, the parent(s) adopt older infants and children who may have suffered early neglect, loss, and/or traumatic family disruptions (McKenzie, 1993; Reitz, 1999). These include post-foster placement adoption, international adoption, and skipped-generation kinship adoption. In other situations, families are engaged in a new form of adoption, referred to as "open adoption," in which the doors between the birth parent(s), their biological child, and the adoptive parent(s) remain open to some degree (Gritter, 1997; Wegar,

1997). In this volume, we consider each type of complex adoption and the ways in which it is differentiated both from traditional adoption and from other types of complex adoption. As we shall see, each form of complex adoption poses unique questions for parents, children, clinicians, and researchers.

When a child is conceived and born through one of the many new forms of ART, the parents may have experienced a long and difficult road to parenthood before the arrival of their much wanted infant. Those who rely on forms of ART as pathways to parenthood have encountered many biological and/or social barriers to parenthood. Indeed, married couples, single adults, and gay and lesbian couples may, for a variety of reasons, use ART in the process of becoming parents. In order to understand the experience of ART, practitioners must consider the ways in which the realization of infertility and the loss of an anticipated and valued sense of parental identity can create psychological crises for individuals and couples in diverse family situations (Burns & Covington, 1999; Leiblum, 1997). Clinicians working within the field of ART must recognize that decision making regarding its use is strongly shaped by access to the technology, personal values and belief systems, and experiences of loss and societal discrimination (Leiblum, 1997; Miller, 1992; Patterson & Chan, 1999). Among the most difficult issues are those associated with the use of sperm and ova donors and/or the assistance of a gestational/surrogate birth mother.

While complex adoption and ART can be differentiated along many important dimensions, these pathways to parenthood share common themes that are also central to the study of human development and to discussions regarding the role of children and family life in society. The relative balance of genetic, biological, social, and psychological factors on human development is of primary importance in considering complex adoption and ART as pathways to family formation. Both complex adoption and some forms of ART require families to think through the ways in which "nature" and "nurture" interact to shape personality, behavior, and psychological development. In addition, the emergence of complex adoption and ART as pathways to family formation has occurred during a time of great social and political change regarding the definition of "who is a parent" and what it is that constitutes a "family."

While families formed through complex adoption and ART share much in common with all parents and children, there are also ways in which these family narratives are unique, poignant, and compelling. We believe that by studying the experiences of complex adoption and ART from the perspectives of both parents and children, clinicians and researchers can develop a better understanding of the strengths, special challenges, and intervention needs related to these new forms of parentage. As importantly, it is our hope that the study of the many facets of complex adoption and ART can be utilized to inform the broadening definition of "family" in ways that will serve to increase understanding of the diversity of family life in our society. Indeed, many current racial, cultural, political, and socioeconomic issues are central to the emergence of complex adoption and ART as pathways to family formation. Thus, clinicians and researchers working in this field of practice must consider multiple dimensions of diversity in both problem definition and in the development of intervention services.

The range represented by families formed through complex adoptions and the use of ART reflects the increasing diversity of family life in our society. As family structures have become more diverse, developmental researchers have studied the experiences of both parents and children in nontraditional families (Hetherington & Parke, 1999; Lamb, 1999). *Nontraditional ways of building families have greatly multiplied, but children still have basic developmental needs of being wanted and loved, in environments in which they receive attuned and empathic care commensurate with their maturational age.*

A primary goal of this volume is to consider the similarities and differences between various types of complex adoption and ART, and the importance of these differences for the development of collaborative interventions designed to support children and families. This chapter presents a conceptual framework that can be useful to practitioners in considering the many challenges associated with these new forms of parentage. It consists of the following sections:

- An integrated conceptual approach to practice: developmental, ecological, and ethnographic perspectives.
- Complex adoption and ART in context: Changing patterns of family formation and family life.
- Relevant insights from the study of traditional adoption.
- Family narratives: The parents' view and the child's view.
- An overview of the chapters.

AN INTEGRATED CONCEPTUAL APPROACH TO PRACTICE: DEVELOPMENTAL, ECOLOGICAL, AND ETHNOGRAPHIC PERSPECTIVES

Three perspectives are interwoven throughout this book in our efforts to consider the effects of complex adoption and ART on child and family development. The integration of developmental, ecological, and ethnographic perspectives is necessary because the influence of complex adoption and

ART on child and family development reverberates across the lifespan for parents and children alike. Individual, familial, and social factors combine to particularize the experience for individual children and families. The diversity created by this matrix of factors requires that practitioners be able to combine an understanding of basic developmental processes with an appreciation of the ways in which child and family well-being are affected by the many social systems with which the family transacts. In addition, practitioners must develop competence in working with different clients in ways that support their capacity for self-determination, independence, and optimal developmental outcomes. The ethnographic perspective can support the clinician's ability to elicit and attend sensitively to the stories of families whose experience lies outside the mainstream and/or the clinician's frame of reference.

The Developmental Perspective

As will be discussed more fully in Chapter 2, developmental research has made important contributions to our understanding of risk and resiliency in childhood, and to the development of clinical interventions with children and families. A broad-based understanding of human development is an important aspect of the knowledge base needed for practice in this area. An understanding of risk and resiliency, and the processes by which children grow and develop, can help clinicians in assessing client strengths and vulnerabilities. In particular, a developmental model guides the clinician to focus on multiple areas of development and on how individual, familial, and social system factors are working to support or impede developmental competence in a particular child. In addition, developmental knowledge can help clinicians to identify gaps that may exist between expected lines of development and difficulties a particular child may be experiencing in physical, social, emotional, or cognitive growth, and to think through relevant points of intervention.

Increasingly, developmental research has focused on more diverse populations of children and families. This research has been important because it shows that multiple pathways to development are possible and that while early life experiences are an important determinant of child well-being, development itself remains "plastic" or open to change in more supportive circumstances. Across contexts, the presence of attachment relationships has emerged as a central protective factor and determinant of emotional, neurobiological, intellectual, and physical growth of children. Thus, we examine in this volume the ways in which family structure combines with the life experiences associated with complex adoption and ART to influence patterns of attachment and relational capacity in the developing child.

In complex adoption, where children are likely to have experienced early traumatic beginnings, important questions are raised about patterns of risk and resiliency in early life and the centrality of attachment relationships to a child's growth and development. The ways in which the absence of attachment relationships poses risks to the child, the potential for recovery in the context of new attachments, and the special challenges associated with the formation of attachment relationships following traumatic loss are central to this discussion. In the case of ART, where children generally have the benefit of continuous caregiving from birth, other psychosocial challenges frame the family context in a variety of ways.

The Ecological Perspective

As proposed by Bronfenbrenner in 1979, and expanded on since that time by other authors, the ecological perspective recognizes the importance of the multiple systems that come to bear on individual and family functioning (Allen-Meares, 1995; Bronfenbrenner, 1979; Webb, 1996; Zigler & Hall, 2000). Rather than viewing the child's development as unfolding solely "from the inside out," the ecological perspective encourages us to remember that cultural, social, demographic, familial, and individual factors combine to influence the child's trajectory of growth and development.

The emergence of new forms of parentage reflects great change in the "ecology of family formation and parenthood," and requires practitioners to consider the many social and cultural influences on the life experiences of these families. Because families formed through complex adoption and ART are, in many cases, forging new pathways, it is important that practitioners effectively use their knowledge base but remain open to the unique experiences and diversity within this special, growing population of children and families.

Ethnographic Theory and Clinical Practice

The narratives of the families we discuss often include many elements of loss, discontinuity, and difference. Broken attachment relationships, for example, may be experienced as a biographical discontinuity and often precipitate a major identity crisis for adults and children (Borden, 1992; Cohler, 1982; Shapiro, 1995). Moreover, the subjective narratives of children and parents in nontraditional families may be unvoiced, untold, and known only to family members themselves. "Subjugated knowledge" refers to the hidden knowledge of what it is like to live outside the cultural mainstream. These stories are often unexpressed in clinical work because both parents and children may not realize that this part of the family history is relevant to the circumstance that led them to seek treatment.

Insights from ethnography, psychoanalytic theory, and clinical practice provide understanding of the importance of narrative expression for the resolution of grief, mourning, and adaptive recovery (Borden, 1992; Freud, 1957). In this sense, an ethnographic approach can be helpful to clinicians in working with nontraditional families whose unique formation is outside the mainstream and who feel "different." Both children and parents may have to cope with special circumstances of loss, biographical discontinuity, and prejudice. Their subjective experiences are often not revealed to others because of the very personal nature of their stories and possible feelings of stigmatization.

Ethnographic theory suggests that parents and children are the "experts" in the subjective experience of their more painful family histories. As we have already noted, parents and their children reveal their inner stories through different verbal and nonverbal modalities. Clinicians who work with children and adults need to be informed by and sensitive to the very different processes by which each person within the family communicates his/her subjective internal feelings, and the ways in which unique cultural, ethnic, and personal history affect the forms of narrative expression.

While clinicians may have a general understanding of the stressors on parents in nontraditional family life, ethnographic theory suggests that an empathetic "informed not knowing" clinical approach is helpful. The clinician must respect parents' and children's "expert knowledge" of their own subjective family experiences. This story may include anger, resentment, grief, mourning, and identity confusion—emotions that often reflect an experience that is the private and personal knowledge of the individual who feels "outside" the mainstream culture. *Telling this part of the story while receiving the empathy of the listener is helpful in mourning the past losses that were often invisible to others, and in constructing a more positive personal identity* (Shapiro, 1994; White & Epston, 1990).

The following case vignettes illustrate the importance of an integrated conceptual framework that includes individual, familial and social factors in the development of assessment and intervention models for practice in complex adoption and ART.

Vignette 1

A gay couple became foster parents to an infant who was HIV positive and had spent his early months as a "boarder baby" in an urban hospital. The couple faced multiple challenges in coping with the child's physical and socioemotional needs. Their efforts to become permanent adoptive parents for this child were stymied by the bias of laws that only permitted married, heterosexual couples to adopt children.

Vignette 2

A married couple decided to utilize sperm donation as a pathway to becoming parents. Although they both wanted a child, the birth of the child precipitated a psychological crisis for the father, who did not want the child to discover that they were not biologically related. This secret weighed heavily on the parents, interfered with open communication, and adversely affected relationships within the family.

Vignette 3

A couple who had spent several years going through infertility treatments, without success, decided to adopt a child from Romania. While they were aware that the child might have experienced severe medical and psychological neglect in the orphanage, they believed that their love and willingness to provide a variety of resources would make up for the child's early history. However, they were unprepared for the severity of the child's developmental problems, which included severe sleep disorders, separation anxiety, and difficulty in attachment relationships.

Clinical work in complex adoption and ART requires that the practitioner attend to the unique history of the family and the social milieu in which it lives. Clinicians must be able to integrate an awareness of the developmental needs of young children, the influence of a range of ecological factors, the difficulty families may have in talking about the circumstances of family formation, and family members' unvoiced fears about its impact on their child. Throughout this book, we use case vignettes and case examples to illustrate our approach to practice.

COMPLEX ADOPTION AND ASSISTED REPRODUCTIVE TECHNOLOGY IN CONTEXT: CHANGING PATTERNS OF FAMILY FORMATION AND FAMILY LIFE

The experiences of families formed via complex adoption and ART are strongly influenced by social attitudes, historical circumstance, scientific developments, and the demographic structure of contemporary society. By the end of the 20th century, these factors had sharpened our view of the importance of families to adults and children alike. The new forms of parentage that we are considering have emerged from the combined circumstances of the greater social acceptance of emerging family structures, changing cultural norms, and scientific discoveries that provide new opportunities for family formation.

The traditional notion of the two-parent "nuclear" family within a heterosexual marriage is no longer the dominant model of family life in the United States (Mintz & Kellogg, 1988, Lamb, 1999). Rather, families of divorce, blended families, single-parent families by choice, gay and lesbian couples, and households headed by grandparent(s) present new models of family life and now represent a rather large component of the various family structures (Lamb, 1999). The increasing diversity of new models of family life has afforded researchers and clinicians the opportunity to discover multiple contexts and pathways that can support positive developmental outcomes in children. Their observations provide an important base for our discussion of the needs of children in families formed via complex adoption and ART.

The strong desire for parenthood endures in our changing world. In all societies, family formation and parenthood hold deep cultural and symbolic meaning (Erikson, 1950; Murray, 1996; Zelizer, 1985). For some women and men, having a child is one of the most profound experiences in life, an important turning point in the life cycle that can provide a sense of personal fulfillment in the feeling of being emotionally connected to their past heritage and to future generations (Benedek, 1959; Chodorow, 1978; Erikson, 1950). When, for various reasons, an individual or couple cannot have children, the prospect of childlessness may be experienced as a deep existential loss (Domar, 1997).

In previous eras, medical and/or social barriers to parenthood often stymied the wishes of infertile couples, single intentional parents, or gay and lesbian couples for a child. *The idea that each individual has the right to experience the gift of parenthood has been increasingly acknowledged in the broader culture and has led to a greater acceptance and respect for various forms of nontraditional families* (Lamb, 1999; Macklin, 1994b). For example, until recently, there was little acceptance or support for single parenthood. Changing social contexts and new scientific advances in human reproduction have combined to support the efforts of a diverse group of families to consider complex adoption and ART as routes to parentage. Nevertheless, many nontraditional families still experience a level of prejudice and discrimination that makes it hard for them and their children to feel acceptance by the broader world (Gadsden, 1999; Gibbs & Huang, 1999).

The Emergence of Different Forms of Complex Adoption

A historical perspective helps in understanding the significant shift from traditional adoption practices of adopting infants at birth to the current models of complex adoption (Reitz, 1999). Important social issues have influenced the rise of complex adoption and the relative decrease of traditional adoption at birth, including: the broad breakdown in family life for many families unable to provide protective care for their children because of poverty, illness, substance abuse, AIDS, and other disruptions; the resulting numbers of children placed in the foster care system (Chase-Lansdale & Vinovskis, 1995); the needs of these children for permanent homes (Adoption and Foster Care Analysis and Reporting System [AFCARS], 2000); and the number of individuals and couples who seek to form a family (Evan B. Donaldson Adoption Institute, 2000).

- The number of intentional parents seeking to adopt a healthy infant at birth far exceeds the number of available infants. The shortage of healthy infants available for adoption at birth is a result of many factors. For example, the rate at which women relinquish their infants for adoption has been decreasing since 1965, especially among white women. In 1965, 19% of white women who were pregnant gave up their infants for adoption at birth, but by 1988, this rate decreased to only 3%.Very few families of color have ever released their children for adoption at birth (Evan B. Donaldson Adoption Institute, 2000).
- The reasons that fewer women are giving up their children for adoption at birth may be related to the changing views of society toward the rights of single parents to keep and nurture their children, and to the increasing social acceptance of nontraditional families (Wegar, 1997). In addition, the advent of birth control and the right to abortion has resulted in fewer babies being born to women who are not ready to have a child. The decreasing number of available infants has made the wait as long as 7 years to adopt a healthy infant. Many eager intentional parents are now adopting a child through the newly emerging forms of complex adoption in which the wait for a child is much shorter (Evan B. Donaldson Adoption Institute, 2000).
- Families now can adopt children in circumstances that are quite different from the past practices of traditional adoption of infants at birth. In the past, adoption practices were more likely to include and reflect preferences for matching ethnic, racial, and religious characteristics of infants with those of their adoptive parents. In addition, closed adoptions that sealed the identity of the birth parents from the child, and the preference

for parental characteristics such as the "two-parent nuclear family," no longer prevail in adoption practice (Reitz, 1999). In complex adoption, children are often older when adopted and usually have had traumatic early preadoptive histories. Adoptive families represent a far more varied set of parents: older parents; grandparents in kinship adoption; parents of mixed racial, ethnic, and religious heritage; parents who may be single parents by choice; and gay and lesbian couples (Adoption and Foster Care Analysis and Reporting System [AFCARS], 2000).

• The number of children available for complex adoption is increasing in the United States and abroad. Indeed, the number of children entering the public foster care system in America doubled between the early 1980s and the year 2000 (Adoption and Foster Care Analysis and Reporting System [AFCARS], 2000). Of the 547,000 children in foster care in 1998, 115,000 children were eligible for adoption, but only 30%, or 36,000, found permanent homes that year. The remaining 80,000 children join the increasing number of children who await adoption in the foster care system (Adoption and Foster Care Analysis and Reporting System [AFCARS], 2000).

• Many of these children have been removed from their families of origin because of a severe breakdown in their family life and the corresponding risk to their emotional and physical safety. Often, they have suffered early neglect and/or abuse, multiple family disruption, and loss. Moreover, in extended foster care, the children who wait may suffer accumulative risks as they experience multiple models of care in foster homes and remain in prolonged states of family impermanence. A disproportionate number of these are children of color, and special concerns exist because many of them stay in foster care for long periods of time (McKenzie, 1993). Adoptive parents must often deal with the severe repercussions of the early traumatic preadoptive history on the social, emotional, and cognitive development of their child (Paret & Shapiro, 1998).

• Transcultural adoptions add to the complexity of new adoption patterns. Children are becoming available for adoption from institutions in other countries because these societies cannot provide the necessary care for abandoned and orphaned children. In 1997, approximately 14,000 children were adopted from abroad by American families. These children often need intensive medical and psychological help (Holt International Children's Services, 2000; Reitz, 1999). In addition to the many losses of culture, language, and caregivers at the moment of transition to their new environments, over time, the children may face challenges in trying to integrate their complex dual ethnic and cultural family heritage (Grotevant & Kohler, 1999; Lamb, 1999; Webb, 1999).

• Open adoptions permit birth parents to take some initiative in choosing the adoptive parents for their child and negotiating some form of continuing communication or relationship with the child and the adoptive parents. This form of adoption has emerged for many reasons. The realization that closed adoptions may not always have been in the best interests of members of the adoptive triad has influenced adoption practices to move toward more openness in general (Wegar, 1997). Furthermore, the shortage of infants available for adoption at birth helps birth parents feel more empowered, and many choose to have greater involvement in the future of their child.

Some benefits are clearly present in open adoption. As in traditional adoption, open adoption allows for the possibility of an early relationship between the infant and adoptive parent. This relationship is conducive to the establishment of a satisfying interaction between parent and child (Benedek, 1959). However, when contacts with the birth parents remain open, difficulties may sometimes occur. The adoptive parents must provide the child with a strong sense of family identity while still maintaining knowledge about and perhaps contact with birth parents. This creates a new form of extended kinship family in which both the birth and the adoptive parents must keep the needs of the child in mind when establishing a reasonable set of relationships between the families (Wegar, 1997).

The Emergence of Assisted Reproductive Technology

In 1978, the first baby was born through the clinical application of a new ART, known as *in vitro* fertilization (IVF). This generally refers to a group of medical procedures that involve the fertilization of an ovum outside of the human body in a laboratory procedure, followed by its successful implantation in the mother's womb. This procedure has allowed many infertile couples, and other intentional parents, to bypass the traditional method of conception and to overcome certain medical or structural barriers to parenthood. In subsequent years, many new methods have been developed to treat both male and female infertility, and the psychological and emotional experiences of the potential loss of biological parenthood.

Increasingly, individuals in diverse family circumstances are utilizing ART as a pathway for overcoming social and biological barriers to having a child. There are approximately 2.1 million infertile families in the United States. Various ART procedures are used by approximately 15% of those American couples who have fertility problems (The Institute for Science, Law, and Technology, Working Group, 1998), and by many single mothers by choice, and gay and lesbian couples (Lieblum, 1999; Miller, 1992). Approximately 75,000 infants are born annually through the use of ART (The Institute for Science, Law, and Technology, Working Group, 1998).

The biological, social, and psychological issues raised by the new forms of reproduction have created an important new field of clinical practice with families and children. The new advances in ART have also raised many important social, ethical, psychological, and legal questions regarding the definition of family (Andrews, 1999; Levine, 1990). For example, the use of ART procedures can allow a child as many as five parental figures in his/her birth history: a genetic father who provided the sperm; a genetic mother who provided the ova; a gestational mother who carried him/her to term; and the psychological parent(s) who intend to nurture the child throughout life.

The psychological parents may have difficulty coping with the realities of shared parentage; therefore, supportive counseling that allows parents to reflect upon the symbolic meaning of collaborative parenthood is often essential to help them arrive at decisions that feel comfortable and support attachment to their child. The careful exploration of underlying feelings about infertility and the important decisions regarding biological and psychological parenthood can help form the basis for the formation of strong attachments between parents and infants, and the development of a strong sense of family identity. Of particular difficulty is the family decision of whether to tell their child about his/her complex birth heritage.

Not all forms of ART or IVF are biologically complex in that many couples can have their own genetic children. Practitioners, however, must be sensitive to the strenuous efforts and the psychological, social, economic, and physical costs of treatment. Although approximately one-third of infertile couples will achieve a pregnancy (The Institute for Science, Law, and Technology, Working Group, 1998), many couples face many treatment trials and disappointments. For others, who decide to form their child through collaborative parenthood, many important decisions need to be made regarding the choices in the use of ova and sperm donors, and a gestational birth mother. In addition to competent medical care, these families may need a range of supportive services, including education, guidance, and various modalities of therapy both during medical treatment and following the birth of the child.

The intentional parents who use ART often form a deep psychological commitment to the idea of parenthood and the wish to nurture a child well before actual conception, gestation, or birth. This subjective commitment becomes the core basis of family identity, and counselors must integrate their general knowledge of therapeutic work with children with the special dynamics of ART in family formation. The parents' ability to form an unconflicted relationship with their child and to accept the circumstances of the child's special birth heritage serves as the basis for helping the child to feel valued and accepted. Special family structures, such as single or same-sex parents, add complexity to the family narrative. The parents must deal with the issues of difference regarding the child's birth history, the realities of collaborative parenthood (which often is not shared with others), the potential differences in family structures, and the resolution of their own loss and ambivalence that may still exist.

Extensive literature exists on traditional adoption of children at birth (Brodzinsky & Schechter, 1990; Brodzinsky, Smith, & Brodzinsky, 1998; Reitz, 1999), but the emerging forms of complex adoption and ART described earlier raise new clinical questions and often require special clinical approaches. While general themes emerge within the distinctive contexts of each form of complex adoption and ART, every family is unique, and each child's developmental pathway must be understood in terms of his/her specific history. The diversity of parents and their use of new forms of parentage combine to create a complex set of social and psychological issues for these nontraditional families. In using ART, intentional parents may have to deal with not only their own psychosocial responses but also new legal and ethical questions that evolve relative to collaborative parenthood.

RELEVANT INSIGHTS FROM THE STUDY OF TRADITIONAL ADOPTION

Many themes from the study of traditional adoption are relevant to our conceptualization of complex adoption and ART. In particular, the literature on traditional adoption has focused much attention on the relative contributions of biology and nurturance to the child's unfolding development, and to the ways in which adoption shapes the development of family identity and attachments within the family. Themes of attachment, loss, and identity formation echo through the life experiences of families formed via both complex adoption and ART. Among the other most salient themes drawn from the literature on traditional adoption are the following:

- *The importance of the parental sense of "entitlement" in relationship to the role as parent.* Many adoptive parents grapple with the issue of "entitlement," which refers to the parental perception that they have the "legal and emotional right to parent their child" (Reitz & Watson, 1992, p. 125). In some forms of complex adoption and ART, even when the legal status of parents is clear, a range of psychosocial issues may contribute to parental uncertainty regarding their status as the primary caregiver. Not feeling "entitled" may interfere with parents' capacity to claim fully their parental role. In situations of complex adoption and ART, barriers to entitlement may derive from the unique processes of family formation.

- *The many factors that may influence the degree to which parents desire, or are able, to be open about the family history.* Unresolved ambivalence and loss, shame, or the belief that the extended family or social environment is prejudiced may negatively influence parents' ability to communicate openly. Clinicians tend to agree that parents must come to their own decisions as to how they will handle the most sensitive questions of birth heritage with their child (Epstein & Rosenberg, 1997). Empathic responsiveness to the child's questions about his/her birth history supports trust and openness in communication that serves the family well over time (Grotevant, McRoy, Elde, & Fravel, 1994). Parents must be able to decide on some mutually consistent approach to dealing with issues of birth heritage, privacy, and the nature of the family narrative.
- *The need of parents to be able to accept differences between themselves and their children.* While this is true for all families, it may be especially important when parents perceive their child's differences as stemming from a lack of biological relatedness. The ability to accept his/her differences is central to the child's sense of being valued. In this regard, practitioners may be able to help parents see and accept the child they have, and keep in mind his/her unique developmental needs and requirement for support, love, and understanding.
- *The parental capacity for self-reflection is central to their willingness to reach out for therapeutic help when needed.* Clinicians need to develop a therapeutic relationship that supports the parents' ability to work through difficult issues on behalf of their child's long-term development (Epstein & Rosenberg, 1997).

These insights from traditional adoption literature are relevant to the families that we discuss. However, the issues become even more complex given the special origin of the family and its potential impact on family dynamics.

FAMILY NARRATIVES: THE PARENTS' VIEW AND THE CHILD'S VIEW

Themes of attachment, identity, and loss are woven through the life story of every family but are more sensitive when families are formed through complex adoption or ART. In these families, parents must weave the threads of their unique psychological, social, biological, and historical experiences into a coherent and meaningful narrative. The construction of a narrative that includes the many social and biological intricacies of family history is necessary to the formation of a shared family identity and the child's development of his or her own core identity (Grotevant & Kohler, 1999). The parents' ability to construct a coherent narrative and to share it over time with their child has an important impact on the child's emerging sense of self, the view of his/her place in the family, and beliefs about his/her relationship to the external social world (Grotevant, 1997).

It is often hard for parents to construct a comfortable family narrative when painful and sensitive issues remain at the core of family formation. In complex adoption and ART, the history of family formation has many unusual pathways and can be difficult to reconstruct, and even more difficult to tell. For example, the traumatic early preadoptive experiences of children from foster placement and the painful, but often invisible, biopsychosocial issues that may exist in collaborative parenthood may pose emotional barriers to the parents' ability to construct a coherent family narrative for themselves or for the purposes of sharing with their child(ren).

As children with unique family histories mature, the meaning of early history will be understood with increasing complexity as it is revisited over the course of various developmental phases (Brinich, 1990; Brodzinsky & Schechter, 1990; Grotevant & Kohler, 1999; Kirk, 1964; Reitz, 1999; Sorosky, Baron, & Pannor, 1989). Children in complex adoption may find it painful to talk about their early history. The real facts may be conscious but the emotional experiences may be remembered only in unspoken affects such as sadness, insecurity, and doubt about being cared for or wanted. Often, it is hard for the parent(s) to address this aspect of their children's early history for fear of raising anxiety for both themselves and their children. Parental efforts to protect their children may inadvertently result in children being left "alone" with their preverbal and unspoken affective memories.

When the family history differs from "mainstream" family models, prejudice and family isolation often become part of the subjective experiences of children and parents. In this sense, the family narrative may be subjugated, unvoiced, untold, and unshared with others. This unvoiced family narrative can have consequences for the relationships between parents and children as well as between the family and the wider social environment.

As with all children and families, parents and children can develop different internal narratives about their families and selves over time. Indeed, during childhood and adolescence, the differences between parental and child narratives often serve as important points of self-definition and exploration for developing children.

In complex adoption and ART, children will develop their own explanations and fantasies about their early life experiences. The emotional life of children is often experienced not in words but in behavior, and in the ways in which children relate to people in their lives. When they are unable to identify and/or articulate feeling states, children may have bodily and affective memories of preverbal experiences. Thus, their "narrative," or description of important events, themes, and relationships, is often told through action and affective reactions rather than through verbal reconstructions. Parents may be confused by behavior and emotions that seem out of context with regard to actual events. By helping parents understand the ways in which young children think about and encode early life experiences, practitioners can support parents' abilities to recognize that children's emotions and behavior at times are related to past memories rather than current circumstances (Gardner, 1991).

For example, children's early experiences can sometimes be inferred from the quality of both their adaptation to relationships with caregivers and their play. Children adopted following a history of broken attachments may have difficulties in forming new attachment relationships because they fear rejection and loss. By contrast, children who have been cared for by empathetic parents since birth, as is possible in ART, may have a more positive narrative of early experience. Nevertheless, they may internalize the unresolved ambivalence of parents who have not worked through their conflicts around infertility or collaborative parenthood.

Of the many aspects of development that are relevant to the study of complex adoption and ART, the interwoven themes of attachment and identity formation are primary. For young children who have experienced multiple trauma and family disruption, the road to recovery after adoption is often difficult. Stressful early experiences may have interrupted development in many spheres. Sometimes these children, with fragmented life histories, get "stuck" in the difficult task of constructing a coherent sense of self. Identity formation is an ongoing process in all children, but the risk to identity coherence in the children we discuss can be high because of the degree of disruption and loss in their life histories. Grief and mourning can occur across their lifespan, and their lifelong subjective narratives may carry painful memories of figures and experiences in their past (Hoopes, 1990).

Children in families formed through ART may feel that they are "different" even though there may be no visible sign that their birth history is unusual. This may be especially true when parents have experienced discomfort about the birth narrative of their child. Often, as children enter the broader world of school, questions about family origin arise. Sometimes these questions precipitate a crisis for the family, especially regarding secrets and the untold story. Parents often seek clinical advice, and clinicians become aware of the multilevel psychological issues that emerge for parents and children in telling this narrative.

Clinical practice with children that utilizes a biopsychosocial perspective in assessment and treatment can be enhanced by an ethnographic perspective. The clinician then becomes the "informed but not knowing" listener to the deeply subjective knowledge of the child's unique experiences of nontraditional family heritage. For some children, one of the most emotional issues is the realization that they may never be able to know and feel the love of their genetic parents. These feelings are expressed in children's age-related capacities to communicate their internal world. The clinician's therapeutic approach to children's revealed subjective view becomes an important part of children's capacity to find acceptance, to mourn, and to experience the possibility of hope.

OVERVIEW OF THE CHAPTERS

Chapter 2. Developmental Perspectives and Clinical Issues in Complex Adoption

We discuss the importance of developmental theory to clinical practice in complex adoption. A broad developmental framework is essential to the understanding of the impact of early trauma and loss on the development of children and the special implications for their relationship with their parents. While open adoption presents different parameters, the integrated developmental, ecological, and ethnographic approach is equally important in understanding the issues families face. A summary of the importance of a developmental approach to assessment and treatment is also included.

Chapter 3. The Adoption of Children Following Foster Placement

This chapter places social, psychological, and policy issues of post-foster placement adoption in historical perspective. We discuss the acute needs of children who have experienced severe early trauma, neglect, and multiple separations. A major focus is on the difficulties children face in the adaptation to adoptive parent(s) and the implications for practice with both parents and children. New issues surrounding transracial adoption are discussed at length, particularly potential psychological impact and the public policy debate. A case illustration describes the impact of early neglect on a 6-month-old child and the special parenting tasks involved in helping her recover. An assessment outline is provided to assist clinicians in integrating the preadoptive history of a child with treatment planning.

Chapter 4. The Impact of Delayed Adoption: A Case Study

This chapter presents a long-term case of a boy adopted after 6 years of uncertainty about permanent placement. The case documents the psychological stress and anxiety precipitated by the long delay and the ongoing threat of losing the primary attachment figure, his foster mother. The case demonstrates the effects of early neglect and multiple separation on ego development, presenting the process of treatment in detail.

Chapter 5. International Adoption and Family Formation

Here, we describe the physical, psychological, and experiential hardships of children awaiting international adoption. For most of these children, poverty, neglect, and institutional care can present high risks to their physical, cognitive, and psychological development. The adopting parents are not necessarily prepared for the degree of emotional and physical delay in the children they will encounter. These children have their own distinctive adjustment reactions to adoption, with varying capacities for recovery. Case vignettes illustrate the slow recovery from early neglect and biographical discontinuity, and the role of treatment in helping both parents and children. We also consider the experience of transracial and transcultural issues that impact the child at the time of adoption and throughout development.

Chapter 6. Skipped-Generation Kinship Care: Grandparents and Their Grandchildren

We discuss the rising number of grandparents who are taking care of their grandchildren following family breakdown. The role of kinship care is placed in historical perspective. Skipped-generation adoption is especially prominent in African American and Latino families, although kinship care occurs in all ethnic and racial groups. Often, grandmothers must cope with their own poverty and illness as they try to provide family continuity for their grandchildren. Clinical vignettes describe the variety of difficult preadoptive histories of these children, the emotional consequences of family disruption on children, parents, and grandparents, and the extensive family needs that ensue for each generation.

Chapter 7. Open Adoption: Family Attachments and Identity Formation

This chapter reviews the sea change in adoption practice. Open adoption has evolved because of the growing concern over the impact of sealed records, laws, and the resulting permanent cutoff between birth parents and their children. In open adoption, birth parents have the opportunity to take some initiative in choosing the adoptive parents for their child and negotiating some form of continuing communication. The meaning of adoption to birth parents, adoptive parents, and children is discussed, and the pros and cons of open adoption are explored. Clinical evidence suggests that while certain problems exist, particularly in the establishment of secure family boundaries, the absence of "cutoffs" between children and their birth parents can have beneficial effects on all members of the adoption triangle. Clinical vignettes illustrate the many dimensions of the issues we discuss, and three models of open adoption practices are described.

Chapter 8. Social and Scientific Changes in the Formation of Families

We describe the many forms of ART developed during the last 20 years. These methods, especially IVF, have enabled many infertile couples, single parents by choice, and gay and lesbian families to overcome social and biological barriers to parenthood. Collaborative parenthood, through the use of ova or sperm donors, or the assistance of a gestational birth mother, has broadened the concept of the family beyond traditional legal, biological, and cultural perspectives, and emphasizes the role of psychological parenting and the subjective meaning of family identity. New ethical, legal, and psychological issues are reviewed.

Chapter 9. Family Identity and Emerging Psychological Issues

The chapter addresses the psychological meaning of infertility and the emotional dimensions of infertility treatment. In particular, we consider the choices that parents must make in deciding on various pathways to parenthood, such as the use of collaborative parentage with ova and sperm donors and/or the assistance of gestational birth mothers. These forms of parentage raise many difficult questions. Men and women have different underlying feelings about infertility and its treatment. Often, families need therapeutic help in reaching a consensus about decisions such as whether to tell their children or extended families. Although these new pathways to parenthood can be very satisfying, they can also set in motion complex family dynamics. Case vignettes illustrate some of the conflicts that can emerge for children and parents.

Chapter 10. Single, Gay, and Lesbian Parents: New Family Perspectives

We review the increasing diversity of American families and the social and scientific changes that expand the choices of single parents and gay and lesbian couples. The chapter discusses the relative impact of these nontraditional family structures on the developmental pathways of their children. While each family has to address special concerns regarding the children's development in the context of single or same-sex parenthood, we suggest that the quality of caregiving overrides the specific nature of family structure. These families, however, often face discrimination and special burdens in meeting the social and psychological needs of their children. Case examples illustrate the many special issues that arise.

Chapter 11. A Clinical Look at Knowing and Telling: Secrets, Lies, and Disillusionments

This chapter uses clinical vignettes to illustrate the crises that may develop when children are caught in the dilemma of family secrets. The secrets may prevent parents from resolving ambivalent feelings related to their children's birth histories. We describe the therapeutic process by which the parents begin to resolve their ambivalence and the ways in which communication can be restored to the developmental advantage of the child.

Chapter 12. New Forms of Parentage: Summary and Implications for Practice, Training, and Research

The primary goal of this chapter is to consider the ways in which our understanding of new forms of parentage can inform therapeutic work within this emerging new field of practice. The chapter also informs a wide range of practitioners, such as child welfare workers, social workers, psychologists, physicians, lawyers, and teachers, who may be involved with important concerns of parents and children at various points in their history. In addition to new approaches to direct practice, we discuss the implications for education, training, and research.

In summary, ethnographers who study family narratives discuss the three strands of cultural and personal experiences that combine to form the core basis of individual identity: the influence of the broader culture within which the individual lives; the more immediate ethnic or special group with whom the family most identifies; and the particular intimate experiences of the individual within his or her immediate family (Myerhoff, 1978). In this volume, we explore all three levels of experience that influence the social and psychological lives of children and parents who live together in new forms of families.

2

Developmental Perspectives and Clinical Issues in Complex Adoption

Developmental research has made important contributions to clinical work with children and families by increasing our understanding of the nature of human development and the processes by which children grow and develop. In addition to providing an overview of normal development, a developmental perspective has allowed us to establish an important framework for our understanding of risk, resiliency, and the etiology of emotional difficulties in childhood (Chethik, 2000; Cicchetti & Cohen, 1995; Davies, 1999; Fraser, 1997; Freud, 1981; Webb, 1996). Our knowledge of developmental processes in childhood is therefore an important resource for practitioners focused on the support of developmental competence in children and families. A developmental perspective can be especially valuable in helping clinicians understand the gap that may exist between the expected normal lines of development and the difficulties a child may be experiencing in the spheres of social, emotional, and cognitive growth (Freud, 1981).

Increasingly, the study of human development has broadened to include more diverse populations and, in particular, the study of children at risk (Cicchetti & Cohen, 1995; Vondra, Hommerding, & Shaw, 1999). This body of literature demonstrates that multiple pathways to developmental competence are possible and that the particular social ecology, or cultural milieu, of a child combines with individual and familial characteristics to influence important developmental outcomes (Belsky, 1984; Fraser, 1997; Webb, 1996). This literature is relevant to practitioners who work with nontraditional families and are faced with new questions with regard to child and family well-being.

Developmental and clinical researchers have explored, for example, the risk and protective factors in special populations of children and families. Research on subjects such as single parenthood, divorce, child care, early motherhood, childhood stress, and the effects of poverty has focused on the processes by which these characteristics influence developmental outcomes in children (Eth & Pynoos, 1985; McLoyd, 1990; Shapiro, Mangelsdorf, & Marzolf, 1995; Webb, 1999). Across these special populations of children, researchers have continued to identify the presence of secure attachment figures as an important protective factor (Masten, Best, & Garmezy, 1990). Conversely, disruptions in primary attachment relationships have been shown to present important risks to early development.

The importance of attachment relationships to the positive emotional and developmental growth of children is a central theme that emerges across populations in both traditional and nontraditional families. The kinds of complex adoptions described in this volume represent a special population of children and families in which early attachment has been disrupted and new attachments have been formed. The literature on the dynamics of complex adoption (i.e., the adoption of older infants and children, and open adoptions) is sparse and only just emerging. The developmental research in traditional adoption, however, is a base that can inform the field of practice with children and parents brought together via new forms of family formation. The extensive literature on traditional adoption is based on a developmental approach to child well-being and focuses on areas such as the internal psychological meaning of adoption, the impact of adoption on identity formation, and the influence of the child's adoptive status on longer term adjustment (Brodzinsky, 1993; Brodzinsky & Schechter, 1990; Brodzinsky, Smith, & Brodzinsky, 1998; Hoopes, Alexander, Silver, Ober, & Kirby, 1997).

The adoption literature is grounded in two aspects of developmental research that have been basic to our conceptualization of child outcomes: *the importance of biological or genetic influence on special attributes of the child, such as temperament and physical characteristics*, and *the role of nurturance, or attachment, on human development*. Children in traditional adoptions generally have the benefit of continuous caregiving from their psychological parents. The quality of empathetic care in this kind of stable and continuous "holding environment" supports early development in ways that provide a foundation for later resiliency (Garmezy, Masten, & Tellegen, 1984; Winnicott, 1965a). We now understand that these early caregiving experiences continue to shape brain development in early life in ways that blur the traditional boundaries between nature and nurture (Perry, Pollard, Blakley, Baker, & Vigilante, 1995; Shapiro & Applegate, 2000; Siegel, 1999).

COMPLEX ADOPTION

Complex adoption, as defined in this book, involves two broad adoption contexts: (1) the adoption of older infants and children from settings such as foster placement or institutional care; and (2) the adoption of infants through open adoptions in which the birth parents have a relationship with the adoptive family. These forms of adoption present not only new opportunities for both children and parents but also challenges to the processes of family formation.

The psychological adaptations of children in complex adoption have not been studied extensively, and systematic clinical reports are just emerging. These reports reveal the difficult developmental sequelae for children with traumatic preadoptive histories and the idiosyncratic process by which they may begin to establish attachment relationships with their adoptive parents (Castle et al., 1999; Downey, 2000; Goldberg, Gold, & Washington, 1997; Paret & Shapiro, 1998). It is clear, however, that both children and parents in complex adoption face many obstacles in the process of establishing secure parent–child relationships. *It is generally thought that the age of a child at the time of adoption and the quality of his/her early care have particular importance for the child's emotional and physical health status at the time of adoption and the nature of his/her future adaptation to the adoptive family.*

Adoption of Older Children

The first form of complex adoption is the adoption of older infants and children whose preadoptive histories may have included neglect, trauma, and multiple disruptions. This form of adoption includes both international adoption and the adoption of children who have been in the foster care system. The number of such adoptions has been growing rapidly, and the adoptive parents may be known foster caregivers, new adoptive parents, or kinship family members (Evan B. Donaldson Adoption Institute, 2000). While the quality of care in institutional or out-of-home care varies widely, many of these children will have experienced substantial emotional and/or physical neglect and child abuse. Thus, trauma, loss, and disruption are themes that almost certainly characterize the early life experiences of these children.

These early preadoptive experiences may result in developmental delays in the important spheres of social, cognitive, and emotional development. As a consequence, the adoptive parents of vulnerable children often seek help in understanding and responding to the difficulties both they and their children may encounter. Common presenting problems at the time of adoption include the child's internal emotional fragility, difficulty in forming trusting relationships, evidence of extreme separation anxiety, and significant developmental delays. In addition, at the time of adoption, many children have difficulties in homeostatic regulation that present many caregiving challenges, including primary problems in sleeping, eating, sootheability, and the regulation of affect (Paret & Shapiro, 1998).

In fact, however, relatively little is known about these children's subjective experiences, the different levels of risk related to the amount of time in impermanent care, the caregiving challenges faced by their adoptive families, or the lifelong symbolic meaning of their early experiences to themselves and their adoptive parents. In Chapters 3–6, we explore in depth specific aspects of post-foster-care and international adoptions, including the meaning of transracial and transcultural adoption to children and parents, as well as adoptive parents' difficulties in helping their children recover from the internal fragility that often remains for years.

Open Adoption

The second broadly defined form of complex adoption is open adoption, in which a child is adopted at birth by the intentional caregiving family. In this context the birth parent(s) take some role in choosing the adoptive parents, with the mutual understanding that they can in some way continue to remain in touch with their child (Wegar, 1997). While this form of adoption has many positive characteristics, such as the opportunity for adoptive parents to become involved as caregivers *at birth*, little is known about the impact of this family structure on the child's developing sense of identity. The problems that parents and children encounter in open adoption are different from the challenges of post-foster care or international adoption. In open adoptions, the birth parents can choose the adoptive parents, and the adoption most often occurs at birth, although, in most states, the birth parent(s) have the right to take some time to rethink their willingness to give up the baby. If the adoption does not go forward, the intentional parents may experience a sense of great loss, as they have already come to believe the baby is theirs and often have developed a relationship with the birth parent(s). If the adoption proceeds, the adoptive parents have an opportunity to begin a continuous parental relationship with the neonate.The infant can begin to establish a qualitatively good attachment relationship with the adoptive parent(s) from birth, and this will be an important contribution to good developmental outcome. The adoptive parent(s), however, will need to establish strong family boundaries while maintaining with the birth parent(s) a constructive relationship that is in "the best interest of the child." In Chapter 7, we address the complicated set of relationships that can develop and the range of emergent issues.

This chapter presents an overview of the ways in which a developmental perspective on child well-being can help clinicians understand the special issues in complex adoption. In particular, the recent conceptualizations of childhood trauma and its influence on developmental well-being are salient to our discussion of complex adoption, as they shed light on the difficulties children may have in overcoming early deficits and establishing new relationships with parental caregivers (Webb, 1999). In addition, a multisystemic perspective on risk and resiliency in childhood is central in informing practitioners in the use of effective assessment and treatment strategies that help children progress in different spheres of development (Fraser, 1997).

This broad developmental perspective can help clinicians understand the many complex social, cultural, familial, genetic, and environmental factors that contribute to the developmental status of the growing child. The material presented in this chapter is intended as a conceptual foundation for social workers and other professionals who practice in this area. In particular, it is meant to increase clinicians' diagnostic understanding and broaden practitioners' views of the possible routes to intervention in response to concerns of parents and children in complex family structures.

A DEVELOPMENTAL APPROACH TO COMPLEX ADOPTION: A TRIPARTITE PERSPECTIVE

Many observations from developmental and clinical research have expanded our understanding of the clinical issues often encountered in work with special populations and children at risk (Fraiberg, Adelson, & Shapiro, 1975; Masten et al., 1990). An understanding of children's psychological development over time can combine with an ecological awareness of their sociocultural milieu to inform clinicians of important areas of assessment and strategies for intervention. Assessment spheres include the following developmental perspectives:

- The impact of diverse sociocultural contexts on children in complex adoption.
- The concept of developmental lines and the assessment of delayed development.
- The history and effects of primary attachment relationships.
- The history and trauma of disruption and loss.
- Special issues in identity formation in complex family structures.
- Interactive environmental and biological risk factors, such as prenatal exposure to alcohol and drugs.
- The nature of infant temperament and other biological factors.

A broad conceptual developmental framework is critical in assessing the course of developmental vulnerability in childhood and the nature of both risk and capacity for resiliency. A primary characteristic of a developmental approach in assessment is the recognition of potential gaps between the chronological age and maturational age as represented by developmental achievements in various spheres. Consideration of the preadoptive history of the child and multiple biopsychosocial factors in his/her early years may help explain any apparent developmental delays. This knowledge is critical in constructing strengths-oriented, effective assessment and treatment plans (Webb, 1996).

Among the most important shifts in our understanding of child development is the acceptance of the idea that the child's social surround, or social ecology, is a strong determinant of developmental outcomes. This stands in contrast to the idea that development is driven forward primarily by internal characteristics of the child. Research from fields as diverse as social work, psychology, public health, medicine, sociology, and anthropology confirms the anecdotal understanding that single factors are rarely unique determinants of global developmental outcomes. Rather, biological, psychological, and sociological factors combine to influence developmental outcomes and well-being. This tripartite view of development is referred to as the "biopsychosocial perspective" (Webb, 1996). It describes the ways in which interrelated psychological, social, and biological factors combine either to protect or impede developmental competence (Masten, Hubbard, Gest, Tellegen, & Garmezy, 1999). This perspective is important to practitioners as they make diagnostic assessments, assess risks, formulate a dynamic understanding of the problems, and plan for related interventions.

Practitioners must be careful to balance their assessment of risks and strengths within those contextual factors thought to influence developmental outcomes. For example, the experience of persistent poverty poses a clear risk to developmental outcome but does not determine developmental well-being on its own. Rather, the experience of persistent poverty combines with related factors such as parenting, single parenthood, access to medical care, nutrition, housing, and education in ways that substantially influence child development (Chase-Lansdale & Brooks-Gunn, 1995; Thomson, Hanson, & McLanahan, 1994; McLanahan & Sandefur, 1994). Using this perspective, the assessment of a child at risk may more clearly delineate what has been missing or traumatic, and what specific treatment objectives may be most helpful. For example, children who have been adopted internationally are likely to be suffering from unmet health needs, and their lethargic behavior may be indicative of both illness and neglect due to long-term institutional care. Both the physical and emotional needs require attention.

Likewise, the well-being of a child who is adopted post-foster placement cannot be fully understood by focusing on a single factor such as early experiences of abuse or neglect. Rather, practitioners must assess a complex array of both risk and protective factors that may have existed in the preadoptive environment and how the influence of these factors may be manifested in the child's current behavior and emotional life (Davies, 1999; Fraser, 1997). The tripartite perspective therefore involves the integration of biological and genetic factors, as well as sociocultural and psychological dimensions of the child's experience.

THE TRIPARTITE PERSPECTIVE AND CLINICAL ISSUES

The Interactive Dynamic of "Nature and Nurture" on Child Development

Historically, researchers have understood "nature" and "nurture" to be dichotomous variables. Classified under the construct "nature" have been factors such as intelligence, health, temperamental style, and the genetic origins of mental illness. Factors such as the caregiving environment, parenting behavior, and social context have been clustered under the construct of "nurture." Researchers now understand that "nature" and "nurture" interact in a recursive manner and are related sets of influences on development (Nelson & Bloom, 1997). The boundary between "nature" and "nurture" can be permeated by factors such as the quality of caregiving relationships or the holding environment that surrounds the developing infant and young child (Siegel, 1999; Winnicott, 1965a).

For example, with regard to the current research on the ways in which environmental factors influence brain development in early life (Shapiro & Applegate, 2000; Siegel, 1999), adoption research has traditionally focused on the heritability of factors such as temperament and the genetic transmission of factors relating to mental illness (Cadoret, 1990). Later in this chapter, we present a more detailed discussion of infant temperament and factors associated with prenatal health and development.

In *all* adoptions, issues of similarity and difference between parents and their adopted children have symbolic meaning to children and parent alike (Brodzinsky et al., 1998; Hoopes, 1990).When children are adopted in the new forms of complex adoption, the problems of sifting out what accounts for developmental attributes is even more complex. Trauma may have occurred *in utero* or after birth via a combination of biological and environmental factors such as poor nutrition, inadequate health care, exposure to substance abuse, or early neglect. When children have experienced early trauma, it is hard to know how to evaluate their true "temperament" or natural "abilities," since they may have developed maladaptive, defensive coping mechanisms that interfere with positive development. Parents who attribute to children damaging, heritable characteristics may become pessimistic about the possibilities of recovery. Sometimes they fear their child becoming like his or her unknown birth parent(s). In open adoption, the known birth parent can help the adoptive parents better evaluate the potential influences of heritable characteristics and nurturance on their child's development. These are difficult, ongoing worries that emerge over time, at different phases of the child's development.

The Sociocultural Context of Development

Ecological systems theory has made important contributions to the study of child development (Bronfenbrenner, 1979). One of its major tenets is the idea that individuals *transact* with their external social environment in a variety of ways, at multiple systems levels (Bronfenbrenner, 1979). In this context, human behavior and development are embedded within, and influenced by, larger institutional, cultural, and social contexts. Such understanding is particularly salient in examining emerging social issues such as complex adoption. For example, the experience of parents who adopt older children, children with special needs, children from other countries, and children from other racial, ethnic, and religious groups, is shaped by cultural norms, values, and beliefs with regard to the core meaning of family and the acceptance of new family structures (Bartholet, 1993). In this regard, for example, long-term research on the outcome of transracial adoption has found that prejudice and bias have negative effects, especially on self-esteem and ethnoracial pride in transracially adopted sons (Feigelman, 2000).

A Multidimensional View of Development

A strengths-oriented approach to the experience of children in diverse families is supported by research suggesting that *development unfolds not by one common pathway but by alternative routes in a variety of contexts* (Cicchetti & Cohen, 1995; Zigler & Hall, 2000). This perspective is important because it addresses the breadth of individual differences that can occur within a population. This view is also central to our ability to think about the nature of cultural variation in development, as well as the nature of plasticity, or the capacity for growth and change. These ideas have special importance for practitioners working with diverse populations and children who may have experienced difficult early beginnings.

For example, the idea that development proceeds along alternative pathways can be utilized by practitioners to conceptualize the ways in which a variety of family structures, such as those described in this volume, can organize to support adaptive competence in infants and children. Nevertheless, despite family differences and styles of caregiving, all children share a universal need to be loved and wanted, and require a certain basic context for early social caregiving to help them develop their capacities for intimate relationships and functioning in the broader world. The *quality* of early care is seen to be importantly related to the capacity for attachment relationships and overrides the particular impact of diverse family structures or cultural styles of caregiving on developmental outcome (Lamb, 1999; Pruett, 2000).

THE SOCIAL AND CULTURAL SURROUND OF THE CHILD: IMPLICATIONS FOR PRACTICE

Cultural and societal changes shape the values, belief systems, and norms a society holds regarding the nature of childhood, the structure of family life, and the role of children in both families and society at large (Aries, 1962; Zigler & Hall, 2000). Practitioners who are able to place the experience of complex adoption in important sociocultural contexts improve their ability to practice in three interrelated ways:

1. *It is important that practitioners have a historical view of adoption that enables them to consider how social, economic, cultural, and demo-*

graphic changes shape the experience of complex adoption. Many social, demographic, and cultural trends have combined to shape the experience of complex adoption as a way of family building. The number of healthy infants available for adoption at birth has declined dramatically, resulting in a growing discrepancy between the number of intentional parents wishing to adopt and the number of infants available. At the same time, an increasing number of children in the foster care system in the United States and in institutional care abroad are awaiting adoption. As a result, more intentional parents are willing to consider diverse forms of complex adoption (Evan B. Donaldson Adoption Institute, 2000). Cultural changes in society reflect a more accepting view of family diversity both in regard to the range of potential parents considered eligible to adopt and the adoption of children who do not match the religious, ethnic, or racial characteristics of the parents (Lamb, 1999; Sullivan 1995b).

The nature of complex family formation thus requires that practitioners be able to apply their sensitivity and training to issues of cultural diversity that affect adopted children within families. Inherent in many forms of complex adoption are racial, ethnic, and cultural differences between intentional parents and their adopted children. Many authors have written extensively about the ways in which an appreciation of these differences can inform frameworks for assessment and practice (Gibbs & Huang, 1999). The experience of children adopted internationally is an example of the difficult shift that occurs when children go from one caregiving context to another vastly different one. Many of these children come from group care settings such as orphanages, foster homes, or hospitals, and in the transition must adjust to a new language, a new cultural milieu, and parents whose conceptions of caregiving differ greatly from those represented in their previous environments. The loss for the children relates not only to their early caregivers but also to the social context of their lives, including familiar smells, foods, objects, other children, and style of play and interaction. As children become older, awareness of difference can become an issue in identity formation; children become more clearly aware of the loss of both their indigenous cultural identity and birth parents. Many adoptive parents of transracial children are developing ways to help their children resolve issues of ethnic, racial, and cultural identifications over time (Dewan, 2000).

2. *The nature of complex adoption requires that practitioners bring sensitivity and cultural understanding to issues of diversity and the ways in which cultural differences shape important contexts for child development.* As Lieberman (1990) points out, beliefs about parenting, the nature of childhood, and the importance of the parent–child relationship are culturally grounded to some degree. Other beliefs about the role of professional

helpers and the origins of mental health and illness are also central to the practitioner's ability to work across issues of cultural diversity (Gibbs & Huang, 1999). Increasingly, this requires that practitioners be not only culturally aware in a general sense but also open to individual differences within cultural groups. Such a stance helps the practitioner avoid errors associated with overgeneralizing and stereotyping (Gibbs & Huang, 1999). Assessment tools such as the "culturagram" described by Congress (1994), can help practitioners to think about the influence of culture and perceived cultural differences on family functioning. Specifically, the culturagram can be utilized to consider variables that influence degrees of assimilation to the dominant culture and individual differences among family members in this regard.

Increasingly practitioners are called upon to provide guidance, support, and treatment to minority kinship caregivers, for example, and need to listen to the perspectives of these adoptive parents and come to understand their view of the needs of children. Often, adoptive kinship parents are grandmothers who face extensive financial and health care needs, and are grieving the loss of their own children. The process of developing a working alliance that recognizes their beliefs about child raising and respects their positive efforts to support their children under difficult circumstances is critical. Without an empathetic acceptance of the cultural and personal views of the grandparents, the practitioner may not be effective in aiding the family in the use of new developmental perspectives that may be helpful to the grandchildren in their care (see Chapter 6).

3. *An understanding of the ways in which our view of childhood and child development has changed in the last century has important implications for methods of assessment and intervention.* The idea that changing societal norms and values influence the experience of important life events is represented in Elder's (1998) work on the life course. Elder utilizes the term "cohort effects" to describe the way in which norms, values, beliefs, and expectations that exist at a given point in history influence our experience of major life events and exert psychosocial influence on development itself. For example, the practice of international adoption is a relatively recent phenomenon that reflects social and political changes both abroad and in the United States.

Current social views of childhood represent important changes in the philosophy of childhood and ways we understand children's behavior and developmental needs (Aries, 1962). The concept of *adultmorphism* refers to a tendency to think of children as miniature adults. The modern understanding of childhood as qualitatively different from adulthood reflects both societal change (e.g., longer expectable lifespan, changing roles of children in the family) and the emergence of concepts such as maturation and adaptation, which are central to many 20th century theories of child development (Hetherington & Parke, 1999). Awareness of maturational differences between children and adults is central to understanding the meaning of a child's behavior in a particular phase of development. For example, because childhood depression is often manifested by different symptomatology than that found in adults, it was once believed that children did not experience depression. Thus, many important opportunities for early assessment and intervention were lost.

Work in the field of complex adoption requires a knowledge base that includes an understanding of general concepts central to child-focused work and the ways in which work with children differs in both substance and process from work with adults (Chethik, 2000; Gardner, 1991). In this regard, the developing knowledge base has enlarged our understanding of the different treatment strategies that are useful with infants, toddlers, latency-age children, and adolescents. This understanding is also important in the assessment of children adopted at different ages and from very different circumstances.

EARLY EXPERIENCE AND THE PSYCHOLOGICAL WORLD OF THE CHILD

From a variety of theoretical perspectives, researchers have described the importance of the early caregiving, or holding, environment as a context for infant and child development (Ainsworth, Blehar, Waters, & Wall, 1978; Bowlby, 1969; Spitz & Wolf, 1946; Steele, Steele, Croft, & Fonagy, 1999; Vaughan, Egeland, Sroufe, & Waters, 1979; Vondra et al., 1999; Winnicott, 1965a). From this multidisciplinary literature, a shared understanding posits that normative social, cognitive, and affective development in infancy and early childhood occurs most optimally in the context of consistent and responsive caregiving, provided by a single caregiver or a small group of caregivers.

In terms of the emotional life of the child, one of the most significant developmental lines is the emerging capacity for human relationships (Fonagy & Target, 1998a; Greenspan & Porges, 1984; Stern, 1985). The genesis of the child's capacity for human relationships begins before birth and is nurtured in the context of the developing child's earliest relationships with primary caregivers (Schore, 1994; Siegel, 1999). These primary relationships change throughout infancy, toddlerhood, latency, and adolescence as development continues in multiple spheres. The quality of the psychological tie and relationship between parent and child is critical in helping the child to master successive maturational phases of development. Trauma and loss can interrupt the child's capacity to move forward successfully, as he/she may not have the internal organization or adaptive capacity to withstand age-related experiences of anxiety and grief. This may be especially true if the child has experienced loss or disruption with regard to primary caregivers (Bowlby, 1969).

Winnicott (1965a) describes the early caregiver–child relationship as a holding environment that provides the basis of a healthy psychic infrastructure and the development of a sense of trust. Because children in complex adoptions may have experienced repeated or sustained disruptions in early caregiving relationships, they may be at risk for developmental disturbances. Infants and young children rely on primary caregivers for the modulation of anxiety and other states of emotional and physiological arousal. Traumatic separations, losses, and, in extreme cases, child abuse and neglect preclude the experience of being "psychologically held." Furthermore, work in cognitive neurobiology describes how the sustained experience of such early trauma can precipitate changes in the developing brain that predispose the child to further vulnerability (Perry et al., 1995).

Children in complex adoptions may have experienced repeated or sustained disruptions in early caregiving relationships and be at risk for attachment and developmental disturbances (Ainsworth et al., 1978; Fraiberg et al., 1975; Paret & Shapiro, 1998; Perry et al., 1995). Infants and young children who cannot rely on primary caregivers to help them cope with anxiety and other states of emotional and physiological distress often develop coping styles, or adaptations, that may interfere with mastery of developmental goals and the process of establishing new and important attachment relationships with others (Fonagy & Target, 1998a; Freud, 1966). Thus, it is important that practitioners have a solid understanding of the nature of early caregiving relationships, including a history of the quality and stability of attachment relationships, so as to understand the developmental and relational difficulties experienced by the child in the present.

Since the 1960s, a multidisciplinary research base has documented the importance of early interaction between infant and caregiver, and reveals a wide array of early neonatal and infant sensory and perceptual competencies. This body of research stands in contrast to the prior notion that infants are born as a type of *tabula rasa,* or blank slate, and without the reflexive, sensory, and perceptual competencies that prime their readiness for social relatedness and interaction. Current understanding of infant development shows that infants are indeed active participants, albeit not symmetrical partners, in their earliest relationships. Research on both attachment and temperament describe the ways in which characteristics of the child combine with factors such as the psychological health and characteristics of the parent and a confluence of environmental factors to shape the caregiving context (Belsky, 1984).

ATTACHMENT RESEARCH AND IMPLICATIONS FOR PRACTICE

Attachment research has expanded our understanding of the importance of positive early care. This knowledge base can help practitioners provide informed preventive and tertiary care services. The earliest studies of what is now termed "attachment" showed that both human and animal babies show severe developmental disturbance if separated from their attachment figures (Bowlby, Robertson, & Rosenbluth, 1952; Harlow, 1958; Spitz & Wolf, 1946). These disturbances were evident even if the infants' physical needs for nutrition and warmth were met. Thus, infants who lack the opportunity for meaningful attachments are at risk for serious developmental difficulties.

Among the earliest scholarly works describing the importance of stable and continuous attachment relationships were the descriptive reports of Spitz and Wolf (1946), Freud and Burlingham (1944), and Bowlby et al. (1952). These reports carefully described the grief-stricken reaction of children separated from their primary caretakers under conditions of stress, such as war-related violence and childhood hospitalizations. Until that time, the internal meaning of the primary attachment figure to the child was not clearly understood or appreciated. Specifically, these early studies laid the foundation for further investigation into the ways that stable access to primary attachment figures supports the ongoing ego development of the young child.

Ego function refers to the overall capacity of a person to integrate different spheres of the psyche in order to deal with the realities of the external world. All children, for example, have to cope with their internal feelings, the demands of the external world, and the gradual mastery of new developmental tasks. Ego function can be described as the "command post" for integrating the important affective, social, and cognitive spheres that encompass the core of human life (Blank & Blank, 1974). Thus, the disruption of primary attachment relationships can be associated with some disturbances in the "command post" that present challenges to ego function and the adaptive capacity of the child; depression and anxiety may follow.

Bowlby's (1969) work on attachment and loss created an ethological conceptual frame for understanding the role of primary attachment relationships in human development, providing the theoretical frame for the empirical study of attachment (Ainsworth et al., 1978; Cassidy & Shaver, 1999). This view of attachment understands the parent–infant or parent–child relational system as organized to achieve the dual developmental goals of security and external exploration of the environment. During the first years of life, children develop internal representations, or internal working models, of their important attachment relationships (Fonagy & Target, 1998a). The development of a secure sense of the other and the self supports the child's psychological investments in the external world of objects and people.

Thus, "securely" attached infants are able to seek and utilize proximity to the caregiver when distressed to modulate emotional arousal and to see the caregiver as a "secure base" from which to explore and gain mastery over the external world (Ainsworth et al., 1978). Conversely, "insecurely attached" infants are understood to represent infant–caregiver dyads that are not organized to achieve consistently the dual goals of emotional modulation and exploration (Lyons-Ruth, Bronfman, & Parsons, 1999). Classified as "insecure/avoidant," "insecure/resistant," or "disorganized," these attachment patterns are associated with a range of suboptimal developmental outcomes (Davies, 1999; Solomon & George, 1999; Steele et al., 1999). The classification of "disorganized attachment" was created when researchers found clusters of parent–child dyads that could not be reliably classified by one of the three existing patterns (Cassidy & Shaver, 1999). Infants classified as "disorganized" show the greatest insecurity in that their attachment behavior is confused and inconsistent. These infants may display unusual postures or engage in behaviors such as "freezing."

Work in the cognitive neurosciences provides an additional empirical base for the importance of attachment relationships to developmental well-being (Schore, 1994). This research suggests that it is through the process of forming attachment relationships that important aspects of brain development continue in early life (Siegel, 1999). Specifically, the neurobiological substrate of the developing child's capacity for affect regulation, or the modulation of emotions, depends in part on caregiving that is empathetic, consistent, and infused with understanding of the mental life of the child. Within the context of such a caregiving environment, children themselves develop the capacity for empathetic understanding of emotional states, tolerance of emotional arousal, and the basis for an optimistic sense of self.

Practitioners can use this understanding in the assessment and treatment of children who have not had the benefit of secure attachment relationships. When a supportive environment does not exist and the attachment relationship has been disrupted for a period of time, the infant may experience severe stress and develop behavioral mechanisms for coping with poorly regulated interactive experiences. In her work, Selma Fraiberg (1987a) described the emergence of infant defenses such as gaze aversion, withdrawal, aggression against the self, hyperactivity in infants and toddlers, or extreme separation anxiety. While these defenses may function temporarily to relieve internal anxiety states, they clearly limit the infant's opportunities for either the proximity or exploration needed to promote developmental competence.

In summary, children who are adopted following foster care, or institutional care, are likely to have experienced environments that contain risk factors for social, emotional, and cognitive development. They may have deficits in their capacity for attachment relationships and possess a limited capacity for important exploration of relationships and the external world. Such infants may also be impaired in important capacities such as the ability to self-soothe, and to problem solve, to articulate feeling states or to utilize language and important relationships to modify emotional life and experience. Adoptive parents, therefore, may be faced with caring for children who experience internal states of disorganization and anxiety, and are narcissistically vulnerable, as they may have established a very negative picture of themselves. Often, new adoptive parents are overwhelmed as they realize the extensiveness of their children's needs in many spheres of development.

A common example of difficulties may be found in the attachment behavior of children who move from one foster placement to another. In such cases, the child's fear of abandonment and rejection, or even of being loved, may precipitate behavior that undermines the process of forming new attachments to potentially more available caregivers. For example, some children may provoke rejection not only to test the commitment of their new caretakers but also to experience an intense relationship with the "other." It is important that practitioners and adoptive parents understand how early caregiving experiences shape the child's sense of self in general and how the child has internalized the meaning of relationships in particular. Adoptive parents may need much support and guidance, and practitioners must provide an empathetic and informed therapeutic holding environment for the family and the child. The process of recovery is uncertain and occurs over a long period of time. The child's development does not progress in a linear fashion, and as new questions emerge, therapeutic work can be characterized by periods of both progress and regression.

SPECIAL ISSUES IN IDENTITY FORMATION AND COMPLEX ADOPTION

Identity formation is a continuing process that has its roots in earlier stages of development and growth (Cote & Levine, 1988; Erikson, 1950; Josselson, 1987; Kroger, 2000). Identity has been defined as "the stable, consistent and reliable sense of who one is and what one stands for in the world" (Josselson, 1987, p. 10). The process of identity formation requires children to evaluate the ways in which their own attitudes, beliefs, and goals are similar to or different from those of their parents and other important aspects of their psychosocial surround as represented by peer relationships, other adults, and other institutions, such as neighborhood, school, and community (Blos, 1967; Josselson, 1987; Marcia, 1994; Stevens, 1997).

While the early literature on identity development was primarily psychodynamic in nature and focused on adolescence as a particularly salient developmental phase, Erikson broadened this perspective by including the psychosocial aspect of identity development (Blos, 1967; Erikson, 1950). More recently, authors have addressed the ways in which gender and cultural differences require a broader conceptualization of identity in order to describe the various possible pathways from childhood to adolescence (Gilligan, 1982; Kroger, 2000; Phinney & Rosenthal, 1992; Stevens, 1997).

Among all adolescents, there is great variation with regard to their ability to engage actively in a process of evaluating their degree of identification with parents and others (Cote & Levine, 1988; Josselson, 1987; Marcia, 1994). Many children have a hard time resolving conflicts with parental figures; therefore, they may experience great difficulty in the process of differentiation. Children who are adopted often have additional stress in the processes of identity formation because of the symbolic meaning of loss they endured over time, and the challenge to achieve a coherent and integrated identity especially in transracial or nontraditional families. Adopted children have dual sets of parental figures—the adoptive parents, whom they know, and birth parents, whom they may know only through fantasies and emotional representations (Brinich, 1990; Hoopes, 1990; Lifton, 1994). For all adopted children, having to live without knowledge of their roots may bring a sense of genealogical bewilderment that can undermine efforts to "claim" their own identity (Lifton, 1994). This process may be further complicated for children adopted at an older age, such as in complex adoption. These children may have affective memories of their lives with their birth parents and also have experienced multiple disruptions of early caregiving relationships. The discontinuities and loss of early relational figures may have resulted in unstable internal representations of self and other, making the process of identity formation more difficult.

For children who have been adopted, the process of coming to terms with loss and rejection by birth parents can persist over time. Anger, resentment, and loss may temporarily hinder the children's ability to form their own identity (Brinich, 1990; Hoopes, 1990). In complex adoption, children may get stuck, as they are frightened of identifying with past and present parental figures. In post-foster or post-institutional adoption, children's sense of self may already have been challenged by earlier abandonment and trauma, and they may be stymied in efforts to formulate an optimistic sense of themselves and their future. For these children, the process of identity formation in adolescence may reach a crisis, as they may be unsure if they will be able to establish long-lasting intimate relationships. A return of separation anxiety may make it more difficult to consider psychological separation from their parents.

Children who have been in foster care and experienced severe trauma, neglect, or abuse may have very disturbing memories and/or fantasies about their biological parents. At some level, they may believe they played a central role in their own mistreatment or abandonment. This child's eye view of separation from biological parents can become a lifelong part of a negative identity and sense of self. For some children who have extreme difficulty moving forward, therapeutic assistance may help them to work through their complex feelings regarding their birth parents, their adoptive parents, their sense of self-blame and shame regarding the perceived abandonment that led to the adoption, and the concerns they may have about being able to integrate disparate family roots and parental figures into a coherent narrative.

The literature on adolescent identity development in children of color in general (Brown, 1990; Phinney & Rosenthal, 1992; Stevens, 1997) and in biracial children in particular, can help us understand the special issues in identity formation for transracially adopted children (Gibbs, 1987; Williams, 1999). Several authors have discussed the challenges posed to minority children in identity formation due to the need to integrate multiple cultural reference groups in the contexts of discrimination and the European American worldview (Gibbs, 1987; Stevens, 1997). For transracially adopted children, this process may be further complicated when external negative bias and prejudice joins with their own negative identity. They may feel pressure to reject one part of their heritage in order to resolve ambivalence and achieve a greater level of comfort (Gibbs, 1987).

In transracial adoptees, therefore, the process of identity formation may be even more complicated than for other adoptees, and it is important that the child's steps toward identity consolidation be supported by his/her parent(s). Feigelman (2000) has found that when transracially adopted children live in integrated communities, the conflicts some of them feel are abated and they find it easier to construct an identity that fits with their own sense of themselves. It is important, therefore, that parents and practitioners consider the ways in which the children's wider social surround is supportive of their effort to integrate various aspects of the self. In Chapter 3, we explore the special issues faced by adolescents in transracial adoptions.

Finally, as with all children, adopted children have their own temperamental characteristics that may be very different from those of their parents. Adoptive parents may react in different ways; sometimes conflicts emerge regarding the choices their children make. Open adoption, in which children may know their birth parents, offers them known parental figures with whom they can identify to some extent. While the psychological parents have the primary relational tie with them, children may perceive themselves to "be more like" one or the other birth parent. Knowing the birth parents can help to give children an opportunity to accept their own attributes and temperament. In this sense, children can more realistically both identify with and differentiate from the important persons who are relevant to their sense of who they are, and who they will become. Of course, often, children may be beset by feelings of loyalty conflict and fear of disappointing one or the other of their parental figures. It is helpful to the adopted child's ongoing efforts at identity formation if both sets of parents are able to offer supportive environments that communicate acceptance of the child's own attributes, his/her inherent nature, and the need to consolidate his/her own identity (Brodzinsky & Schechter, 1990; see Chapter 7).

THE INTERACTIVE RELATIONSHIP BETWEEN BIOLOGICAL AND PSYCHOLOGICAL DEVELOPMENT: IMPLICATIONS FOR PRACTICE

Temperament

Temperament, as a construct, refers to an individual's general style of responding to the world. Temperament is usually described by its behavioral manifestations along many dimensions, such as level of activity, rhythmicity, distractibility, intensity, stimulus threshold, mood, and capacity for persistence (Lemery, Hill-Goldsmith, Klinnert, & Mrazek, 1999). Research on infant temperament sometimes factors these characteristics into clusters identified as easy, slow-to-warm-up, and fussy/difficult temperamental styles (Chess & Thomas, 1991; Goldsmith, Hill, Buss, & Lemery, 1997; Kagan, Arcus, & Snidman, 1994). For example, an "easy" baby might be one who is well regulated, has an overall positive emotional tone, and can move from one state of alertness to the next with relative ease. In contrast, a "fussy" baby might be one who is difficult to soothe, has a hard time establishing regulated patterns of eating and sleeping, and is very sensitive to changes in stimuli such as light, sound, and temperature.

In addition to a focus on the classification of infant temperament, researchers have studied the degree to which temperament is a heritable characteristic and the relevance of the match or mismatch in caregiver–infant temperamental styles. One view of infant temperament, which suggests that individuals inherit various concentrations of neurochemicals associated with different aspects of temperament (Kagan et al., 1994), conforms to the anecdotal belief that temperament is a heritable characteristic.

The assumption is sometimes made that because temperament is a heritable characteristic, biologically related parents and children are more likely to exhibit a "good match" of temperamental styles. However, temperamental mismatches occur in both biological and nonbiological parent–child relationships, and all parents must work to understand the particular style of their children and related caretaking needs. The applied value of the "goodness-of-fit" concept goes beyond a description of parent–child temperamental styles to include the parenting skills associated with the ability to achieve a regulated pattern of relational interaction despite differences in temperamental style (Chess & Thomas, 1991).

In the case of complex adoption, when a child is adopted after having experienced periods of trauma, it can be difficult for families and practitioners alike to differentiate the child's inherent temperamental characteristics from symptoms of the trauma itself. If contact with the practitioner is initiated by the parents when the child's behavioral symptoms have become overwhelming, it is important to understand whether the parents view the child's difficulties as driven by *inherent* characteristics (i.e., temperament) or as resulting from a combination of life experiences. A careful assessment of how the parents view their child's temperament is important and should be coupled with independent observations of the child and a review of other factors, both social and biological, that could be causal in the behavioral manifestation of developmental difficulty.The parents' explanation of the origin of their child's problems is an important entree into exploring the degree to which parents are accepting of their child as he/she is, as opposed to how they may have hoped he/she would be. Increasing parents' fuller understanding and acceptance of their child is a worthy goal of child-focused treatment.

The concept of maternal self-efficacy has to do with how mothers perceive their own competency in being able to care for a developing child. Mothers' feelings about their effectiveness as parents shape their parenting behavior (Donovan & Leavitt, 1992). In situations of complex adoption, where the relationship between adoptive parents and their child is being formed following a history of disrupted, broken, or fleeting attachments, the child's adaptation may cause the parents to feel less than adequate. Often, they feel stymied in their efforts to comfort and discipline their child and seek guidance about how to ameliorate the sequelae of the child's difficult early experiences.

It is particularly important to help parents to formulate a more informed understanding of the interactional dynamic of innate characteristics of the child and environmental factors that influence his/her behavior (Benedek, 1959). In understanding their child's capacities and developmental status, they may feel more competent to try new approaches in caregiving. Many children present a challenging caregiving environment for adoptive parents because they may be initially unresponsive to caretaking efforts and thus a challenge to adoptive parents' sense of competence or efficacy.

Prenatal Exposure to Risk: Infant Health and Challenges for Caregiving

Development during the fetal period is driven by a complex matrix of factors. In addition to the genetic endowment of the fetus, development during this period is strongly influenced by both direct and indirect indices of maternal health and behavior. Factors such as maternal stress and social support, access to nutrition and medical care, the biological mother's overall health and well-being, and maternal behaviors such as the utilization of illicit drugs as well as exposure to other teratogens (e.g., lead, radiation) influence fetal development (Hetherington & Parke, 1999). Many adoptive parents of children in complex adoptions are told very little of the early neonatal and postnatal history of their child and the risks that might be involved. This is important information as infants who have been exposed to early risk often experience serious symptoms that may last for a long time.

A teratogen may be defined as any factor known to influence fetal development negatively. Such a factor is said to have a teratogenic effect. A common example is the effect of cigarette smoking on fetal development and neonatal health. It is believed that 20% of all incidents of low birthweight occur primarily because of nicotine exposure *in utero* (Carter & Larson, 1997). Prenatal exposure to teratogenic influences can have a range of negative sequelae on the developing fetus and infant. As with other stages, researchers believe that critical periods of development exist during fetal development. Thus, teratogenic exposure will have differential effects on the developing organism depending on both the level and time of exposure. Because neurological fetal development is so rapid in early pregnancy, early awareness of pregnancy and purposeful avoidance of teratogenic agents are important to the developmental well-being of the fetus and neonate. A good example of this is research describing the influence of folic acid deficiency on spinal cord development and the development of spina bifida. By supplementing the diets of pregnant women early in the pregnancy with adequate amounts of folic acid the rate of spina bifida can be greatly limited.

Prenatal exposure to teratogenic drugs may have both immediate and long-term consequences for developmental well-being (Chasnoff, Anson, Hatcher, Stenson, & Iaukea, 1998). Infants exposed to such drugs prenatally are more likely be born prematurely (e.g., < 37 weeks' gestational age) and/or with low birthweight or be small for their gestational age. Both prematurity and low birthweight are associated with a variety of potentially serious complications that interfere with the regulation of respiration, sleep, and feeding. This dysregulation may in turn be associated with the emergence of difficulties such as failure-to-thrive syndrome. Prenatal exposure to teratogens is also associated with the emergence of fetal alcohol syndrome, sudden infant death syndrome, and a variety of central nervous system disorders (Chasnoff et al., 1998).

Drug-exposed infants may require extraordinary care and a longer period of time to establish a consistent pattern of sleeping and eating. These infants may appear to be temperamentally "difficult" because of their sensitivity to stimuli and a marked difficulty in the modulation of sleep–wake states or states of emotional arousal. Social interaction patterns may be difficult to establish because these infants may have significant difficulty with eating (e.g. problems with sucking, vomiting) and other atypical interaction patterns marked by an absence of eye contact and muscle tone (e.g., rigidity). These children may be more difficult to hold and comfort. As development continues, drug-exposed children may more likely be characterized as displaying increased activity levels, increased impulsivity, delayed language and social development, and difficulties with auditory and visual processing (Carter & Larson, 1997).

It is important that parents, other caregivers, and practitioners become familiar with the range of sequelae associated with prenatal exposure to a variety of teratogens. Such knowledge not only facilitates an accurate assessment of neonatal and infant health but also can help to identify the caretaking challenges associated with such sequelae. This is particularly true in light of research suggesting that the effects of teratogenic exposure can be ameliorated by a sensitive caretaking environment or, alternatively, intensified by an environment that lacks sufficient nurturance.

PRACTICE WITH CHILDREN IN THE FIELD OF COMPLEX ADOPTION

Developmentally informed practice is based on the understanding that childhood difficulties occur in the context of growing up (Chethik, 2000; Lieberman, 1990). Thus, practitioners must have a dual focus in the assessment and treatment of children. Children's behavior and emotional lives must be considered in terms of both their current level of functioning and later developmental competence. This takes on particular meaning in work with children who have experienced either acute or chronic trauma in their caretaking environments and may be delayed in social, emotional, and/or cognitive development (Pynoos, Steinberg, & Wraith, 1995). For example, in complex adoptions, new adoptive parents often report the difficulty they have in establishing a rapport with their child, and may not understand that his/her withdrawal from expressions of love represents a style of coping developed under extreme stress. In the context of therapeutic work, it may be possible to help the child adapt to a more nurturant environment and develop more positive relationships.

Child-focused practitioners must also consider the ways in which age-related differences between children and adults shape the processes of assessment and intervention (Chethik, 2000; Freud, 1965). For example, young children typically lack the cognitive and verbal capacity to articulate emotional states such as sadness or excitement. In the therapeutic environment, they are more likely to express their emotional lives through the language of action and play (Webb, 1999). And the overwhelming dependency of young children on their caregivers requires that practitioners involve the parents as "colleagues" in their work on behalf of the young child. Because primary caretaking relationships define the context for development in early life (Chethik, 2000; Schore, 1994; Siegel, 1999), one way to consider the influence of the child's primary interpersonal relationships on well-being is via the conceptual frame of developmental lines (Freud, 1965).

The concept of developmental lines is central in work with children (Freud, 1981). As first conceived by Anna Freud, the concept of developmental lines refers to the child's unfolding maturation with regard to various aspects of relational capacity and ego development (Freud, 1965). Since that time, researchers have utilized the idea of developmental lines to describe the trajectories of maturation that occur in many spheres, such as emotional, cognitive, social, physical, and language development. In assessment and intervention, it is important that practitioners assess the child's developmental status across all lines of development and explore the dynamic relationship between his/her preadoptive history and current developmental status in each sphere. Development across lines may be either synchronous or uneven within a given child; that is, a child may show great vulnerability in one sphere of development but great strengths in others. Often, the adoptive family may find it helpful to know the child's relative strengths so that together they can achieve a sense of satisfaction in relation to achievement in various spheres of development.

During the 1980s, there emerged a field of study focused on the integration of developmental research and the study of psychopathology. Named developmental psychopathology, it involves the investigation of the origins, course, changes and continuities in maladaptive behavior over the lifespan (Hetherington & Parke, 1999). The basic tenets of this discipline reflect many of the advances in developmental theory and clinical research over the last quarter century. Because this field is closely involved with the study of risk and resiliency across the course of the lifespan, it is an important conceptual foundation for work with children whose caregiving environments have been disrupted and/or for whom the caregiving context is characterized as being "at risk." Thus, many of the complex family structures described in this volume can be considered from this perspective.

Cicchetti and Cohen (1995) describe the basic themes of developmental psychopathology. First, developmental psychopathologists assume that indicators of psychopathology occur in a developing organism (Cicchetti & Cohen, 1995). An important implication of this assumption is that practitioners must consider the cost of children's particular coping strategies and behavioral organization to their ongoing development and well-being. For example, if a child has experienced several broken attachments with primary caregivers, he/she may develop an avoidant or highly resistant behavioral organization that poses further challenge to the development of other attachment relationships. Caregivers in such a situation must be helped not to personalize the child's behavior but to sustain their efforts to connect with him/her. Second, it is the perspective of developmental psychopathology that the studies of normative development and psychopathology as disciplines can recursively inform each other. For example, Cicchetti and Cohen (1995) describe research on the developmental well-being of children in

Romanian orphanages. It showed that children who experience disruption in one developmental domain are more likely than other children to exhibit difficulties in other domains as well (Kaler & Freeman, 1994). This research confirms the idea that developmental lines tend to be interdependent and also shows that it can be difficult to predict the trajectory of development.

Third, the discipline of developmental psychopathology examines early precursors, or risk indicators, of later developmental disruption and psychopathology. This kind of research is particularly important to the development of sophisticated prevention efforts and is thus relevant to those interested in supporting strengths and preventing developmental difficulties. This literature has shown that while some behavioral manifestations of developmental difficulty appear early and tend to be consistent, other symptomatology may be ameliorated by the progression of development itself. For example, when a child experiences a shift in caretaking context that is characterized by the loss of shared language, as might be the case in international adoption, the emergence of shared communications with the new caregiver(s) may serve to ameliorate the child's distress.

And finally, developmental psychopathologists recognize that there is more than one pathway to both normal and "abnormal" adjustment over the course of the lifespan. This extremely important idea serves to challenge monolithic views of development and provides a conceptual basis for the study of multiple developmental contexts. As has been noted, developmental research shows that multiple factors interact to shape developmental processes. The kinds of psychological, political, and sociological changes underlying complex family formation require researchers and practitioners to broaden their view of "family" and question anew assumptions about the impact of early experience.

Practitioners who work with children must balance ideas generating from a deterministic belief in the role of early experience with hopes for change via the processes of altered situational characteristics and therapeutic intervention. Indeed, explanatory models of development suggest that many patterns are possible and that a broad range of developmental patterns exists among healthy populations of children and families (Cicchetti & Cohen, 1995).

A focus on the role of early experience must also be placed in the context of our understanding of the many phases of development in infancy, childhood, and adolescence. While many developmental theories are epigenetic in nature, meaning that each phase of development is considered to be, in part, dependent on mastery of earlier phase-specific tasks, it is also now understood that development remains "plastic" to some degree throughout childhood (Nelson & Bloom, 1997; Zigler & Hall, 2000). Thus, practitioners and researchers have the dual task of assessing both current developmental status and risk, and the kinds of intervention or prevention experiences that may function to ameliorate risk or repair developmental disruption. In this regard, a strengths focus assesses not only developmental risk but also the confluence of strengths and supports in a given child and family.

II

Complex Adoption

3

The Adoption of Children Following Foster Placement

The increasing number of children in the foster care system in the United States reflects the many difficult social problems in our society. Entry into the foster care system is the result of not only the vulnerability of individual families but also the lack of adequate social and economic support available to both families in poverty and vulnerable children and parents. Therefore, clinicians and practitioners who work in the field of child welfare must focus on the matrix of individual, familial, and social factors that combine to increase child and family vulnerability.

The adoption of a child from foster care often takes place after the child has had to cope with early trauma, multiple losses, and family disruptions. While adoption provides children with the external stability of a permanent family, their preadoptive histories often leave them with a certain degree of internal fragility (Paret & Shapiro, 1998). The child's difficult early beginnings add to the complexity of adoption, as the transition to the care of adoptive parent(s) is often shaped by the child's view that relationships with caregivers are easily broken. Thus, it may be difficult for the parent(s) and child to begin to establish a relationship that provides for the child a sense of permanent family belonging.

Researchers and clinicians who study adoption at birth discuss the shared fate of the adoption triad (Brodzinsky & Schechter, 1990). In all adoptions, the birth parent(s), the child, and the adoptive parent(s) experience a significant loss because of the break in the thread of biological relatedness between parent and child (Kirk, 1964). Yet in traditional adoption, the adoptive parents and the young infant have the opportunity to develop an attachment relationship within the earliest months of the child's life, and within a context that provides for continuity and stability of care. However, infants, toddlers, and older school-age children who are adopted post-foster placement may not have had the benefit of spending their infancy and early childhood within a protective circle of family care. Rather, their early relational experiences may have been characterized by episodes of neglect, trauma, disruption, and loss. Often, a combination of individual, familial, and social factors combined to hamper the ability of their parents to provide the "good enough" caregiving associated with positive child development outcomes (Winnicott, 1965b). In addition to individual and family vulnerability, children in foster care and their families of origin are more likely to have experienced the direct and indirect influences of poverty and discrimination.

For a variety of reasons, by the late 1990s, over 500,000 children were living within the public foster care system in the United States (Adoption and Foster Care Analysis and Reporting System [AFCARS], 2000). The child's initial entry into foster care and the length of time spent in care awaiting permanent placement or family reunification are associated with a complex set of individual, familial, and societal factors. For example, contextual factors such as poverty and lack of access to preventive care are associated not only with higher rates of entry into foster care, but also with barriers to eventual family reunification.

As we shall see in our discussion, it is important that practitioners become adept at recognizing individual differences among children in foster care. For example, variation with regard to early history, reasons for entry into the foster care system, length of time spent awaiting permanent placement, and the number of moves a child experiences within the system may combine to shape important developmental outcomes and the quality of adjustment within the adoptive family. These factors also can inform the nature and extent of a broad range of needed services.

The rising number of children in the public foster care system who are awaiting adoptive homes is of particular concern because of the potential negative effect on their psychological, cognitive, and emotional development. The unmet needs of children in the public foster care system can be overwhelming and often require the cooperation of interdisciplinary teams. Child welfare workers, social workers, psychologists, doctors, lawyers, and judges have important roles to play in providing direct services to children and families, and in advocating for policies that support the care of all vulnerable children, both within their families of origin and within the foster care system (Adoption and Foster Care Analysis and Reporting System [AFCARS], 2000). Often, a developmental perspective is central to the practitioner's ability in assessing a wide range of unmet needs and in providing intervention services (Webb, 1996).

This chapter begins with a brief review of the current status of children in the foster care system in the United States. Our primary focus is on the many barriers to permanency planning for children in foster care that exist, especially for minority children. These children are disproportionately represented in the foster care system and may face unique obstacles to either family reunification or adoptive placement. More broadly, we address the psychological ramifications of early trauma and loss, and the nature of problems that can occur for the child and parent in the transition from foster care to adoption. We present a case vignette that illustrates the importance of understanding a child's life experiences prior to placement as a way to gain insight into the child's developmental status upon entry into foster care and/or transition to an adoptive family. An outline is included of some important factors to consider in reviewing a child's pre-foster care or preadoptive placement. This outline can be used in conjunction with attention to the child's wider social surround to inform assessment and intervention planning.

CHILDREN IN THE FOSTER CARE SYSTEM

"Foster care" is defined as a living arrangement in which a child resides outside his or her own home, under the case management and planning responsibility of a child welfare agency. These living arrangements can include relative and nonrelative foster homes, group homes, child care facilities, emergency shelter care, supervised independent living, and nonfinalized adoptive homes. Almost by definition, children who have been placed in foster care are more likely to have experienced disrupted or unstable care.

The barriers to a family's ability to provide safe and protective care are often related to a number of social as well as personal problems. Socioeconomic factors such as poverty, social isolation, institutional discrimination, single parenthood, and father absence can combine to create extraordinary challenges and barriers to successful parenting (Cox, 1999; McKenzie, 1993). In addition, specific problems can interfere with parents' ability to use prevention and treatment services in ways that support either keeping their family together or achieving family reunification after initial placement of the children into out-of-home care. Such problems may include drug abuse, AIDS, mental illness, and/or the psychological fragility of the parent(s). Moreover, these burdens can be cumulative and undermine the family's ability to provide protective and emotional care of their children. Many of the children in foster care have emerged from families who have experienced a number of such crises (Chase-Lansdale & Vinovskis, 1995).

States have various practices, but in general, a child is placed in foster care when a court or protective services agency determines that a family cannot provide a minimally safe and emotionally caring environment. In other situations, the parents themselves may be too ill, either physically or emotionally, to care for their child, and foster placement is arranged (McKenzie, 1993). In the United States, both federal and state laws discourage removal of children from their families unless necessary to ensure safety. Placement in foster care is an extreme step taken only when a child is in immediate danger, or when attempts to help the family to provide a safe environment have failed. Still, sensitivity to the legal rights of biological parents is balanced in the courts with the knowledge of the damaging and sometimes fatal effects of severe neglect and psychological and physical abuse in the parental home (Mintz & Kellogg, 1988). Under current law, professionals who see children (e.g., doctors, nurses, teachers, social workers, and therapists) have a responsibility to report abuse and neglect. Furthermore, the state and local child welfare agencies are responsible for intervening on the child's behalf by investigating the charges and taking protective action if it is thought to be necessary.

The Federal government has squarely placed responsibility for the monitoring of the safety and survival of children within the State Departments of Health and Human Services. Social workers, psychologists, psychiatrists, welfare workers, lawyers, judges, and other professionals, who work with children at various points in the placement process, have to make difficult judgments as they seek to make informed decisions during all phases of foster care placement, potential adoption, and effective intervention.

In the United States, the number of children in the foster care system doubled between the early 1980s and the year 2000. In the year 2000, there were 547,000 children in the public foster care system compared to only 262,000 children in 1982. The number of children in the public foster care system at any moment in time is the result of a complex set of factors (Adoption and Foster Care Analysis and Reporting System [AFCARS], 2000). While over time, the demographic profiles of those who enter and exit foster care are roughly matched, significant differences may arise in any short period of time. Moreover, available data do not distinguish between children who enter the system for the first time and those who may have experienced multiple entries and exits from the system. Therefore, great care must be taken in interpreting the available data (Spar, 1997).

The growth in the foster care system results from not only an increased number of children entering the system but also an increase in the number of children waiting to be adopted or anticipating family reunification. Of the approximately 115,000 children who were eligible for adoption in fiscal year 1998, for example, only 36,000 or just over 30% were adopted (Adoption and Foster Care Analysis and Reporting System [AFCARS], 2000). Unfortunately, many of the children waiting to be adopted, the "children who wait," spend an average of about 3½ to 4 years in foster care (Adoption and Foster Care Analysis and Reporting System [AFCARS], 2000; McKenzie, 1993). Often, the psychological development of these children is further strained by the time spent in "family limbo" (Paret & Shapiro, 1998).

While children of all ages and ethnic groups enter into foster care, children of color are overrepresented in the system as a whole. In 1999, 43% of the children in the foster care system were African American, 36% were white, 15% were Hispanic, and 6% were Native American/Native Alaskan, Asian/Pacific Islander, and other backgrounds (Adoption and Foster Care Analysis and Reporting System [AFCARS], 2000). The disproportionate representation of children of color in the foster care system reflects, among other things, the fact that children of color are overrepresented in families of poverty. They are more likely to live in the most economically disadvantaged urban and other areas that are underserved by social support systems. Indeed, rapid increases in foster care have occurred in states with major urban areas, such as California, Illinois, New York, Michigan, and Texas (Spar, 1997). Many of these children are in formal kinship foster care, and these arrangements account, in part, for the rapid rise in skipped-generation adoption (Cox, 1999; see Chapter 6).

Some patterns of entry into and out of the foster care system can be associated with particular parental illnesses, such as AIDS or substance abuse. Parents who have AIDS still face a future of uncertainty even as medical treatments are becoming more effective in extending life. Although, new medical treatment approaches have given parents new personal hope and have drastically reduced the number of children born with AIDS, children of parents with AIDS are more likely than other children to need a period of foster care. The prospect of loss still casts a long shadow on the life experiences of these families and their children. The care of children who have lost parents through chronic illness such as AIDS can be a challenging and emotional undertaking; often this care undertaken by dedicated foster parents and grandparents (Joslin, 1999; Levine, 1990).

An analysis of the Adoption and Foster Care Analysis and Reporting System [AFCARS} data (2000) that relate to the public foster care system reveals the following trends:

- The percentage of children under age 1 entering the public foster care system has been increasing.
- Younger children, such as infants and toddlers, are likely to be adopted within a year of entry into foster placement.
- The average age of initial removal from a parental home is 4 years, 1 month.
- The average length of stay for older children in the public foster system is estimated to be about 3½ years, and most of these children become eligible for adoption at the age of 8.
- Of the 36,000 children who were adopted in 1998, about 65% were adopted by their unrelated foster parents, 15% by kinship relatives, and 23% by families they had never known.
- The number of children who wait for an adoptive home is rising. In 1998, for example, 70% of the children eligible for adoption were not placed and remained in foster care. Although the foster care system was designed to provide "temporary" care, all too often the care becomes semipermanent, and many children spend almost 4 precious years in temporary care (Adoption and Foster Care Analysis and Reporting System [AFCARS], 2000).

Defining the Best Interests of the Child

In their groundbreaking book, *In the Best Interests of the Child: The Least Detrimental Alternative*, Goldstein, Solnit, Goldstein, and Freud (1996) put forth three principles that place the *developmental needs* of the child at the center of permanency planning once a child is referred to child welfare:

1. The importance of maintaining the relationship between children and their primary psychological parent.
2. The importance of family continuity and stability.
3. The negative impact of extended time in foster care without a permanent home.

The primary goal of permanency planning reflects the strongly held belief that parents should be given every chance to regain their children and reunite the family (Sanchirico & Jablonka, 2000). Often, however, the courts have great difficulty coming to a determination as they try to balance concern for parents' rights with concerns for the needs of children. Historically, the rights of families in the United States to raise their children have always been counterbalanced by the community's social standards regarding appropriate parental care. These community standards, however, have shifted over time.

While American society has always sanctioned the authority of institutions to intervene and remove children from their family's care for a variety of situational, relational, or other reasons, the criteria for deciding when and how to intervene reflects a shifting set of strongly held and culturally grounded beliefs. These beliefs mirror society's changing views of the nature of childhood, the developmental needs of children, and the role of children in our society (Chase-Lansdale & Vinovskis, 1995; Mintz & Kellogg, 1988; Murray, 1996; Zelizer, 1985). For example, in the world of the early Puritan settlements in New England, children could be removed from their homes if their fathers were seen as not having acceptable moral character. In the 18th and 19th centuries, it was unacceptable for unwed mothers to rear their own children, and often informal kinship "adoption" occurred (Mintz & Kellogg, 1988). During the generations of slavery, African American families had no legal rights to maintain an ongoing relationship with their children. Most birth parents could not claim their children as their own since they were seen as the property of the slave owner and could be removed from their parents at will (Painter, 1996).

Changes in the philosophy of childhood and the ways in which we think about the development of children has had an important influence on decision making regarding the care of vulnerable children. Until recently, the idea that children might miss their families, or that parents might mourn the loss of their children, was not considered. Our understanding of the meaning of "the best interest of the child" standard indicates our current beliefs regarding the importance of attachment relationships and protective family care to the emotional and developmental life of the child (Chase-Lansdale & Vinovskis, 1995). Various streams of influence, including new research, have raised the consciousness of policymakers regarding the need to protect the child from extraordinary stress related to familial and/or environmental factors. Early neglect, abuse, and long-term experiences without a permanent home have been identified as risks to development (Pynoos et al., 1995).

The case studies of children who leave foster care at age 18 without having been adopted reveal that they have severe social and emotional difficulties that often result in their spending time in detention centers or prison upon leaving the foster care system (McKenzie, 1993). Recent reports of children who remained in foster care for long periods during childhood, without ever having been adopted, reveal that they were poorly prepared for adulthood. One-fourth of the boys were in jail within a year; many girls were mothers at the age of 17 and on welfare. Many other boys and girls experienced a multitude of psychological and medical problems, including AIDS and substance abuse (Sengupta, 2000).

Addressing the many problems of long delays in adoption, President

Clinton introduced the Adoption and Safe Families Act of 1997 (Public Law 105-89), which offered monetary awards to states that found ways to hasten permanency planning and increase the rates of post-foster care adoption. Although there is general agreement that children need a permanent home as soon as possible, this may at times mean that the birth parent(s) may not have had sufficient time to recover from the circumstances and long-term exposure to risk associated with the child's initial removal. An often ignored aspect of discussions around family reunification and the current trend toward faster permanency planning is the limitations of current knowledge regarding treatment approaches to problems such as drug addiction and mental illness.

In Figure 3.1, we see President Clinton presiding at a ceremony to celebrate the accomplishments of the Adoption and Safe Families Act at the White House on September 24, 1999 (McNamee, 1999). At his side is Brian Keane, who, through the efforts of the program, found a home after spending many years in foster care. President Clinton himself spent many years separated from his mother as a young child. We can infer from the

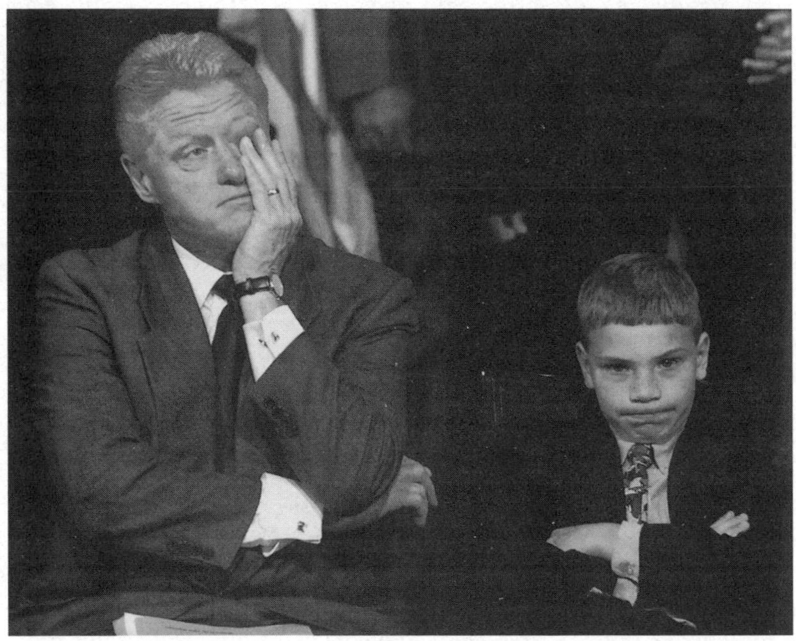

FIGURE 3.1. President Clinton and Brian Keene at a White House ceremony recognizing important changes in adoption practice, September 24, 1999.

expressions on both their faces that this event, which recognized the importance of a family to a child, had profound meaning for them.

Child welfare advocates must work with the courts to establish protocols that can help resolve the abyss that many children experience in protracted delays regarding adoption when family reunification is not possible. A recent study has suggested that if a child advocate or caseworker is assigned to oversee the child until permanency planning is achieved, the length of time is shortened and the number of different placements is curtailed (Calkins & Millar, 1999). Some states now initiate concurrent planning and make contingency plans even before the court's evaluation of reunification is completed (Reitz, 1999). In making these decisions, the grief and loss of the birth parents is often of concern; these parents will need professional help to come to terms with the court's decisions. In some situations, the birth parents can continue to have some form of contact with their children over time, in a sense, entering an open adoption relationship with the adoptive parents.

EMERGING ISSUES IN TRANSRACIAL ADOPTION

Until the 1960s, adoption practices in the United States emphasized the placement of children in racially matched homes (Reitz, 1999; Alexander & Curtis, 1996). However, many social, political, and demographic changes have led to an increase in the practice of transracial adoption. The Civil Rights movement of the 1960s, the increased number of children available for adoption internationally, and the larger number of minority children awaiting adoption in foster care are all associated with the more recent increases in transracial adoption. In addition, the greater social acceptance of families of diversity and nontraditional families has furthered the willingness of many families to adopt children whose racial or ethnic heritage is different from their own. Still, the practice of transracial adoption remains highly controversial. In 1972, the National Association of Black Social Workers (NABSW) issued a statement protesting transracial adoption on the grounds that it may be associated with important obstacles to development for minority children (Howard, Royse, & Skerl, 1997). Researchers, clinicians, and advocates continue to evaluate the potential benefits and costs of transracial adoption for children, families, and society (Brooks & Barth, 1999; Hollingsworth, 1997; Reitz, 1999; Simon, Alstein & Melli, 1994; Taylor & Thornton, 1996).

In 1994, a Federal law, the Multiethnic Placement Act (MEPA), was passed. This law prohibited agencies that received Federal funds from denying individuals the right to become adoptive parents on the basis of race, color, or nationality.The primary goal of MEPA is to shorten the length of time thousands of children spend in foster care by removing barriers to adoption based on policies of racial and/or ethnic matching (Reitz, 1999). As originally written, MEPA did allow the cultural, ethnic, and racial characteristics of the child and the intentional parents to be considered in placement decisions, but only in terms of the capacity of the intentional parent to support the overall well-being of the child (Hollingsworth, 1997). This qualification, however, was removed by an amendment to the act, Removal of Barriers of Interethnic Adoption, in 1996, and race can no longer be a factor in considering the merits of adoptive parents.

Earlier policies, such as the Indian Child Welfare Act of 1978, represented efforts to recognize the importance of cultural and ethnic heritage in child placement decisions. In this regard, critics of MEPA suggest that the legislation does not adequately respond to the potential losses in ethnic and racial heritage that can occur when children are taken out of their communities. Moreover, important questions remain about the many societal factors that create the disproportionate number of children of color in the foster care system in the first place. These factors include problems such as poverty and lack of support for families and children of color.

Protracted cycles of poverty are associated with increased rates of child abuse and neglect, inadequate access to basic medical care, periods of malnutrition, and a range of developmental difficulties (Chase-Lansdale & Brooks-Gunn, 1995; Hollingsworth, 1997; McKenzie, 1993). Thus, children of color are more likely to be exposed to circumstances that may result in their entry into the public foster care system. Institutional discrimination and culturally insensitive practices may prevent children and families of color from receiving adequate preventive and intervention services. More effective services and a reduction in barriers to service utilization might strengthen families and either prevent initial entry into foster care or result in more timely placement decisions (Hollingsworth, 1997).

The debate over whether to promote transracial adoptions is thought by some to represent the problems in over simplistic terms. Often, the importance of permanency is pitted against concern for the protection of the child's racial and ethnic identity. Both opponents and proponents of transracial adoption agree that enhanced and more effective efforts at permanency planning for children of color are important. But differences of opinion emerge as to the factors most responsible for the overrepresentation of children of color in the public foster care system and the availability of foster and adoptive parents of color.

Transracial adoption is only one of a wide variety of strategies needed to help decrease the number of children of color in the child welfare system (Alexander & Curtis, 1996). Other useful strategies might include the search for better prevention and treatment to increase the chances for reunification of children with their families, and support for new efforts both to encourage more kinship adoptions and increase our understanding of the economic and social issues that may account for the barriers to family well-being. Furthermore, the practice of categorizing all children of color who have experienced long periods in foster care as having "special needs" status may inadvertently create barriers to adoption, since this term connotes children with special physical, mental, and emotional vulnerabilities. Finally, a reevaluation of the fee-driven services for adoption completion is necessary because these fees may deter families with fewer resources from adopting.

Outcome Research on the Psychological Impact of Transracial Adoption

The most important question at issue is the potential impact of transracial adoption on the developmental adaptation of the child over time. Opponents pose the following question: Is there a risk that the child will feel marginalized both in the majority society and within the minority community because of his/her distinctive difference? Will this marginalization lead to cultural confusion and identity conflict? Those who support transracial adoption, however, cite research findings over the last three decades that reveal generally positive developmental outcome. They also contend that adoption is far superior to extended institutionalization (Feigelman, 2000).

Long-term outcome research has compared children who grew up in inracial and transracial adoptive families (Brooks & Barth, 1999; Feigelman, 2000; Shireman & Johnson, 1986; Vroegh, 1997). These studies focus on characteristics such as the self-esteem, ethnoracial identity, school achievement, physical and mental health status, and behavioral functioning of adopted children (Brooks & Barth, 1999; Rosenthal, Groze, Curiel, & Westcott, 1991). This research, admittedly, is not definitive and has some shortcomings because of the high attrition rates of families and the homogeneous family structures of participants in the studies. Moreover, the few existing studies focused on children adopted at a young age and, thus, do not take into account the potential impact of the traumatic early histories of older children (Simon et al., 1994). Nevertheless, the findings of these long-term studies show consistently encouraging outcomes over time.

Brooks and Barth's (1999) analysis of the adjustment of 224 adoptees sheds some light on specific variables in transracial adoption. Their analysis was based on a comparative survey of outcomes for adopted Caucasian, Asian, and African American children. The Caucasian children were adopted by same-racial families (inracial adoptees), and the Asian and African American children were adopted into multiracial families (transracial adoptees). Their findings, summarized below, add to our understanding of the special needs of children and the concerns of parents in both inracial and transracial adoptions.

The study revealed that over 70% of the adopted daughters in all racial groups were rated as having good adjustments, while both Caucasian and African American sons had more adjustment difficulties growing up. Developmental outcome scores were based on school achievement, behavior problems, and the assessment of functional health and impairments (Brooks & Barth, 1999). Thus, gender seems to be an important factor in positive adjustment in both inracial and transracial adoption (Rushton & Minnis, 1997).

This is true in the general population as well. The analysis also assessed the degree of conflict over ethnoracial identity in transracial adoptions. Ethnoracial identity was rated on the basis of discomfort or pride in ethnoracial appearance and the children's identifications with their ethnoracial birth group. Approximately 60% of the African American daughters and sons identified themselves as black despite having attended predominantly white schools. These children also expressed more pride in their racial heritage compared to the Asian children in this study. This may relate to the adoption history of the Asian children in terms of cutoff from their birth culture through international adoption. Significantly, African American daughters expressed a high degree of pride in their appearance and were also less likely to experience discrimination than African American sons (Brooks & Barth, 1999).

Feigelman (2000) found that experiences of discrimination and societal racism presented the greatest risk to adolescent and young adult outcomes for African American adopted children, especially men. The findings reveal, for example, that discrimination and any resulting discomfort about appearance can complicate the experience of adoption and have a negative effect on development, especially for African American boys.

These outcome studies point to the need for education, guidance, and support for adopting families when early difficulties emerge. It is painful for adoptive parents to cope with bias in the broader community. Some recommendations have emerged regarding the role of parents. The willingness of adoptive parents to respect and support the racial and ethnic identity of their child is linked to the child's achievement of ethnoracial pride and identity. Parents can help their children by encouraging them to establish friendships that are meaningful to them, including identification with same-race friends (Silverman & Feigelman, 1990). Living in racially integrated neighborhoods has been found to provide an optimal context for social development. Finally, parents, and teachers, and other professionals, can help these children learn adaptive skills to cope with discrimination.

Vroegh (1997) suggests that racial identity and self-identification is not a static concept and changes over time as children conceptually understand what race means to them. "Racial identity, like other aspects of identity, appears to be complex and fluid, changing constantly over time" (p. 568). A family that can offer both strong parental support and a positive attitude that supports the child's opportunity to develop a sense of ethnic identity can provide a beneficial environment for him or her. Often, parents find these issues extremely painful and need professional help.

Practitioners are often called upon to provide help to adopted children, especially adolescents with adjustment problems. Children who have experienced many levels of "difference," including family disruption, prejudice, and transracial family life, have a unique set of distinctive, meaningful experiences that they may not have voiced to others (Grotevant, 1997). In the process of developing an integrated sense of identity, it is important for children to be able to voice their many feelings and views about their history, family, and the prejudice of the mainstream culture. Clinicians who can be empathetic in listening to the painful aspects of children's life narrative can provide an opportunity for them to mourn the many difficult circumstances related to loss and prejudice, and to develop effective coping strategies. In working with transracial families, practitioners need to allow themselves to confront their own potention biases and prejudices. A clinician who can establish an empathic therapeutic relationship is providing a holding environment that enables children to express their subjective experiences of complex family issues, and this understanding may help them construct a firmer sense of their own identity, agency, and self-worth.

THE TRANSITION TO FOSTER CARE AND ADOPTION: ASSESSMENT ISSUES

Children adopted from foster placement are a diverse group in terms of age, the nature of their early experiences, ethnic and racial backgrounds, the length of time spent in foster care, and the particular contexts of their adoptive families. As we stated at the outset, some children will be adopted by known caregivers (foster parents or kinship relatives), whereas others will have adoptive parents they do not know. The preadoption history of children affects not only their cognitive and social development but also their adjustment to adoptive parent(s). This is true whether or not the child is adopted by a known or unknown caregiver, as the relationship between parent and child takes on new meaning when the child becomes a permanent member of the family (Paret & Shapiro, 1998). An assessment of the child may be most helpful to parents in understanding his or her needs during the transition.

Adoptive parents are also a very diverse group of people. Some families are more traditional. Others are nontraditional and may be single parents by choice, or gay and lesbian couples. Each family dynamic will be different, and parents will face specific problems in resolving the transition to adoption. All adoptive parents may be unprepared for the encounter with complex developmental problems and the difficulty the child may have in responding to their care. The case vignette that follows (Shapiro & Gyzinsky, 1989) illustrates the special caregiving needs of a young infant in her first move to foster care. When and if this infant transitions to permanent adoption, this part of her history will need to be taken into account. The case was chosen because it represents the extreme impact of early neglect and the difficulties presented to the foster parent(s).

Case Vignette: The Preplacement History and Developmental Status of 6-Month-Old Sandra

Sandra was referred to protective services for evaluation at the age of 6 months because the public health nurse was worried about her poor health status and life-threatening situation. Sandra's mother, Ms. D, a single parent, was depressed and addicted to drugs and alcohol. She had some psychotic features and was unable to provide basic safety or care for Sandra and her two siblings. Sandra suffered from "failure to thrive," multiple episodes of pneumonia requiring hospitalization, and delays in all spheres of development. She was finally referred to protective services when hospitalized because of an untended illness, and failure to thrive had worsened. In the hospital, she began to gain weight. She was placed in "temporary" foster care to ensure her health and safety, and to allow time to evaluate her mother's treatment needs and develop a treatment plan.

Over a series of weeks prior to placement, the nurse had been observing Sandra at home, offering support, suggestions, and medical assistance to her mother. Sandra was most often left alone on a couch, undressed and untended, and when she whimpered, Ms. D directed the two older children, ages 4 and 6, to feed her. Ms. D seemed to be in her own world. The house was chaotic, and her mental health status was fragile. She needed treatment that the public health nurse could not provide.

In the referral request, Sandra was described by the public health nurse as a passive, limp, unresponsive child who seemed indifferent to the approach of others who tried to engage her. Her passivity and muted affect was evidence of her state of aloneness in her earliest months. Emotionally devoid of a range of affect that one might expect of a 6-month-old, she did not smile, was lethargic in her movements, and seemed indifferent to the approach of others.

At 6 months of age, most babies can anticipate parental actions; engage in baby games; show joy, surprise, fear, and disappointment; and express their feelings to influence external actions, such as preference for their psychological parent (Emde & Sorce, 1983). They can also enjoy playing with others and exploring toys and other objects. Like other children with similar histories of neglect, however, Sandra's interest in the social world around her was limited. Developmentally, she was far behind her chronological age and showed no evidence of the experience of play or interactions with others. She was behind in sensory motor development. She did not attempt to reach for a toy that was offered, did not have midline organization (i.e., she did not bring her hands together), and had poor trunk and neck control, perhaps because of a lack of physical holding. A silent baby, her vocalizations were muted and not socially reciprocal if they did occur.

Diagnostically, one needed to question whether the developmental retardation was due to the impact of illness or other organic factors, or the emotional neglect and general deprivation in her original home. Thus, the limits of Sandra's potential improvement were unknown. She needed a devoted, sensitive, and knowledgeable foster parent who could tolerate and understand her initial lack of responsiveness.

Sandra's foster parent(s) would need guidance and support to help her begin to regain her health. She needed care from a sensitive caregiver who could woo her into a relationship with a caring parental figure. A child like Sandra may begin to recover over time with good foster parenting. However, if and when a shift to another home occurs, she may lose ground and regress to her former withdrawal. Yet in this and similar situations, it typically takes many months before a determination can be made about the potential for reunification with her birth mother, or a recommendation for permanent placement. Thus, Sandra's preadoptive history of early neglect, separations, and the potential for multiple disruptions would profoundly affect her emotional and developmental status at the time of permanent placement, whether in an adoptive home or in reunification with her birth mother (Shapiro & Gyzinski, 1989).

Sandra's mother requires special treatment and the provision of concrete resources. Unfortunately, many communities do not have such services available; even when treatment is possible, Sandra's mother's recovery may take many years. This conflicts with Sandra's needs for a permanent placement. These kinds of poignant questions are often at the heart of judicial decisions about the termination of parental rights.

This case vignette illustrates the impact on development when a child has experienced early impoverishment of caregiving relationships. This basic early relationship contributes both to the child's capacity for normal developmental growth and the emotional depth of his/her child's life. Sandra's passivity and nonresponsiveness illustrate her lack of experience with human interactions. The early holding environments of children before entering foster care often includes medical, social, and caregiving risk factors, as we have seen in Sandra's preplacement history. Table 3.1 summarizes some of the important dimensions in assessing a child's preplacement history. Such an assessment can help in thinking through placement and treatment decisions.

EARLY TRAUMA, LOSS, AND MULTIPLE DISRUPTIONS: IMPLICATIONS FOR CHILDREN AND ADOPTIVE PARENTS

At the time of adoption, parents often face a number of serious issues that interfere with the establishment of relationships with their children. Many parents report that in the transitional phase to adoption, their children may not be responsive to their outreach. Infants like Sandra, who never experienced an adequate reciprocal relationship, need the help of their parents to begin to participate in the to and fro characteristic of responsive and empathic care. The child's developmental age might be much younger than his/her chronological age, and the parents may have to find the right level of interaction and sensitively pace their attempts at engagement. They must become thoughtful observers of the baby's responses and be attentive to signals and emotional reactions. Infants can begin to give cues about their needs, the level of intensity of attention they can tolerate, and what gives them pleasure or pain. As Stern (1985) suggests, it is through predictable and sensitive interactions that the child begins to develop a sense of trust in the other and a sense of personal agency. As the child shows signs of preference for their parents through smiles and reaching out, and the parents'

TABLE 3.1. Preplacement History: An Assessment Tool for Placement and Treatment Planning

- *The child's age and health status at the time of adoption and reason for permanent placement*

- *The child's birth history*
  The birth family members and primary caregivers
  The prenatal history of the child
    The birth mother's prenatal medical care
    The prenatal health environment: maternal drug use during pregnancy, maternal nutrition, teratogenic exposure
    Prematurity or full-term delivery
    Birthweight and weight for gestational age
    Labor and or delivery complications
  Health status at birth and special problems: muscle tone, level of alertness, readiness for sucking, neurological status

- *Reasons for removal from birth family*
  Age of child at first removal
  Reasons for referral to protective services and/or foster care
  Medical health status of infant at time of removal (e.g., failure to thrive, chronic or acute illness, or injury)
  Psychological and developmental status: cognitive, social, and emotional development and signs of emotional trauma or neglect
  Length of time between referral to protective services and entry into foster care

- *The transition to first foster care home*
  Child's age
  The child's initial adjustment to foster care and relationship to foster care parent
  The quality of child care in the foster home
  The length of time in foster care home
  The health and emotional status of the child at the time of leaving

- *The long-term foster placement history of the child*
  The number of separations and placement experiences
  Precipitating reason for each move
  The child's developmental status at each move
    Age
    Physical and emotional health status
    Adjustment across spheres of development
    Child's relational capacity
  Differences in social, cultural, and emotional style of care between homes

- *The child's coping style*
  The child's behavioral and emotional reaction to separations and to new caregivers
    Approach–avoidance
    Emotional withdrawal
    Aggressive/rejecting behavior

(*continued on next page*)

TABLE 3.1. ***(continued)***

The nature of coping mechanisms that help the child overcome frustration and anxiety
The availability of a primary relationship to help the child cope with loss and distress

- *Assessment of the child's strengths and vulnerabilities*
  Special strengths in cognitive, social, and emotional development.
  Evidence of emotional resiliency or fragility
  - Self-esteem issues
  - Primary ways of communicating thoughts and feeling
  - Quality of relationships with peers, teachers, and adults
  - Behavioral problems
  - Reality testing
  - Capacity to cope with stress

An assessment that considers these historical experiences of the child and gives an integrated overview of the child's psychological and health status can be the basis of a treatment plan for the child and a framework that can help the adoptive parent understand the child's needs. This developmental assessment can assist the practitioner and the parent(s) to "start where the child is" in setting treatment goals and pursuing appropriate caregiving strategies. Overall, the health and age of the child at first disruption are primary considerations.

sense of being valued is heightened, this leads to more positive interaction with their child. This process takes considerable time but furthers the attachment relationships between parents and children.

When parents adopt an older child with an extensive history of early trauma and loss, it often takes great effort and an even longer time to establish a trusting relationship. The long years spent in uncertain family circumstances bring their own costs to the child's emotional life. For those children who are eventually adopted, the entry into a permanent family does not easily erase the internal fragility that may have resulted from the years of "family limbo" (Eth & Pynoos, 1985; Paret & Shapiro, 1998; Pynoos et al., 1995; Webb, 1999). Research findings confirm that children who have experienced multiple trauma and family disruption are at a developmental disadvantage in physical, behavioral, social and psychological domains (Brinich, 1990; Cicchetti & Cohen, 1995; Hoopes, 1990; Shapiro & Applegate, 2000; Winnicott, 1965b).

In forming a relationship with an older child, parents must keep in mind the ways in which the child's relational history may have negatively shaped his/her views of the trustworthiness of adults and the consistency with which they will show love and concern. The child may feel that relationships with others are easily broken and characterized by uncertainty, disappointment, rejection, and indifference. These children often feel betrayed by "the adult world" that did not value them; often, these perceived injuries lead to intense anger that is hard to control. In addition, the child's view of him/herself may be damaged. He/she can experience intense feelings of self-blame for the predicament and the multiple perceived "abandonments" by others may lead to a diminished sense of self. When a child has experienced long periods of impermanence, he/she may feel a lack of personal "agency," a sense of helplessness, rootlessness, and lack of self-confidence (Triseliotis & Hill, 1990). In this regard, children who have been without a parent who was able to "keep the needs of the child in mind" may feel that life "happens" to them, and that they may have no influence over others or over their own destiny. The voice of such children is lost and, in many situations, they develop an artificial way of being, hiding the real self and real feelings.

The child may cope with the loneliness and pain by denying the need for adults. The defensive adaptation of withdrawal, for example, may be protective in the immediate situation but is likely to prevent children from being able to form new relationships with adoptive parents who are eager to be close to them (Festinger, 1990). Although some children withdraw, others may have significant behavioral problems. For example, they may be aggressive, rejecting, and defiant even when parents reach out to them. These children may be testing their parents' commitment to them. It is also likely that they have great difficulty modulating feelings of anxiety and anger, and cannot easily recover their emotional equilibrium (Shapiro & Applegate, 2000). Often, these children do not feel connected to others, and their behavior is a symptom of depression and helplessness.

At school, the children who act out may be identified as noncompliant, oppositional, and indifferent to authority figures. When children have experienced stable and empathetic caregiving, the authority of adults is for the most part experienced positively and as helpful to their needs and ongoing development. Children who feel they have been disregarded do not trust that others care about their well-being, or that anyone can improve their situation. Their attempts to experience mastery and regain a level of personal control and agency may first appear in behaviors that are either aggressive or defiant. For adoptive parents, these behaviors can cause extreme anxiety, worry, and frustration. It may be helpful for both parent(s) and child to realize that through the sensitive efforts of both family members and professional helpers, change is possible but may occur only over an extended period of time and effort. In addition, it is important for both practitioners and parents to remember that change is not likely to be linear.

Rather, as development continues and the child faces new tasks, it may be necessary to revisit his/her early history.

Young children can have intense grief reactions following loss and separation from parental caregivers. The depth of loss can be experienced as sadness or a deeper depression that can disrupt development (Bowlby, 1969; Spitz & Wolf, 1946). For children who are already vulnerable because of the loss of a birth parent, the experience of multiple separations from different foster care parents can have devastating consequences. For example, a toddler who was separated from his foster mother on whom he had come to depend was sad, withdrawn, and hard to reach when he was returned to her care some months later. He had regressed in speech and language, and for a time refused to respond or interact with her. Another child, who had spent years in five different foster homes, was abusive and angry with his new adoptive parent, to an extent that was almost intolerable for her. It is hard for parents to realize that the promise of their love does not quickly alleviate the suffering of the child. The child needs to express his/her grief and anger and can experience relief through the efforts of the parent to give comfort, but often the pain does not ease quickly. Time, empathy, and stability may help build better emotional functioning.

Older adopted children carry the memories of their early histories and parental figures with them. The meaning of abandonment and loss changes over the years, and sometimes true mourning occurs only when they are much older and understand more fully the finality of loss (Webb, 1993). These memories, which include the affective experience of early loss, can be reevoked at different developmental phases and by evocative circumstances. When a child reexperiences feelings of grief at a later date, his/her parent(s) can become discouraged. But recovery is not a straight line for these children, and parent(s) must realize that as their children experience life transitions, they will likely revisit the conflicts, losses, and anxieties of the past.

Because the child's concept of time is very different from that of the adult, the length of time without a permanent family is critical to the well-being of the child (Chethik, 2000). Unlike adults, children experience time in relation to their immediate wishes and needs, and not in relation to its actual passage (Freud, 1965). Depending on the age of the child, the separation from the psychological parent can feel intolerable, even if the actual separation is brief (Bowlby et al., 1952; Robertson, 1953). An older child, who can anticipate time, can still tolerate only brief separations from a primary caregiver before experiencing intense anxiety. Once attached to an adoptive parent, any separations may still precipitate intense anxiety. Parents often note that transitions such as moving to a new home, or brief separations for an evening, can cause the old fears and anxiety to return. Under these circumstance, parents may not realize that anxiety underlies disruptive behavior such as the emergence of anger, threats of self-injury, or excessive clinging.

The affective meaning of long-term foster care was revealed in a study of 52 young adults who were adopted following foster care (Triseliotis & Hill, 1990). The image of fostering they carried with them was "temporariness" and "moving on," and conveyed the feelings of anxiety and uncertainty, and lack of control over one's life. On the other hand, adoption evoked different images for these children: intangible feelings of "belonging," being the family's "real child," being part of the family, not feeling left out, having a family for life (Triseliotis & Hill, 1990).

These observations demonstrate how children may internalize a sense of their place in the world. Belonging to a permanent family affects their sense of identity in a positive way, and gives them a firmer sense of who they are, and of being valued. The external reality of the child's family experience interacts with the developing internal view the child has of him/herself. The voices of the adopted children studied by Triseliotis and Hill reflect their awareness of the positive meaning of permanency and the importance of belonging to an enduring family.

While children adopted from foster placement are identified as being developmentally "at risk," they show varying patterns of adaptation and degrees of resilience. Some fortunate children may have received warmth and attuned care from persons who made a real connection with them in situations of family impermanence (Anthony, 1983). Some children have more resilience, and their strengths may reflect more adaptive defensive styles of behavior that helped them cope with traumatic early experiences (Fonagy & Target, 1998a). Both adoptive parents and practitioners must understand the child's internal world in the context of his/her preadoptive history and support the child's strengths while addressing internal vulnerabilities with sensitivity and understanding. Despite the long-term sequelae of delayed permanence, children who are adopted following early trauma do have a chance to use their new family relationships to recover and overcome the previous barriers to development (Feigelman, 2000).

SUMMARY

The care of vulnerable children is an important area of public policy. It is embedded in the context of the society's values and the resources provided for services. Many thousands of young children are in the public foster care system awaiting permanent placement, and children of color are overrepresented in this group. While laws have been instituted to promote faster resolution of permanency planning, too many children still remain without a permanent home. The Adoption and Safe Families Act of 1997 (Public Law 105-89) provides new resources for states that meet certain standards in placement planning. Other efforts are being made to expand the number of potential adoptive parents by including grandparents, kinship relatives, older and single parents, and gay and lesbian couples (Sullivan, 1995a). The solution to the difficulties described in this chapter lie not only in the assessment and treatment of individual children, their birth parents, and the adoptive families, but also in the development of social policies and practices that better identify and serve the needs of vulnerable children in our society. Intervention strategies with families who have multilevel needs require both direct and indirect service strategies (Johnson, 1999).

The children adopted from foster placement have experienced multiple levels of environmental risk and often suffer delays in physical, cognitive, social, and emotional growth. The cumulative effects of early family trauma, multiple separations, loss of caregivers, poor attachment histories, lack of basic protection, neglect, and abuse all take their toll. Each child has his/her own special affective memory of early traumatic experiences and loss, even though he/she may not remember the actual facts. Early caregiving experience affects the child's view of him- or herself, and the view of what to expect from others, including parental figures. Often, children who have suffered early neglect, abuse, and multiple separations develop cynical and negative views about not only their own self-worth but also the worthiness of adults. They often cannot easily trust adults to care about them, and this view is likely to be transferred to the adoptive parents who wish to nurture them as well as to society as a whole.

Adoptive parents have the poignant and challenging task of helping their children recover from the scars of the past. They need to be informed about their child's history and the ways in which these experiences have affected his/her capacity for relationships with others. The children are likely to need lengthy periods of time to develop a beginning relationship with their adoptive parents; to "transform an alien adult into a parent and to feel that he/she has a secure existence within the mind of this new parent" (Cohen, 1996, p. 300).

Many older children who have experienced early traumatic histories are frozen in their development, as they may not have a strong sense of their own self-worth and are unable to cope with their confusion and fears about separation, individuation, and identity formation (Anthony, 1983).

They may not have developed positive coping strategies to help them modulate their impulses or modify strong emotional reactions to disappointment and frustration. Parents may need to help their children achieve self-control and develop more effective adaptive structures through a combination of limit setting and conveyed empathy.

Because of the circular reciprocity of emotional give and take, a growing attachment can result between parent and child. In some ways this process parallels the earliest years of infancy within an attuned relationship. Parents may not realize the extent to which children carry forward the scars of the past. For those children with the most devastating preadoptive experiences, adoptive parents face enormous challenges in helping them recover from all they have endured. The needs of the children are multiple, and parents can gain support from therapeutic assistance, including education and guidance to help them cope with the burdens of care. Often, parents also need support and therapy to cope with their own reactions to their child's ambivalent and often conflicted feelings. Although parents may wish to help their children resolve issues from the past, this often cannot be done quickly. Still, Feigelman (2000) suggests that over time, children may indeed be able to internalize a more positive sense of self and relationships with others.

For the child, a therapist can offer a new relationship based on empathy, acceptance, and sensitivity. The new relationship does not erase the memories of the past, and at each developmental phase, new therapeutic work may be needed. These children will continue to revisit the past, to mourn their losses, and to struggle with the establishment of a coherent identity. Through a therapeutic holding relationship, and with the patience and love of their parents, even traumatized children may reconstruct a more positive sense of self-worth and realize the pleasure that comes from emotional acceptance and understanding.

4

The Impact of Delayed Adoption

A Case Study

This chapter describes the developmental dilemmas of children in long-term foster care whose permanent placement is delayed for years. Developmental theory and clinical research postulate that the psychological risks to children who face the continuous threat of loss of primary attachment relationships are significant. The detailed account of Matthew's case illustrates the effects of early neglect, abuse, and multiple separations on ego development.

In recent years several remarkable legal cases have focused on the complex questions that arise in protracted foster placement (Clay, 1997). This chapter discusses the psychological development of Matthew, who was taken from his birth mother at 13 months because of physical and emotional neglect. For the next 6 years, Matthew lived intermittently with the same foster mother. At the discretion of the state child protective services, he was repeatedly returned to his birth mother for days or even months, until the court finally ruled in favor of Matthew's adoption by his foster mother. The primary focus of this chapter is the psychological meaning to this child of early neglect and abuse, and the continuing threat of separation and loss of one of his primary caregivers.

From the time that he was first removed from his biological mother, Matthew lived in a fragile and splintered "holding environment." His life had little stability, as he was repeatedly and unpredictably shifted between two very different families. Matthew shares this traumatic history with other young children in foster placement. But his situation was unusual; he had only *one* foster mother, who eventually adopted him, and when he was 4, his foster mother sought help and arranged for him to be in psychotherapy. It is rare to have a child with Matthew's history in long-term, weekly psychoanalytic psychotherapy.

Our discussion draws on 3½ years of clinical work to describe the disruption in Matthew's development, caused by a severely erratic and unsafe external world in which his primary attachment was at risk. Matthew's inner world, especially his object relationships, ego development, emerging autonomy, and capacity for adaptation, was under strain at each developmental stage. His developing identity was also affected by the reality that, like many children in foster placement, he had to deal with two different maternal paradigms and two different ethnic and cultural backgrounds: His family of origin was Hispanic and poor; his foster mother was Caucasian and middle class. Despite the gravity of his situation, therapy provided Matthew with a safe holding environment in which he could express his feelings, question his experience, and develop a capacity for insight and self-reflection. This chapter also considers special issues in foster placement cases: the role of the therapist as a new object; the necessary modifications to traditional therapeutic processes, especially in a private practice setting; ethical and legal issues; and the significance of developmental issues for child welfare policy and practice and judicial determinations.

THEORETICAL PERSPECTIVES

Researchers, clinicians, and theorists agree on the critical importance of the primary relationship(s) between a young child and his/her parental caregiver(s), and the importance of attuned care as the foundation for the child's psychological development (Ainsworth, 1979a; Bowlby, 1969; Spitz & Wolf, 1946). Donald Winnicott (1965b) conceptualizes the earliest parent–child relationship as a "holding environment" and emphasizes the importance of empathy, continuity, stability, and safety to the well-being of the child. Being held in an embrace of safety is essential in nourishing the development of a healthy intrapsychic structure and a sense of trust. Clinical experience and retrospective studies show that early separation and loss, particularly when coupled with neglect and abuse, tend to cause extreme anxiety and disrupt normal developmental pathways (Bowlby, 1973; Freud, 1965; Redl, 1966). Neurobiological research in the 1990s described how early traumata affect atypical changes in the developing brain (Perry, 1994; Perry et al., 1995). All children must cope with anxiety as they move through the sequence of developmental phases, but when turbulence becomes intolerable, they may be overwhelmed by anxiety and develop atypical defenses that are adaptive in the immediate crisis but aberrant in the long run (Fraiberg, 1987b; Freud, 1966). These children are in danger of developing cognitive, social, and affective problems (Eth & Pynoos, 1985).

Children in foster placement usually experience multiple separations and live in two or more psychological worlds with very different maternal images. They oscillate between qualitatively different holding environments, ranging from "good-enough mothering" (Winnicott, 1965a) and "average expectable environment" (Hartmann, 1939) to frightening, erratic conditions. In Winnicott's framework, the child internalizes the qualities of the holding environment and retains either a feeling of safety or a sense of fragility. Winnicott (1965) suggests that if trauma occurs at the stage of absolute dependency, a caretaker self may develop and the infant, and then the child, will have the capacity to go through the motions of interpersonal relationships, but these encounters will be with the false self that serves to hide the true self.

The development of a basic sense of trust in others (Erikson, 1950) and the capacity to sustain homeostasis are essential for a healthy personality. Joseph and Anne-Marie Sandler (1978) consider mother–infant interactions to be the context for the earliest self- and object-representations, providing the basic building blocks for the representation of the self and object over time (Sandler & Sandler, 1978). Daniel Stern (1985) and Heinz Kohut (1972) link the development of empathetic trust in early object relationships to the emergence of a robust sense of self that helps to sustain homeostasis in the face of anxiety, disappointment, and loss (Kohut, 1972; Stern, 1985). The four major psychoanalytic models—drive, ego, object, and self—are in agreement that the nature of intimate relationships, the structure and strength of the ego, the quality of identifications, and the development of self-esteem are shaped by the nurturing experience in the early years of life (Pine, 1990).

Clinical research suggests ways in which psychoanalytic developmental theory can be helpful in the treatment of traumatized children. Selma Fraiberg and her colleagues developed a model of treatment that takes into consideration impairment in the capacity for trust and its repetition in other relationships (Fraiberg, Adelson, & Shapiro, 1975). They stress the importance of an empathetic therapeutic holding environment for both child and parents. Their model incorporates developmental guidance and supportive psychotherapy, as well as interpretative psychotherapy where appropriate (Seligman, 1994).

Goldstein et al. (1996), in their important work on the best interests of the child, highlight three major points for courts to consider when making placement or custody decisions: (1) the significance of the psychological parent; (2) the importance of stability and continuity; and (3) the negative impact of extended time in permanency planning. They argue for timely decisions based on the least detrimental alternative for the child (Goldstein et al., 1996; Goldstein & Goldstein, 1996). Matthew's experience demonstrates the effect on a child when these three principles are not observed.

THE EARLY SPLINTERED HOLDING ENVIRONMENT

Matthew was first removed from his birth mother's care at the age of 6 weeks, when the police suspected that she, Ms. Rivers, was selling drugs. The police noted that the house was "filthy" and "unsafe," and that the children were neglected. Matthew was placed in an overnight foster care facility with his 5-year-old brother, Bobby. The children were returned to the mother the following day, when she agreed to attend a drug treatment program.

Ms. Rivers expressed the wish to keep Matthew but she could not meet his day-to-day physical, emotional, or safety needs, nor was she able to avail herself of the treatment services offered to her. After Matthew's first removal, Ms. Rivers asked the state several times to place the children temporarily with others so that she could pursue various personal plans, such as joining the National Guard. These requests were refused. When Matthew was 13 months old, his mother's personal life deteriorated further. She entered a facility for drug treatment, and Matthew was placed with a foster mother, Ms. Smith, for the first time. At the time of placement, the caseworker described Matthew as "ill, dirty, frightened, and developmentally lagging." The foster mother noted that, although it was February, Matthew was dressed in a lightweight summer jacket and wore no socks. When Ms. Smith put him in the high chair and started to prepare food, tears poured down his face, but he did not make a sound. The silent crying continued on and off for a few days. Matthew gradually responded to her care and allowed her to feed, bathe, rock, and comfort him. This fragile homeostasis often broke down; Matthew would suddenly become angry, yell, and repeatedly hit a doll on the head with his fist. Ms. Smith thought he might be reenacting something he had seen or experienced.

According to the agency's written reports, Matthew prospered in Ms. Smith's care, and his language developed. By the end of the 2 months he remained with Ms. Smith, Matthew was affectionate, cheerful, and could say "bye, bye," "eat," and "go." At this point, he was returned to his birth mother, who had completed her drug detoxification program. But his situation did not improve. The severity of Ms. Rivers's psychological impairment and vulnerability became more evident to caseworkers and family support agencies when she repeatedly refused direct home help or abruptly terminated other support services. Caseworkers reported that she often became hostile and even threatening.

When Matthew was 18 months old, a visiting caseworker again found the house unsafe, strewn with debris, and the children " filthy" and inadequately dressed. When Ms. Rivers entered another drug program, she left the boys with another addict. Matthew was returned to Ms. Smith. At this reunion, Matthew was a much sadder child. There was a burn scar on his upper thigh; Ms. Rivers claimed that Matthew fell on an iron, but the circumstances were unclear and the doctor was suspicious. Ms. Smith was disturbed by Matthew's state, and this time, it required considerable effort to recover her former connection with him. Initially, he refused to eat and threw the bottle on the floor. Only when she began to sing the lullabies she had sung to him before did Matthew stop crying, and then he clung to her for a long time. The earlier attachment between Matthew and his foster mother was reevoked and began to deepen.

The return to Ms. Smith was the beginning of a painful 5-year process of repeated shifts between birth mother and foster mother. Whenever Matthew left his foster mother for visits with his birth mother, he regressed and was frightened, angry, and clinging upon his return. The psychological intensity of these transitions did not diminish over time.

At 18 months, a time of heightened separation anxiety in all children, Matthew did not possess a reliable attachment figure. The two mothers had very different psychological histories. Ms. Rivers had been known to social service agencies since childhood. Her early history was traumatic. She had been removed from the care of her schizophrenic mother as a child and was placed with a foster family. Although she thought of this family as "her family," she was again given up at the age of 10 and placed in a children's home. From that time on, Ms. Rivers had moved between hospitals, group homes, and shelters, and in late adolescence, she became deeply addicted to drugs. She was not able to hold a job and was on welfare.

At 18, she became pregnant with Bobby and had an intermittent relationship with his father until he died. Bobby was removed from her care when he was found abandoned at the age of 18 months. He remained in foster care for over a year, until Ms. Rivers took him without permission and disappeared for several months. Eventually she brought him to a hospital for an unexplained ingestion of turpentine, after which she abruptly removed him, against the physician's advice. The state agency tried to work with her, but she often threatened caseworkers physically, which resulted in numerous changes in treatment and support services.

At age 23 she gave birth to Matthew. Ms. Rivers was alone, had no relationship with Matthew's father, and could not even provide his name. This had not been the case with Bobby's father and may have contributed to her relative emotional distance from Matthew. Ms. Rivers stated that she had survived the state parental system, but she denied its severe impact on her own development.

In contrast, Ms. Smith, in her 40s, had grown up in a traditional, middle-class, white family and had a professional career. She had been married and had had several miscarriages when her husband died. For several years, she took care of foster children, was well regarded by the state, and managed her job and the children with the help of day care. Until Matthew came to her, all the foster children had stayed for only short periods of time. Her mother and siblings were some support to her, although they questioned the long-term burden she assumed with Matthew. Matthew's return to her at 18 months, and his subsequent long stay, led to the development of a strong mutual attachment. Nevertheless, Matthew was a difficult child to care for, and Ms. Smith repeatedly sought psychological help for herself as well as for him. Understandably, her attachment to Matthew and concern for his future became very strong. As the years went by, the prospect of losing each other became very painful to them both. When Matthew was 4½ years old and it seemed that he would be returned to his birth mother, Ms. Smith decided to adopt a child from a foreign country. Although a new family was being constructed, the issues of separation and loss were dominant, and uncertainty remained for years to come.

Matthew had enormous meaning to each mother, especially since both had experienced significant loss. However, Ms. Rivers's extensive history of loss started at a very early age and impaired her entire development. One can speculate that her limited capacity to sustain an empathetic relationship with Matthew was a reenactment of her own history of abandonment. She could not provide for Matthew that which she did not have. Her defensive denial of pain, both Matthew's and her own, masked the narcissistic fragility and depression that underlay her outer toughness. In contrast, Ms. Smith's losses occurred in adulthood, and she was able to maintain a capacity for empathy and for actively promoting Matthew's developing ego functions.

THE REFERRAL FOR TREATMENT (MATTHEW AT 4 YEARS, 3 MONTHS)

Matthew had been living primarily with Ms. Smith for 3 years when a psychologist consulted by the child protective services recommended that he be reunified with his birth mother. This consultant, Dr. Morris, described her plan as a "high-risk reunification." Her decision was influenced by the dominant case law in the state, which was biased in favor of returning children to their biological parents. She believed that the case law superseded the issues presented by past psychologists, who had stressed the quality and valence of Matthew's attachment to his foster mother and the significance of this attachment for his development. Dr. Morris believed that Matthew had the "resiliency" to handle the loss of his foster mother.

Ms. Smith asked permission from the agency to arrange treatment for Matthew to prepare him for reunification with his birth mother. She was concerned about his symptomatic behavior following the now-required overnight visitations with his birth mother and needed help in handling him. Matthew was having nightmares, wetting himself day and night, and was afraid to be alone in a room. In anticipation of each visit to his birth mother, he became defiant and upset, crying throughout the 2-hour trip with the state social worker. Ms. Smith told the therapist that Matthew had been through many psychological evaluations and clearly had some understanding of his predicament. He seemed eager and willing for the opportunity to tell his story to a "talk doctor."

Matthew came to the first session with his foster mother. He was a handsome, bright, very active 4-year-old with dark curly hair and brown skin. Even before they had fully entered the room, he asked, "Why do I have to go to Bobbymom?" His foster mother explained that he called his birth mother "Bobbymom," while he called her "Mommy." She added that Matthew knew that he would now have more and longer visits with Bobbymom. The therapist told Matthew that she understood his difficult situation and how hard it must be for him to go back and forth.

Matthew began to move rapidly through the room, bringing one toy after the other to show to his foster mother, before settling down at the table to draw a house. He told the therapist that the drawing was Bobby's house, with a road to Bobby's school. Ms. Smith commented that Matthew liked Bobby, and Matthew agreed but said he did not like to stay with Bobby overnight. Then he drew a second house, in which he lived with his foster mother, and the therapist talked about "going back and forth" between the two houses and how upsetting this was to him. (The expression "going back and forth" became a leitmotif in therapy.) He kept asking why he had to go there, and when the therapist put into words the situation of having two mothers, one inside of whom he had grown as a baby, and his present "Mommy" with whom he now lived, he said, "I know, I know! I don't want to go to Bobbymom's." At this point, as though to communicate his turmoil, he went to the dollhouse and, with considerable force, turned every single item in it upside down.

Watching this, Ms. Smith told the therapist that Matthew tended to destroy all the toys he loved most, which was upsetting and incomprehensible to her. To the therapist, this behavior was an indication of his inner turmoil in trying to cope with the impending loss and the unspoken anger that he felt. At times, he would express this anger toward himself, objects that he liked, or the adults who could not protect him. Expressing in words the painful and frightening dilemmas he was facing, the therapist told Matthew she could see that he was troubled by very serious matters, and she would try to be of help to him in the weeks to come.

The first session raised many clinical questions. What defenses were available to a 4-year-old boy to help him modulate the anxiety related to real danger and to primary object loss? Matthew did not understand why he was being sent "back and forth." He had an unusually mature ability to say why he needed help and could express in words his need to remain with his foster mother, but his actions expressed his internal chaos and anger. Although he was coherent in his focus and in his words, at times, his pain and fear broke through. Intense motor activity, rapid speech, and destructive behavior reflected his anxiety and great inner pressure for discharge. This was evident in the methodical, thorough, and angry overturning of the contents of the dollhouse as a representation of his feelings about his threatening life situation. That he had already internalized a sense of vulnerability to impending danger and loss was expressed every time he destroyed his favorite toys.

What was the role of treatment in such a complex situation? Child protective service's plan of separating Matthew from his foster mother and reunifying him with his birth mother was a reality. Therapy might at the very least create a safe environment in which Matthew could share his frightening reality, his feelings, and his fantasies. Matthew had significant internal strengths: he had a talent for expressing himself in words and play and he had a capacity for object differentiation. Although he was frightened of some people, Matthew was able to feel secure with others, which suggested that he could develop a therapeutic working alliance. He trusted Ms. Smith, and this helped him to make a connection to the therapist.

For the time being, Matthew had a safe home with his foster mother, but he faced the impending loss of her every time he had overnight stays with his birth mother. The caseworker took Matthew on these visits despite his panic and severe protests, and he returned from them in an anxious and regressed state. He spoke of dangerous things that happened to him and it was reported by case workers that his birth mother was unable to control or comfort him and sometimes took harsh measures, such as spankings to keep him quiet. The visits were upsetting and trying for both.

The worry for Matthew's safety and well-being became a critical issue in the therapist's concerns and decisions. Because Matthew did not wish to separate from his foster mother, the therapist invited them to come together to the consulting room once a week. To sustain a sense of trust with Matthew was paramount and required constant acknowledgment of the difficulty of his situation and the helplessness that he, his foster mother, and the therapist shared in face of the state's decisions. Within a short time, the therapist better understood Matthew's reactions to the actual danger and volatile realities of his life, and brought these new observations to the attention of the authorities.

INSIGHTS INTO MATTHEW'S INNER WORLD (MATTHEW AT 4 YEARS, 3 MONTHS TO 5½ YEARS)

As treatment began, Matthew revealed the enormous anxiety he was carrying within him. His fear of a final separation from his foster mother dominated his moods. Each time he visited his birth mother, he became more fearful and defiant at home and more anxious about separation. For example, after a 4-day visit with his birth mother, he regressed to an earlier level of attachment. Throughout the session, he stayed close to his foster mother's body, either sitting on her lap or playing at her feet, but touching her constantly. The 4-year-old regressed significantly.

He developed dramatic play in which he was lost and had to be found. He pretended to be a tiny baby, wrapped in a blanket and curled up in a pretend crib, which he constructed from two chairs. He repeatedly verbalized and dramatized his wish to be a baby—Ms. Smith's baby—and to wear diapers. His search for a secure base with Ms. Smith was clear. At times, his play included a sleeping baby who had nightmares and needed to be comforted by his mother. In this play, he asked the foster mother to play the role of mother and the therapist to be the grandmother. It was as though Matthew wanted the therapist to witness the importance of his foster mother's presence to him and understand his longing. Clearly, he wished for permanence with Ms. Smith, and he actually dramatized that she had given birth to him.

In play, words, and behavior, Matthew also began to reveal how much he admired Bobby but how badly his birth mother frightened him. As treatment proceeded, the sessions often started with Matthew describing an event in which he had confronted something very frightening at his birth mother's house. He talked about scary movies he had seen there—*Ghostbusters* and *Dracula*—and the nightmares he had about each. His manner was full of bravado, using swear words and dramatic, aggressive gestures. He bragged of dangerous behavior in Ms. Rivers's house. He opened the window next to the top bunk bed, which he shared with Bobby. This window was on the second floor and had no screen. He started a fire and burned himself slightly. He talked about these things with great excitement. In addition, he revealed that he and Bobby shared a bunk bed with Ms. Rivers's schizophrenic mother, who also acted as their babysitter. Until this time, the grandmother's presence in the home was unknown to the agency.

A pattern developed in the playroom, with frightening material emerging at the beginning of the sessions. Matthew's defensive attempts to master his anxiety included identification with the aggressor, reversal of affect, and turning passive into active (Freud, 1966). His play and behavior were defiant and provocative, reminiscent of his mother's anger and bravado, and included rapid, loud, active movement of soldiers and toy emergency vehicles. He repeatedly tried to take control of the ending of the sessions and to be the "boss" of all that happened in and around the office. But these attempts to master his anxiety were barely adequate, and he often spent the one-third of the sessions dramatizing his wish to be a baby in his mother's lap or playing hide and seek when he knew that he was always visible. In this way, he dealt with not only the fear of losing his foster mother but also his wish to retreat from the frightening problems of his reality.

The therapist's interpretations of Matthew's wish to have some control over all that happened to him helped but were insufficient to stem the waves of helplessness, impotence, and anger that he experienced. His anger was sometimes directed at his two mothers and sometimes at himself as he hit, hurt, or put himself in danger. It had not taken him long to come to terms intellectually with the concept that he was given birth by one mother, who had been too sick to take care of him, and cared for by another. However he could not come to terms with going back to the frightening presence and atmosphere of his birth mother, nor could he deal with the loss of his internalized primary object, his foster mother.

The divided and disparate holding environment created acute separation anxiety for this 4 year old boy. Intense fear of object loss was noticeable at the end of each session, and especially when the therapist went on vacation. Matthew continued to have difficulty falling asleep, and he had bad dreams. He wet his bed and, in the daytime, urinated on the floor. For the first time, he began to run away from his foster mother in a parking lot, placing himself in danger and making her run after him. Matthew expressed his fear before each visit to his birth mother that this one might be "forever." As the overnight visits increased, so did Matthew's symptoms. His adaptive attempts to deal with his world were desperate and painful to observe. Ms. Smith and the therapist communicated the traumatic impact of the overnight visits to the legal guardian and to caseworkers.

RETHINKING THE PLACEMENT PLAN

Two months after treatment began, Matthew's law guardian applied to the court to have the overnight visits stopped, which the court ordered, but daytime visits continued. The reunification plan was still in place, only postponed. A reevaluation of the determination of placement was requested by the child protective services. Dr. Morris, the consulting psychologist, who had previously recommended reunifying Matthew with his birth mother, reviewed the new information supplied by the caseworkers and the therapist. She described Matthew as a child facing object loss, whatever determination was made. Although noting his expressed desire to stay with his foster mother and his extreme anxiety about losing her, Dr. Morris again argued that case law dictated preference for the biological parent and that grounds for termination required proof of serious and enduring emotional and psychological harm. She did not see the proof. She believed that despite Matthew's impulsive, hostile, and aggressive behavior and loss of control before and after visits, he had the resilience to reunite with his birth mother and overcome the separation from his foster mother and the loss of his secure base. Reunification, she noted, would not be too damaging to him if his birth mother would seriously engage in treatment and create a stable home. At this time, Dr. Morris believed that Matthew's birth mother could achieve a higher level of functioning.

The agency made repeated efforts to arrange reasonable, in-depth counseling for Matthew's birth mother, but once again, she could not sustain involvement in therapeutic work. Each therapeutic relationship ended in outbursts of hostility, threats, and anger. Meanwhile, Matthew's development was at great risk. He became more oppositional and defiant. He was confused by Ms. Rivers's alternately reaching toward him and rejecting him. Sometimes she was not home when he came to visit. At times, he did what he could to engage her, kissing her profusely when she agreed to give him something he wanted. At other times, he was provocative and swore or lost control. She might then spank him or wash his mouth out with soap. Matthew felt betrayed by the harsh treatment and her rejection, and did not believe in Ms. Rivers's stated wish to keep him. She now made veiled threats to abduct him, and supervised visits were ordered by the court. Finally, when Matthew was 5, Dr. Morris changed her opinion and recommended adoption by Ms. Smith. Since Ms. Rivers could not sustain counseling to help her with Matthew, who by now was quite a difficult child, how could she help him overcome the loss of his foster mother? Dr. Morris recognized that the years of separation had taken their toll. An attachment still existed between birth mother and son, but it was fragile, fraught with conflict and mistrust, ambivalence and anger.

Dr. Morris hoped that a voluntary open adoption could be arranged. Ultimately, however, Ms. Rivers could not accept the idea of limited supervised visits in this adoption plan and rejected it. The agency now recommended that the parental rights be severed for the purpose of permanent placement and adoption of Matthew by Ms. Smith. It took almost 2 more years for the court to hear the case, make the decision to terminate Ms. Rivers's parental rights, and complete the adoption process. Matthew remained with Ms. Smith during this period.

THE PSYCHOLOGICAL EXPERIENCE OF THE COURT PROCEEDINGS (MATTHEW AT 5½ TO 6½ YEARS)

At an age when most children are transitioning into latency, Matthew was forced to focus on issues so basic and highly charged that he was unable to develop sufficient control over his feelings, which broke through in inappropriate social situations. He did not have sufficient ego strength to modulate his anxiety and aggression. In many ways, he was out of sync with more carefree children. As the trial neared, he had to participate in evaluations by two independent mental health professionals. The birth mother's court-appointed lawyer selected a psychologist well known for his view that children should remain with their biological mothers, especially in cross-racial situations. Matthew's legal guardian requested that the most experienced evaluation team be found. The Yale Child Study Center was selected. Each mother agreed to be seen alone and with Matthew by each evaluator. These evaluations began when Matthew entered kindergarten and lasted through the first semester.

It was hard for Ms. Smith to calm him. Neither he nor anyone could make the process move faster or be assured of the outcome. Whatever the results, he would face loss. At school and at home, his distress was obvious: He was angry; he used foul language and kicked and hit both children and adults. Developmentally, he was falling behind his peers.

But the working alliance of the therapist, Ms. Smith, and Matthew remained strong. The therapist engaged Ms. Smith on the side of the parental ego that could offer protection and comfort to Matthew, and Ms. Smith was able to make use of the guidance offered. She used both the therapist's support to tolerate Matthew's constant testing of her commitment to him and the therapist's interpretations and perspective to understand Matthew's aggressive behavior. All efforts were made to sustain Matthew's positive ego developments, of which there were many: his ability to use words and drawings; his beginning capacity to have concern for others; his growing sense of humor; his voracious appetite for new information; and his capacity for pleasure. He showed signs of internalizing the therapist's approach of finding words to describe his situation.

Ms. Smith and Matthew each brought their worries to therapy in different ways. Ms. Smith might say, "Should we ask Dr. Paret if she can help us with . . . ?" She always tried to maintain empathy with Matthew, even though she might be discussing something that had been extremely upsetting to her. For example, after the Smith family had moved to a new house, Ms. Smith reported that Matthew was scribbling on the walls and smearing excrement. This behavior was interpreted as a defense against his anxiety around separation, as symbolized by the move. He had already experienced innumerable changes of residence with his birth mother.

Matthew joined the conversations in his way. For example, he played on the floor with his Power Ranger dominating all the other action figures and soldiers in an aggressive, controlling manner. Full of energy and pleasure in his role as the leader in charge, he might push the Power Ranger in front of Ms. Smith's or the therapist's face. Ms. Smith perceived this as disruptive and upsetting. The therapist responded to the different meanings of the play. She talked with Matthew about his wish to be in charge of his life in a way that was not possible at the moment. She told him she knew there were many things he wished to control—the amount of time they had for sessions, the borrowing of her toys, the move to the new house, "going back and forth," the fact that they still did not know with whom he would live "forever." She knew that he felt he did not have the power to make sure he would stay with Ms. Smith. She told him that Ms. Smith and she also lacked that power, and this disappointed him and sometimes made him angry at them. But she could reassure him and Ms. Smith that they were all doing their best to help him, and she would list the names of all the professional people he knew who cared about him. In spite of these reassurances, it was clearly terrifying to him that even the grown-ups he trusted most, his foster mother and his therapist, could not control the crucial decision about his future. Matthew expressed intense longing for a father and was angry that this wish, too, could not be granted.

His lack of autonomy was infuriating to him. "I keep telling and telling, I want to stay with Ms. Smith," he said to the evaluators. He regressed again, refusing at times to use the toilet, urinating or defecating when and where he wished. The interpretation was offered that the one thing Matthew himself surely could control was his own body and its functions, and maybe that was why he controlled the time and place of urinating and defecating. In body language and words, he agreed that there was something to this; the behavior abated but remained a sporadic symptom until the judge reached a decision and Matthew knew he would be adopted.

In his sessions, Matthew expressed feelings of guilt and disloyalty to his birth mother. He worried that Ms. Rivers was crying for him, because she always cried at the end of each visit. His own grief was mixed with his fear of returning. Overall, his play and stories reflected a sense that he could not trust Ms. Rivers to protect him. For instance, he said she never made him wear a seatbelt and "always breaks her promises." He felt guilty about his wish to stay with Ms. Smith and tried to justify his desire to save himself. In one of the evaluation sessions with Ms. Rivers, he plaintively told her that he had been with Ms. Smith for 5 years and it seemed to him that she was the real mother and Ms. Rivers was like the foster mother.

The therapist responded to Matthew's disappointment in his birth mother and his guilt about his own wishes. To help him with his feelings that he was a "bad" child, who had somehow caused all this, she tried to put into perspective the idea that his birth mother had been ill when he was small and could not always do the right thing. He deeply wanted to be loved and cared for even by Ms. Rivers, who had neglected him. Matthew said that the one way Bobbymom showed him she loved him was to buy him toys. During this period, he had a particularly insatiable need for toys. He never could get enough to fill what he later called "that empty spot in me." The relief that a new toy brought was transitory. Matthew's self-image was that of a child who was unsatisfactory and deserved to be disposed of and forgotten.

When Matthew was 6, the evaluations were complete, but it was 6 more months before the judge decided to terminate Ms. Rivers's parental rights, thus freeing Matthew for adoption by Ms. Smith. She acknowledged that each mother in her own way cared deeply about Matthew. She took into consideration the testimony about the profound meaning of birth parentage and the complexities of cross-racial adoption in relation to identity formation. But she was especially persuaded by the Yale Child Study Center's evaluation that Matthew should stay with Ms. Smith because of the strength of the attachment Matthew had developed with her. The judge believed that Ms. Rivers's capacity to help Matthew with the loss of Ms. Smith was limited, and that returning him to Ms. Rivers would likely lead to future disruptions and separations for Matthew. She felt there would be serious and enduring harm if, after all these years of not knowing where he would be, he were to lose the only solid base he had.

Matthew was ecstatic when he learned of the judge's decision to allow his adoption by Ms. Smith. He was radiant when he told the news to the therapist, and at home, he shouted out the window to the neighborhood that he was going to be adopted. He stopped wetting and soiling, and his most dangerous behavior abated. During the summer months that followed, he was generally happy and functioned unusually well at a summer day camp and at home, but this quiescent period did not last. He remained extremely sensitive to perceived loss, danger, or narcissistic injury, and gains could be undone quickly, suggestive of Balint's (1968) idea of a basic fault.

EXTERNAL STABILITY AND INTERNAL VULNERABILITY (MATTHEW AT 6½ TO 7 YEARS)

When Matthew entered first grade, he was convinced that he would now permanently live with Ms. Smith; nevertheless, his insecurity and vulnerability were obvious. He was too sensitive to comments from the inexperienced, new teacher and the unknown children in his class. At home and in his sessions, he expressed his inner doubts about himself. He believed that because some children could already read, it would be impossible for him to learn to do so gradually. He often acted "tough" in the classroom and sometimes got into fights. When he was sent out to sit in the hall, he told the therapist that he liked it, because he "could see people come and go." The therapist and Ms. Smith consulted with the teacher, the school psychologist, and learning consultants to formulate a more supportive learning environment for him, and by the end of the school year, Matthew did learn how to read.

In the clinical sessions, Matthew began to express complex feelings about the permanency of his situation with Ms. Smith, and the finality of the separation from Ms. Rivers and Bobby. He often said he missed Bobby. He compared himself to other children in his mostly white school and found himself wanting. He did not like his curly hair or his skin color, and he was teased about his uncircumcised penis. He said he hated the Spanish language. Matthew had connected his guilt and low self-esteem with recognition of society's devalued perception of his racial origin. He was vulnerable to and hurt by comments of other children about his racial origin. This vulnerability was a theme that emerged at different points in treatment as Matthew struggled with his conflicted picture of himself (Hoopes, 1990).

For the first time, he expressed his own ambivalence about Ms. Smith. His concern about each mother—the sadness of Ms. Rivers and the overweight appearance of Ms. Smith—reflected his doubts about his own identity. The therapist now believed it would be more helpful if Matthew had individual sessions, and the new certainty of his placement made it possible for him to see her without Ms. Smith.

In the individual sessions, Matthew's drawings represented questions about his own identity and the dual parental imago he carried. He repeatedly drew an egg-shaped oval that he called ying–yang, a concept that he had learned at school. The oval was divided by a wavy line and each half had an eye in it. The two halves were always different colors, but the two segments fit together to make one whole. This seemed to represent Matthew's attempt to form an integrated whole of his dual realities and developing identity. The same theme was evident in the face of a little boy he drew in an orange circle, with curly hair on top, but scribbled over with jagged brown lines, reflecting his confusion about himself (Brinich, 1990).

He drew other frightening pictures such as Dracula, ghosts, and a blackened house. The therapist commented on how frightening these images might be to a child and asked Matthew if he would like to tell some stories to go with his pictures. He agreed and in consecutive sessions dictated the following three stories about abandonment, the difficulty of trusting, the terror of being alone in the external world, and the wish to survive.

The Mournful Pumpkin
By Matthew

> Once upon a time in a small village there was a mournful pumpkin. The mournful pumpkin lost the other pumpkins 'cause one day all the other pumpkins were stolen except for the mournful pumpkin. The robbers got caught by the police, but all the other pumpkins were smashed. Clip. Clop. Bang. Clip. Clop. Bang. Clip Clop Bang. Bang, bang, bang. All the pumpkins were smashed and the mournful pumpkin decided to run away. He saw a goose. The goose said, "No, you cannot live with me." So the mournful pumpkin walked away from the goose's nest. After a couple of weeks, the mournful pumpkin found a friend. That mournful pumpkin who found a friend had a friend at last. The End.

Matthew had made up his own fairy tale in which the surviving mournful pumpkin experienced pervasive loss and witnessed destruction and violence. He set out on a journey to find a place to live and a friend. Although he succeeded, he was still that mournful pumpkin. Matthew expressed his loss, his determination to survive, and his great need for human attachment. The therapist acknowledged how sad and frightened the little pumpkin was, how he tried to find a safe place and a friend, and how worried he might have been about the other little pumpkins. In the next session, Matthew had an even more painful story to tell.

The Serial Killer
By Matthew Rivers

> Once in a city there was a dark, dark, dark, dark, dark, dark corner. That corner was full of serial killers. Nobody knew who they were because they were dressed up in real people's clothes. One day, one of the serial killers got caught, so another one went out and killed somebody. That serial killer who killed somebody was the Governor. The Governor got arrested. That's why we have a new governor. Who knows? Maybe our governor is another serial killer. The End.

In this story, there are terror-filled secret places where life-threatening injury can occur and no one can be trusted. Even respectable people in authority are suspect. The therapist responded to Matthew's feeling that it was hard to trust anyone or feel absolutely safe. She put into words his feelings that perhaps he did not always trust the therapist. After she raised the issue of trust in the transference, Matthew expressed his fear of his birth mother, explaining that she had had a large knife under her bed and that she might, like Dracula, come back to snatch him.

The erratic early relationship with his birth mother and the inability of the child welfare system to protect him affected Matthew's ability to trust the adult world. His unspoken fear of being killed and his allusions to the fear of his own aggression and badness was revealed in the third story he wrote, which he did not title.

> Once upon a time there were some kids. Those kids went to a fabulous adventure. That fabulous adventure had cut off hands and bloody heads, and everything you saw was disgusting deadness. There was so much deadness you thought you would barf. The end.

When he had the computer printout in his hand, he scribbled over this story with a red crayon. Matthew was preoccupied with fears of annihilation and saw danger everywhere around him and, unlike many children, had few illusions about the security of life. Very bad things could and did happen. He spoke of the frightening places where he had visited his birth mother. Deadness and grief were real possibilities. The therapist put into words his grief as well as his wish to live and go forward. Often, these interpretations were followed by clarifications of reality. Matthew used language well to put his feelings into words and was beginning to have the capacity to differentiate between the past and the present. But his own survival left him with feelings of guilt about Bobby and Ms. Rivers, and what he thought he might have done to them.

The signing of the adoption papers occurred near Matthew's seventh birthday and was a joyful experience. Matthew had invited the therapist to be present saying, "We worked hard for this for such a long time." But once again, the initial euphoria faded and Matthew's sense of loss and inner doubts about himself reappeared. The discussion that follows suggests an assessment of Matthew's developmental status that reveals both his capacity for growth and the difficult psychological sequelae of his first 7 years.

DISCUSSION

The Splintered Holding Environment and the Vulnerable Ego

Matthew's early development occurred in conditions of extraordinarily high risk, including poverty, chaos, maternal drug addiction, and loss (Sameroff, 1989). His circumstances were the antithesis of Hartmann's (1939) "average expectable environment." What capacity did Matthew have as an infant and toddler for coping with these intolerable stresses? When he was first sent to Ms. Smith, she noted that he cried without tears and neither looked at her nor seemed to expect a nurturing relationship. His moments of sadness were an early sign of what he later called "that empty spot" in him. At 18 months, when he returned to his foster mother after a 3-month absence, she noted that she had to work even harder than before to engage him. The absence of a permanent and stable object had resulted in periods of withdrawal resembling anaclitic depression (Spitz & Wolf, 1946). Without expectation that his needs could be met by another, Matthew could only strike out frantically to express his plight. Even in toddlerhood, the beginnings of behavioral difficulties were apparent.

At the age of 4, it was evident that Matthew had developed a strong attachment to his foster mother but the interminable placement process had taken its toll. His fragile ego was insufficient to cope with his mounting anger, fear, and sense of impotence. His defenses were primitive, and he could not tolerate delay or modulate his wishes and feelings. The general insecurity he felt made it impossible for him to fully internalize his foster mother's reassurances. His autonomy was compromised, and he often regressed to earlier phases of development. He was controlling and provocative, identifying with the aggressor. He turned passive into active by reenacting the danger in which he felt he was involved. A high degree of narcissistic vulnerability was evident as he tested the commitment of his foster mother and others.

Despite the fact that external stability was finally achieved when he was 7, Matthew's stories, "The Mournful Pumpkin" and "The Serial Killer," revealed his deep sense of existential grief and annihilation anxiety (Cohen, 1996). Matthew worried about being the victim as well as the victimizer. He had identified with aspects of his birth mother. His false self was a tough guy, swearing and shouting, but his true self was a frightened little boy who felt unworthy and expendable. It was hard for him to sustain homeostasis, and his impulsiveness often broke through. He was overvigilant to unexpected danger. Without constant affirmation of belonging and acceptance, Matthew easily felt rejected or attacked.

As a latency-age child, Matthew was on track developmentally in some spheres but experienced difficulty in others. In the first-grade classroom, Matthew was seen by his teacher as demanding and disruptive. He could not sit still, was often unable to follow directions, and drew attention to himself with his loud voice and clowning. He was easily frustrated and could not expose himself to the risk of revealing that he did not immediately understand how to read or solve math problems. He tried to hide his failures and avoided difficult tasks. His anxiety and low self-esteem interfered with learning new material and making new friends. However, Matthew's capacity for expressiveness through drawing and storytelling brought him recognition and pride. The school requested a full evaluation to explore possible learning disabilities and a differential diagnosis was made of attention deficit disorder. The report revealed that Matthew was in the superior range of intelligence, with strengths in visual processing and integration but some deficits in aural processing. Like many other children with similar backgrounds, his needs could not easily be met in the public school system.

Despite the severe disruptions in his life, Matthew had achieved significant ego strengths. He had a capacity for conceptualization beyond his years, a capacity for reflection, and the ability to put his thoughts and feelings into words and pictures. In his hunger for learning, he had amassed a storehouse of information about the world, albeit with an emphasis on dangers, emergencies, and especially war. In treatment, he was able to give examples from the real world to illustrate the vulnerable nature of his inner world. He developed relationships with the children and adults in his environment and, in general, connected well with people when he was not overwhelmed. In these situations he was a lively, affectionate child with a good sense of humor. But if the memories of early traumatic events were triggered for him, he often unexpectedly lost his composure and self-control. For example, Matthew's behavior suddenly decompensated when the art teacher asked the children to make a collage of themselves as babies; sometimes when he met new people, he found a way to repeat his life story through shocking behavior that resulted in rejection and also set him apart and compromised his social development.

The Role of Treatment

In cases where children have experienced the continuous threat of object loss, psychotherapy can be instrumental in keeping open the developmental pathways. As James Anthony (1983) noted in his study of survivor children, the presence of strong, stable figure(s) is important in helping traumatized children to mediate the impact of their experiences. Matthew had two caring relationships to shore him up—with his foster/adoptive mother and his therapist. In addition, they presented a model of two adults working together to offer him protection and the shared belief that he should have a chance, like other children, to go forward in life. This helped him with his profound survivor guilt.

Matthew engaged in a therapeutic relationship with a new person who responded in a developmentally attuned and empathetic manner. The therapy provided a coherent holding environment, where he could feel understood and safe, and work through his anxieties and conflicts in the language of a child (Hurry, 1998). The way Matthew was able to make use of the therapeutic alliance was remarkable and reflected the trust he had in his foster/adoptive mother.

In cases of children who have been in protracted placement, new parameters arise at every stage of the psychotherapeutic process. The initial working alliance was based on a realistic understanding that Matthew might have to return to his birth mother. It was difficult for the therapist, the foster mother, and Matthew to realize their lack of control over the horrendous situation. Denial was neither possible nor helpful in the presence of the real danger of reunification. The therapist tried to provide a center of reality and exploration, but she also felt she had the ethical responsibility to advocate on behalf of Matthew.

A new phase in treatment began when Matthew became secure in his placement with Ms. Smith. Individual therapy was used to help him approach his feelings about the most hurtful issues of betrayal, neediness, and fear that were at the center of his vulnerability. The sessions were filled with mourning for the past and fear that he could still be hurt in the future. He was able to use interpretive work to differentiate himself from his birth mother. He said he was "stuck," but not as "stuck" as he thought his birth mother was, when he described her as "a grown-up on the outside but a child on the inside." Therapy helped him develop a language for a coherent narrative about himself. He moved from action to verbal expression to reflection and use of interpretation. He could integrate two different feelings at the same time (something that had been too dangerous before). He came to realize that there was a reason for his feelings and behavior and that he could feel better and gain control. Support and developmental guidance were helpful to Ms. Smith. The therapist provided perspective, empathy during trying times, interpretations of Matthew's behavior, and help in limit setting. The therapeutic relationship enabled her to endure her own grief and frustration.

The Legal Issues

The protracted placement process took place within an adversarial system that was indecisive and costly to all involved. The many evaluations and hearings were dominated by significant ethical and legal issues related to the rights of the birth mother and the best interests of the child. Opinions differed within the child protective services, among the psychologists, and among the judges. The relevant case law was biased toward the inherent rights of the birth mother, who stated a wish to regain full custody of her son. Yet the state was obliged to protect Matthew. Another point of contention was the issue of race and transracial adoption, and the impact this might have on Matthew's identity. On the one hand, the birth mother's advocate stressed the importance of Matthew's staying with his birth mother to preserve his ethnic identity. On the other hand, the Yale Child Study Center expert emphasized the greater importance to Matthew's development of remaining with his psychological parent. Stability for Matthew was critical, and the viability of a successful reunification was questioned because, despite the state's many efforts to help Ms. Rivers, she could not assure stability and safety for her child or for herself.

The court's decision for permanent adoption recognized the preeminent need to protect the child physically and psychologically. Unfortunately for Matthew, the system had found it difficult to reach this decision. Lengthy evaluations, the court calendar, and differences of opinion and even ideology all caused delays. For a long time, the plight of Matthew was lost in the bureaucratic process, and the length of the process created new and severe problems for him.

SUMMARY

The case discussed in this chapter is an example of the serious developmental risks to which children are subjected when they face early deprivation and years of uncertainty in protracted foster placement. One cannot lightly take a child from its biological parents, and identifying the best interests of the child, the alternative least detrimental to the child, requires expert diagnostic considerations. The case illustrates the importance of utilizing developmental knowledge to assess the child's primary attachment, his/her psychological status, and the continuity and stability of the environment. Had the principles of preserving the psychological parent, minimizing separations and parental discontinuities, and shortening the time required for decision making been followed, some of the developmental disturbances that we see in Matthew might have been prevented (Goldstein et al., 1996; Rutter, 1990). The clinical material indicates Matthew's strong will to survive, but also his anxious state, his gradual internalization of the fear of primary object loss, his extreme narcissistic vulnerability and hypervigilance concerning danger, abandonment, and annihilation. Treatment was helpful to Matthew in that he was able to strengthen his capacity for object relatedness and self-reflection. The developmental thrust was maintained, and his ability to hope to become an architect and a father is promising. His hopes for the future largely come from the developing security of his relationship with his adoptive mother. Nevertheless, his psychological wounds do not heal easily, and he continues to need treatment.

5

International Adoption and Family Formation

International adoption is both a personal family experience and a political and cultural process. This chapter describes how parentless children from one country are brought together with adoptive parent(s) from a different culture. These unions meet the important needs of both the child and the adoptive parent(s) for a family and are the beginning of a meaningful psychological journey (Kirk, 1964). The complex psychological process of becoming a family through international adoption is filled with hardships and satisfactions. Each country has its own policies regarding the treatment of abandoned and orphaned children, and many children spend their earliest years in institutional care and/or temporary foster placement. The quality of care varies greatly in these circumstances, and the adequacy and the nature of care leaves a special imprint on the child's internal world. Each child also has his/her own psychological and medical history, and the adoptive parent(s) may only begin to learn about the impact of their child's early experiences as the new family begins its journey together (Bartholet, 1993; Castle et al., 1999).

Often children suffer long-term effects from the circumstances of their early institutional care (Provence & Lipton, 1962). The quality of caregiving in the earliest years has an important impact on the child's physical, social, and cognitive development. The length of time the child suffers deprivation in nutrition, medical attention, and responsive social care increases the adverse psychological effects of institutionalization (Castle et al., 1999).

In general, the families bring good will and hope to the act of adoption and believe that by providing a nurturing family environment they may enable the children to have a better life. Some evidence indicates that children can make progress once their health and social environment is improved, but many families soon realize that the children need time and special care to overcome the effect of their early impoverished human environment in the orphanages (Rutter & the English and Romanian Adoptees [ERA] Study Team, 1998). For children who have never experienced a close interactive relationship with a primary caregiver, developing an attachment to parents opens a new dimension of their internal world. Adoptive parents may be unprepared for their child's lack of emotional responsiveness, seeming indifference, and even resistance in the early months of their relationship. The parents often need to cope with both the specific social and cultural circumstances of their child's preadoptive history and his/her undeveloped capacity for intimate relationships.

Over time, many parents of these children seek therapeutic help to cope with the complex family dynamics that develop. This chapter briefly discusses the broad general issues in international adoption and then focuses on the clinical and social issues that arise for children who have experienced severe early deprivation, including their adaptation when they join their adoptive families. Clinical vignettes illustrate the unique experiences of two families who tried to help their children recover from the early trauma that continued to affect their lives.

THE SOCIAL AND CULTURAL CONTEXT OF INTERNATIONAL ADOPTION

As domestic adoption becomes more difficult in the United States, more American families are seeking to adopt a child from abroad. In 1999, 16,396 children were adopted from overseas—a 45% increase in a period of just 4 years. The adopted children came from Europe, Asia, Africa, Central America, and South America. The largest number of children came from Russia (4,348), China (4,101), South Korea (2,008), Guatemala (1,002), and Romania (895) (U.S. State Department, 1999).

That families decide to adopt children from another country is the result of a number of interrelated factors that make international adoption a solution for family building. First, the number of American infants available for adoption at birth has declined, and adoption seekers outnumber actual adoptions by six to one (Evan B. Donaldson Adoption Institute, 2000). Second, an increasing number of American birth parents choose an open adoption for placement of their child, a method that is not attractive to some intentional parents (Berry, 1993). Third, the various policy guidelines in both public and private adoption agencies often discriminate against intentional parents who are older, single, or of the same sex (Sullivan, 1995b). Finally, the average wait for a child in international adoptions is between 6 and 18 months, whereas it can extend to seven years in the United States (Evan B. Donaldson Adoption Institute, 2000).

For some families, the desire for an international adoption is also motivated by altruistic and subjective feelings (Castle et al., 1999). Many intentional parents wish to adopt foreign children who are in a state of great need. Most are in orphanages or other institutional environments in countries with limited resources. In addition to the wish to meet the children's obvious needs for family care, the intentional parents perceive other benefits. The adoption, once achieved, is final, and the possibility of it being contested after the child has come to the United States is almost nil. Although parents are alerted to the possibility that the children may have special medical and developmental conditions, these facts are often vague, and parents hope that their empathy, love, and devotion, together with the provision of good medical care, will solve whatever problems may exist.

The cost of international adoption is high and prohibitive to many families. In 1999, the cost in the five highest sending countries ranged from $12,000 to $14,000, excluding the cost of travel for the parents and child (Holt International Children's Services, 2000). Each country determines its own criteria for the eligibility of children for international adoption and for the selection of adoptive parents. The international agencies acting as intermediaries can be helpful in preparing the forms and applications, and arranging the necessary home study for the family in the United States. The procedures in the native country of the child can be extensive, costly, and anxiety provoking because the adoption is never certain and finalization depends on the decisions of the local bureaucracy (Bartholet, 1993).

In important ways, the adoption policies of each sending country are shaped by its historical needs and cultural norms. These policies may change in response to internal developments. In China, for example, the one-child-per-family policy was intended to moderate the population growth rate but resulted in increasing numbers of abandoned infant girls, which made adoption more desirable to the Chinese government. The harsh political agenda of the Causescu regime in Romania encouraged pregnancy and banned abortion so as to increase the country's population, but pervasive poverty made the burdens of child care impossible for many families, and many babies ended up in institutions (Castle et al., 1999). Other reasons for abandoning children are the lack of acceptance of transracial children, the lack of available financial and medical support, and family illness. Often, children are orphaned and/or abandoned because of the disruptions of war. Some countries make children eligible for international adoption because of the overwhelming number of children and the lack of adequate resources for their care (Talbot, 1998). The policies of certain countries give children with "medical difficulties" higher priority for international adoption. In these difficult circumstances, by the time of adoption, many of these children have extensive developmental and psychological delays (Johnson & Groze, 1993). The social values and economic realities of each country determine the nature and level of medical and psychological care, so that the early care of children in some countries is better than in others (Talbot, 1998).

PHYSICAL HEALTH AND COGNITIVE DEVELOPMENT

In international adoption, as in other forms of adoption, the preadoptive history of the child has a significant impact on his/her well-being at the time of adoption, and more importantly, on the future of the child's adaptive capacities. Contemporary neurological and psychological research highlights the importance of the prenatal, neonatal, and postnatal environment to the child's future developmental well-being (Cicchetti & Cohen, 1995; see Chapter 2). Inadequate nutrition and medical care for the birth parent during pregnancy and a difficult environment for the fetus (perhaps the result of alcohol and substance abuse) increase the probability of a poor outcome, such as prematurity or low birthweight. Both the medical status at birth and the quality of postnatal care form a risk continuum for future developmental health (Hetherington & Parke, 1999). These experiences have clear ramifications for the future physical health of the child and all aspects of cognitive, social, and emotional development.

Extensive differences and variations in early care exist in the five major sending countries (Bartholet, 1993). In Russia and Romania, for example, sparse institutional care is common for abandoned and orphaned children, either because of poverty or perceptions of what constitutes appropriate care. Often, children's age-related needs for individual attention, nutrition, safety, medical care, and stimulation are inadequately met (Castle et al., 1999).

Descriptive reports are now emerging on the psychological, physical, and cognitive outcomes for children adopted from many different countries (Castle et al., 1999; Miller, 1999; Rutter and the English and Romanian Adoptees [ERA] Study Team, 1998; Talbot, 1998). Physicians in the United States are accumulating knowledge about the range of undiagnosed and insufficiently treated medical illnesses that are common in children adopted internationally. For those children who received inadequate medical care in their earliest years, problems include serious conditions such as rickets, malnutrition, fetal alcohol syndrome, parasites, hepatitis B, and tuberculosis (Miller, 1999; Oleck, 2000).

Untreated medical illnesses place children at physical risk and can also cause developmental delay. Many children are ill when their parents first meet them; usually, the adoptive parents arrange for health care immediately. For some of these children, medical treatment and empathetic care produce dramatic improvement. Physically healthy, they can begin to establish an emotional connection to their new parents, and this responsive, interactive experience can help them start on the road to psychological and physical recovery (Johnson & Groze, 1993). Other children may never fully recover and need continuous monitoring and care (Miller, 1999).

More than a dozen medical centers in the United States now specialize in the assessment of medical and developmental problems of children adopted internationally. Many of the children emerging from early institutional care have significant problems in language development, and communication and learning skills. Additionally, severe and mechanistic early care can have an impact on endocrine function, which affects physical development, including the timing of puberty (Miller, 1999; Oleck, 2000). Furthermore, research indicates that early social experience affects the brain development of young children (Perry et al., 1995; Siegel, 1999).

A study by the English and Romanian Adoptees (ERA) Study Team sheds light on the importance of attuned social caregiving to the child's positive cognitive development (Castle et al., 1999). The study evaluated the impact of the quality of care and the length of time in an orphanage for 129 Romanian children adopted before their second birthdays by English parents. The purpose of the study was to evaluate the impact of the following four factors on the cognitive development of the children:

- Quality of food
- Range of physical experiences
- Access to playthings
- Availability of responsive individual care provided by a known caregiver

Conditions in these orphanages were rated as extremely severe, based on the observations by the adoptive families and other independent professionals, including observers from relief organizations and the study team. The observers particularly noted the mechanistic ways in which the children were treated and the lack of individually attuned care.

The children's cognitive functioning was assessed at 4 and 6 years of age, well after they had been adopted. The findings indicate that individual, attuned attention was the most significant predictor of cognitive ability, even more important than nutrition. The length of time the children experienced unresponsive social care was correlated with poorer levels of cognitive functioning at 6 years of age. This evidence points to the importance of early social experience for the future cognitive development of children (Castle et al., 1999). The findings also indicate that even small improvements in individual attention during the first 2 years of life have important implications for cognitive attainment. This supports the findings of other research on the impact of indifferent and mechanistic institutional care on the development of children (Provence & Lipton, 1962; Spitz, 1945; Tizard & Hodges, 1978).

In summary, the growing literature indicates that for children in institutional care, the highest risk factors are length of time in institutional care, stability and quality of individual care, age at the time of adoption, and prenatal and neonatal medical history, including the adequacy of medical treatment.

EARLY DEPRIVATION AND THE CAPACITY FOR ATTACHMENTS

In her article "Attachment Theory: The Ultimate Experiment," Margaret Talbot (1998) described the difficult emotional experiences of children adopted from Romania. Children's initial adjustments into family care were poor, but they had varying degrees of emotional recovery. To assess the children's adjustment, Victor Groze conducted a survey of 229 families who adopted children from Romanian orphanages (Talbot, 1998). Using the parents' own assessments of their children, he classified them into three groups. About 20% were identified as "challenged children," with marked psychological and developmental lags up to 4 years after the adoption. Approximately 60% were called the "wounded wonders"—children who had various developmental lags but were catching up. Finally, 20% were termed "resilient rascals," those who had adapted well without any evident problems.

Groze speculates that before adoption, the care of the children may have varied somewhat in terms of a special relationship some may have had with a caregiver. Resilient children, for example, may have been "pets" of caregivers and received more individual attention (Talbot, 1998), which corresponds with other findings for "survivor children" in chaotic family care or long-term institutional care (Anthony, 1983; Anthony & Chiland, 1988; Provence & Lipton, 1962). While these children's adoptive parents had to provide extensive therapeutic and medical care to help them recover, most of the adoptive parents (78%) thought the adoption had a positive impact on the family, and 97% said they "never thought" of relinquishing their children, despite the hardships of caring for them (Talbot, 1998).

Adaptation to Stress and Long-Term Sequelae

All infants adapt as successfully as they can to their environmental context. When the environment is one of social deprivation, infants cope in ways that minimize psychological pain and discomfort. Adaptive strategies in infancy are primitive and include such behaviors as social withdrawal, gaze aversion, diminished expression of affect, and repetitive, self-injurious behavior. Such responses may be adaptive in the short run as the only defenses against isolation and psychological loss. In the long run, however, these adaptations may be harmful to the capacity for human engagement and cognitive, social, and psychological development (Fraiberg, 1987b). Other serious psychological and health issues can emerge, such as failure to thrive or anaclitic depression (Shapiro, Fraiberg, & Adelson, 1976; Spitz, 1945). Furthermore, early experiences of loss and deprivation can have a profound impact on children's readiness to develop a relationship with the adoptive parents.

Children's Responses to the Adoptive Parents

The clinical vignettes presented here illustrate the early relational problems that can arise between the institutionalized child and the new adoptive parents. Judging from many reports, parents in general are eager to claim their child. The psychological readiness for engagement, however, differs between the intentional parents and the institutionalized child. Children who have already experienced the developmental traumas of institutionalization and early loss often cannot relate to the adoptive parents with any degree of excitement or pleasure. Indeed, they may even fear contact with human beings.

For parents, the joy of meeting their longed-for child is soon tempered by the child's lack of emotional responsiveness to them. They may feel deprived of the anticipated fantasy and joy of having a child, and grieve for themselves and their child. The beginning of a relationship with a child who has had an early history of illness, impersonal care, and multiple disruptions of caregiving is often a difficult, sobering experience.

The Early Relational Experiences of the Child: Attachment Issues

Empirical clinical research and developmental and biological findings help us understand the muted and limited repertoire in responses of adopted infants, toddlers, and preschoolers to the overtures of their new parents. In general, the children have not had the relational experiences that are known to underlie normal social, cognitive, and emotional development. For an older child, these basic earlier social experiences are a necessary precursor to the possibility of engagement with a nurturing other (Ainsworth, 1979b).

Theoretically, the capacity to have a relationship with a responsive other originates within an early relationship of empathetic parental care in which the infant or growing child begins to expect a responsive and reciprocal exchange of emotional feelings, mirroring, and linguistic expressions (Winnicott, 1965b). For example, as parents mold their bodies to hold the baby comfortably, as they engage in the reciprocal dance of movement and vocal exchange, the infant receives and exchanges satisfying moments with the adult caregiver (Stern, 1985). The depth of these experiences in the first 2 years is central to the development of a robust emotional capacity, a versatile expressiveness, and a confident anticipatory trust in the other. Over time, the child internalizes the relational "culture" of the family, adapting to the relational style and dynamics of family life. This affects not only his/her view of what family means but also the internal view of how he/she is regarded by the adults in the family (Anthony, 1981b; Fonagy & Target, 1998). Research on the development of the brain corroborates that early psychological care and stimulation are critical to neurodevelopment and the capacity for language, cognition, exploration, and the capacity to modulate feelings (Perry et al., 1995; Shapiro & Applegate, 2000).

Thus, within a relatively normal parent–child relationship in which reciprocal, attuned interactions occur, repetition of a steady, rhythmic state of response to the child's needs gradually leads to internal structure and effective adaptive responses. The child develops a sense of connection to the parent and shows signs of pleasure, such as smiles, verbal responses, seeking proximity, and imitation. The parent's sense of self-worth and confidence is reinforced by the awareness and joy of being able to provide comfort and satisfaction to the child (Benedek, 1959). Parental empathy with the child and the child's responsiveness and developing trust strengthen the positive quality of the parent–child relationship, which is one of the bedrocks of cognitive, social, and emotional growth (Beebe, Lachmann, & Jaffe, 1997; Ainsworth, 1979b; Freud, 1965).

These optimal social and personal conditions do not exist for children in institutional care who await adoption. Many of these children suffer from various forms of attachment and affective disorders. For some children, the absence of personal, attentive care can result in withdrawal from others and a general state of apathy and medical-like symptoms (Spitz, 1945). Other children actively seek attention but cannot develop a close relationship with a special person.

Parents of older toddlers and latency-age children adopted from abroad often describe them as voracious, emotionally labile, swinging from one mood to another, hard to console, and often subject to severe tantrums (Downey, 2000; Talbot, 1998). These children not only hunger after the fulfillment of earlier unmet emotional needs but also have little experience in dealing with the endings and beginnings inherent in the everyday life of family care. Their routines in the orphanages were often so devoid of periods of change or excitement that they had little experience or help in modulating different states of affect. Their lack of responsiveness resulted in an internalized model of caregivers as emotionally distant, unresponsive, and disinterested (Provence & Lipton, 1962). In some cases, physical illness and medical treatment caused severe pain that may have become associated in their minds with adult caregivers (Downey, 2000). Even where there may have been no physical pain, tiny glimmers of pleasure in human contact were short and disappointing. For these reasons, they will need time to realize that their adoptive parents represent a different model of care, consisting of a close interactive, responsive relationship. At first, some children recoil from this type of closeness. One mother described this well when she said that it took her toddler a full year to let her kiss her. Anastasia, a girl adopted at the age of 9 months, was 5 years old before she could kiss with real feeling (Downey, 2000).

Leaving the Orphanage: Loss for the Child

The adoption from the orphanage is a difficult experience for the child and the parents. Despite the hardships of institutional life, the context of care and the gestalt of the institution have had some meaning to the child. Adoption is often unexpected and frightening, as the child is separated without notice from the only "home" he/she has known. Leaving the institution involves not only a loss of language; routines of eating, sleeping, and being; but also the loss of cribmates and cultural context. This separation disrupts the caregiving gestalt to which the child is accustomed and to which he/she has accommodated and already made certain defensive adaptations. Leaving the orphanage, yet another disruption, may reevoke the first losses in abandonment or separation from the birth parent(s). Like many other children, Anastasia came to America with nothing from her Russian past, not even the clothes on her back. Depending on age, physical health, and emotional resiliency, each child has to find a way of coping with the entry into a totally different surround in the care of a stranger, while grieving over the loss of what was familiar (however inadequate it may have been). Many adoptive parents, emotionally ready to claim their new child, have been hurt by their children's unexpected reactions to them. It is the adoptive parents' challenge to woo the "indifferent" or "rejecting" child into their lives, and to do so in the context of the child's confusion and fear associated with the separation from all he/she has known. Parents are often distraught and frustrated by the range of reactions, such as aggressive, hyperactive, passive, evasive, frightened, and frightening behaviors, they observe as the child enters their family (Downey, 2000; Talbot, 1998). These emotions and behaviors are related to the child's reaction to the loss of moorings and internal deficits in dealing with anxiety, grief, and unmodulated feelings. Some children, like Anastasia, develop bodily symptoms to help them master the helplessness and physical pain that overwhelmed them in the orphanage (Downey, 2000).

Mental health professionals need to learn as much as they can about the preadoptive history of the child in order to understand his/her early relational world and the manifestation of grief and depression related to multiple losses. As we shall see in the clinical vignettes presented below, mourning may occur over a long period of time and be precipitated by events such as birthdays, moves, or the arrival of a new baby (Webb, 1993).

Adoption from the Parents' Point of View

By the time a decision to adopt is made, most, if not all, intentional parents have experienced an unfilled longing to have a child of their own. There are many reasons for adoption, and parent(s) generally have coped with difficult decisions in their search for a child (Leiblum, 1997). In addition, the process of international adoption is complex. Most parents work through an agency and go to the host country when the adoption visit is arranged. Some parents know exactly which child they are to adopt; others may have an opportunity to meet several children and choose one. In the little time they are given to make important decisions and to complete the many steps required in the adoption process, emotions of the parents run very high. They not only face the uncertainty about whether the birth country will approve the adoption, but also they are required to travel to the American Consulate in the host (or foreign) country to apply for a visa that allows the child to enter the United States.

When adopting parents actually arrive in a foreign country, they are confronted for the first time with the specific reality of their child's experience. Parents vividly recall every moment of the first meeting with their child at the institution. Many describe their shock at the first sight of the child's environment, the absence of toys or social stimulation, and often note the lack of a primary caregiver who can tell them about their child. While some parents understand the importance of the physical and psychological impoverishment, they are generally so eager to adopt a child that these concerns are set aside. Many parents talk of falling in love at the first sight of their child, but it often takes a long time for parents to feel that their spontaneous love and affection is returned. An asymmetry may exist between the child's view of the new parents as "strangers" and the adults' view of themselves as "parents." They generally wish to comfort and be accepted by the child, but in many instances, the child aggressively pushes the "strangers" away.

Some parents are so dismayed at the volatile reaction of the child that the adoption plans are forfeited before they return to the United States. In a few cases, frustrated, angry parents, having lost their perspective and control in response to the child's violence toward them, have given up the child (Seelye, 1998; Talbot, 1998). Once at home, parents often have to deal with their own anxiety and exhaustion as they begin to cope with such serious problems as sleep and eating disturbances, tantrums, serious language disorders, and unanticipated breakdowns and fears. Most difficult is the inability to calm their child. These problems temporarily affect parents' self-confidence, self-esteem, and their evolving sense of parental identity (Benedek, 1959).

When it becomes clear that some toddlers and preschoolers have long-term internal problems and adjustment difficulties, many parents realize that far more than their love and devotion are required. They may seek the services of medical specialists, speech therapists, cognitive specialists, preschool and special education experts, and child and family therapists. In each case, even after thorough assessments, therapists and specialists must try to find an approach that fits the specific and often idiosyncratic needs of the child. The dynamics of the child's atypical development requires an interdisciplinary approach to treatment, because of the interrelationship of the child's biological, social, and psychological needs.

On the other hand, parents relate that the children have brought a special fulfillment into their lives. They realize that their parental efforts have provided the children a chance for a qualitatively different life experience than would otherwise have been possible. They take satisfaction in the incremental achievements that occur and especially remark on the importance and satisfaction of the growing attachment that evolves. However, meeting the children's needs for medical care, which can be intrusive and painful, is a particularly difficult parental task. The children, like all children, are frightened but unlike securely attached children, who use their parents as a social reference for dealing with strange or frightening situations, they cannot easily be reassured by their parents (Downey, 2000; Stroufe & Waters, 1977).

Agencies working in the field of international adoptions must address some of the issues related to the lack of preparation of adoptive parents and children. Efforts are made to plan for the parents' first meeting with their child, and the transition and separation from the orphanages and other caregiving centers. Indeed, some progressive agencies organize group adoption trips with language specialists and continue group support after the children are brought to the United States. In summary, the needs of these children and families for support and informed care have become clearer over time. Concern and awareness have given rise to community adoption support groups, with discussion of possible changes in treatment practices (Johnson & Groze, 1993).

A DEVELOPMENTAL FRAMEWORK FOR CLINICAL PRACTICE

Children who are adopted from abroad have had very different contexts of early care. The children's developmental status and their particular preadoptive histories are crucial considerations in formulating an understanding of their needs. Many of the children have experienced emotional neglect and been deprived of adequate nutrition, health care, and sensitive holding. For example, observations in some orphanages abroad reveal that infants often spend most of their time in cribs, restrained by ties (Downey, 2000). Some children may engage in self-stimulating and painful behavior such as head banging, scratching, hair pulling, and biting themselves as a way of coping with lack of human contact (Spitz, 1945; Provence & Lipton, 1962). All children adapt to their experiential circumstances, and for young children in institutional care, adaptations may often include withdrawal and apathy.

At the time of adoption, children are separated from one model of care and expected to adjust quickly to a totally different cultural and personal environment. Some children also experience numerous moves before they join their adoptive parent(s). Initially, it is hard to determine whether their difficulties at the time of adoption are symptoms of behavioral regression related to loss or to the delay in maturational progress related to emotional and physical deprivation.

The children now have an opportunity for more normal relational experiences and the possibility of developing a meaningful relationship with their adoptive parents. But this can be a long and difficult process. Adoptive parents report that they must find a way to engage the child, often at a level far below his/her chronological age. Furthermore, once children recognize the opportunity to have their needs fulfilled by their adoptive parent, they are often voracious to make up for the absence of adequate food, holding, attention, and care. They may need to be with their parents continuously, and separation anxiety can be intense, especially at nighttime. Better health care often results in children having more energy; however, they may have little experience in active play and in modulating impulses. The parents must help their children accept limits and establish new ways to deal with frustration and anxiety. Many of the children have uneven maturational growth, and it is hard for parents to know what to expect and at what level to respond.

Even many years later, early trauma can have an impact on the children's emotional state. Because of their fragile internal world, unexpected stress, disappointments, and frustration in mastering new developmental tasks may overwhelm children. Minor changes and loss may cause regression, often to the dismay of parents. For example, parents who adopted a child as an infant are often surprised at the difficulty the child may experience later on in coping with changes such as moving to a new house or school. As children mature, new issues arise related to their ethnocultural identity and the complex issues related to the separation from their birth parent.

We illustrate the crisis of transition and the long-term dimensions of the developmental problems with two brief clinical vignettes. A developmental framework is used in understanding and conceptualizing the treatment issues of two children, ages 3 and 4, at the time of referral. The reasons for the referrals varied, but in general the parents and the specialists who saw the children feared that persistent behavioral and psychological difficulties were impeding normal developmental progress. The case vignettes illustrate the ways in which family members tried to understand the special needs of their child and "keep the needs of the child in mind." We further address the issues inherent in transracial international adoption related to cultural acceptance and identity formation.

Developmental Recovery of Nikki Following Institutional Care: The Role of Guidance and Parental Support

Nikki's preadoptive history included significant developmental risk factors; early parental loss, physical and emotional neglect, institutional care, and physical illness. Nikki was the seventh child born to an impoverished family in rural Russia. His birth mother died of the effects of alcoholism when he was 8 months old. His father placed him in an orphanage when he was 18 months old. Five months later, at 23 months, he was again uprooted and sent to the United States for adoption. At the time of adoption, Nikki suffered from malnutrition, bowed legs, and intestinal parasites—symptoms seen in many children adopted from Russia (Miller, 1999; Oleck, 2000). Under Russian adoption policy, children with medical problems and those from ethnic minorities had high priority for international adoption.

Mr. and Mrs. Mitchell, Nikki's adoptive parents, who had tried for many years to have a baby through infertility treatment, eventually decided to apply to an international placement agency. Only 4 days later, they were notified that a little boy almost 2 years old was en route from Russia and available for adoption. Although still unprepared for the arrival of a child, Mr. and Mrs. Mitchell decided to meet Nikki at the airport. They met a little blonde boy, extremely thin, with bowed legs and unusual facial features, who had had a traumatic trip to the United States; he was very frightened, upset, and could not be calmed by the people who had brought him.

Mrs. Mitchell remembered that in the airport Nikki seemed to be in his own world, playing with a blue ball and somewhat disconnected from persons around him. He did not respond to her initial soft words and attempts to engage him. Nikki was bewildered by the separation from everything that was familiar to him but his lack of responsiveness to efforts to engage him foreshadowed difficulties with both emotional responsiveness and severe language delays. As they left the airport, Nikki could not cope with yet another transition and a different set of strangers, and he began to lose control of his emotions, sobbing wildly. During the car trip home, his adoptive parents could not reassure him, and his deep sobbing and bodily striking out made it hard to hold him safely in the car. When the Mitchells reached their house he frantically ran from room to room. For the first few days, Nikki ran continuously and avoided his parents' efforts to calm him and touch him.

Mrs. Mitchell did not know how to feed her "running" little boy. She intuitively thought of things that a baby might like and offered him a pacifier, a sippy cup, and a baby blanket, and placed a large bean bag on the living room floor, where Nikki could sit. She found that he could calm himself by being surrounded with these supplies while watching children's videos. Mrs. Mitchell had recognized Nikki's need for the oral supplies and the sense of safety of being wrapped in his blanket. This full complement of oral supplies and holding the soft, physical, nonhuman, large beanbag cushion helped Nikki feel secure. At times, suddenly Nikki jumped up and, as though guided by an internal trigger, ran through the house. Occasionally, Nikki would grasp Mrs. Mitchell's legs and then run off again. She decided to try and hold Nikki even though he protested. She began by holding him tightly and rocking him. The first time, it took 10 minutes to calm him in this way, but over a 2- to 3-week period, Nikki responded in ever shorter periods of time. His calming response gave her hope that he was beginning to look to her for containment of his anxiety.

The parents immediately arranged a thorough medical examination for Nikki, which led to treatment for malnutrition, rickets, and parasites. Below the scale in weight and height for his age, Nikki was diagnosed with failure to thrive syndrome. Various physicians suggested the possibility of fetal alcohol syndrome because of Nikki's facial appearance, but the parents and other specialists thought these features could be related to his ethnic origins. At this time, a thorough medical and developmental diagnosis could not be made. Although Nikki's development was delayed in many spheres, only time, medical treatment, and intensive parental care would reveal how much progress he could make. A major concern was Nikki's poor language development, but it was hard to know whether this was because he was learning a new language or the difficulties were more systemic. Although his physical health improved over time, his early gastrointestinal problems returned occasionally, and the family had to be continuously vigilant regarding Nikki's health.

Both Mr. and Mrs. Mitchell worked full-time but, recognizing Nikki's need to develop a special relationship with them, spent most of the first month with him. By the time a month had passed, they had grown intensely attached to him. When they returned from a holiday with him, his mother was heartened that Nikki remembered the house. They enrolled him in a day care center, so that Mrs. Mitchell could return to work, although they modified their schedules to be with him as much as possible.

Nikki now wanted to be with his parents all the time and separations for day care became increasingly difficult. This was a positive indication of the developing attachment to his mother and father. At the same time, Nikki's frustrations at day care were problematic and related to delays in development. He did not have the internal structure to cope with the complex social world of day care. The center realized that Nikki's emotional and developmental needs might be better served in a group for younger children. He was not used to social interaction and spent much time apart from the group.

At age 2½, Nikki could not express his needs using methods available to many children his age, such as pointing, repeating words, or shaking his head "no" or "yes." When frustrated, he was frantic, at times returning to his earlier pattern of random running and using his body to express his frustration. His parents became worried and wondered if he would ever gain better control over his emotions. The family reached out to many professionals for assistance: medical specialists, speech and language therapists, neuropsychologists, educators, and, when Nikki was 3½, a consultant in child development.

Developmental Consultation with the Parents

The consultant first met Nikki at the Mitchells' home in the evening. The parents had arranged for Nikki to sit in the middle of the living room with his usual supplies—sippy cup, bean bag, cushion, blanket, and toys—to help him remain calm. The family and the consultant gathered in the living room as well to be with Nikki. Within a few moments, and without a noticeable reason, Nikki began racing around the house, seemingly guided by an internal whirlwind. His parents rushed to follow Nikki to protect him from hurting himself in his random frantic behavior. He was not totally disconnected from the adults, as he made brief stops in front of each person in the room.

Over the next weeks the consultant observed that Nikki's ability to maintain a sense of homeostasis was fragile. He had only minimal ability to modulate internal feelings of anxiety and fear. She noted that he seemed to understand his parents' efforts to calm him through offers of alternatives: play and food. He did not have a consistent way of letting them know of his desires. Taking care of Nikki was difficult, as his calmness was disrupted easily and by invisible cues.

The parents told the consultant that the more they responded to Nikki, the more he needed to be close to them. Nighttime was especially difficult, and he fiercely protested being left alone. He resisted falling asleep even if his parents stayed with him. He was hypervigilant about his parents' leaving him at any time. In fact, he was hypervigilant and frightened of many things, especially noises, thunder, and shadows (Perry et al., 1995).

The consultant asked the parents to bring together the medical and developmental information they had gathered, so that she could review these expert opinions. The different medical, speech, and psychological experts who had examined Nikki in the past were puzzled at his uneven development in various spheres of functioning. The greatest concern was for the missing and atypical steps in language development, a problem for many postinstitutional children. Nikki was late in using the pronoun "I" and could not use different parts of speech to communicate his wishes and intentions coherently.

The consultant said that Nikki's recovery was going to be a long-term effort, and his parents would have to observe and respond to the particular ways in which their efforts helped Nikki to learn, to communicate, and to feel secure. She encouraged them to continue to have "conversations" with Nikki through any modalities he enjoyed. She discussed with them the ways in which they were trying to provide attuned care for Nikki, and that while he was responding, he seemed to need much reassurance through physical and verbal affirmation of his efforts. He was showing signs that order and predictability were also reassuring to him, as he was beginning to take pleasure in anticipating events.

The parents found a Montessori preschool whose director took a personal interest in trying to adapt to Nikki's developmental style of learning and communicative ability, so that he could feel understood. The school was based on order, predictability, and a generally peaceful atmosphere to which Nikki responded. He had not had toys as an infant and had missed out on early sensorimotor play and learning. Nikki was encouraged to try new things, such as building with blocks, and was rewarded with praise for his efforts. He responded to the structure of the school and the clear expectations and limits set for him within the empathetic school setting.

The consultant visited the Mitchells' home for several months, observing Nikki with his parents, watching his progress, and providing guidance and support. As crises at home or school emerged, such as the difficulties at bedtime, the parents and the consultant would explore possibilities of alternative methods of coping. At 4, Nikki's improvement was slow but steady, especially his increasing ability to relate to others. Many aspects of speech were still delayed, but Nikki was forming his own pattern of communication with his parents. Their intensive efforts to help Nikki included the kind of early parent–child reciprocity that he had missed in his first years. This attention helped him develop the sense that they were real, predictable, nurturing, and protective people. They helped him learn words through mimickry and play, and to express his wishes verbally or nonverbally, and to accept limits. Nikki experienced pleasure when they understood each other.

Nikki developed an idiosyncratic but substantial ability to communicate preferences and pleasure. He was able to be toilet trained, to be soothed, to have actual emotional exchanges with his parents, and to respond to a curtailed but predictable bedtime routine. Nikki gained significant pleasure in the relationship with his paternal grandfather, who found a way to interest him in tools, and together they worked on projects.

The parents were more able to talk about their own feelings about how much they cared for Nikki, but how hard it was to cope with work, family, and his extensive needs. They hoped that Nikki would be like other little boys and began to realize the tremendous effort required of them to help him progress even a little. They raised many realistic and painful questions. What might they expect for Nikki? What would his speech and language difficulty mean for him, if it did not improve? No one could yet answer these questions.

Mrs. Mitchell told the consultant that she and her husband had not thought in altruistic terms when they applied to become adoptive parents. As they came to know Nikki, they began to feel that they were doing something special for *him*, and they developed a sense of satisfaction in being able to provide Nikki with a life pathway that he would not have had in the orphanage. Mr. Mitchell said, "I know what happens to these babies in the orphanage if they are not adopted—they don't have a chance for a life. At least this won't happen to Nikki. We will be there for him." Both parents realized how much Nikki had changed their lives, and how much their efforts were devoted to his care and their hopes for him. They became involved in a support group with other families who had adopted children from Russia. Members of this group worked together to keep the children aware of their heritage by providing cultural experiences for them.

Nikki at 7

A brief follow-up indicated that Nikki had made significant emotional, social, and cognitive progress between the ages of 5 and 7. He had developed a trusting and close relationship with both his mother and father, and had also made friends in his neighborhood and school. In a special education class in a public school, although he was progressing steadily, he still had difficulties in certain spheres, including speech and reading. His cognitive growth had been steady but his learning style was highly individualized. In language, he could now use pronouns and verbs in full sentences. He did best in subjects in which he could touch and feel objects, and loved to construct and build things. He was involved in athletics and liked swimming and gymnastics. He might join a mainstream second-grade class the next year, with special attention to his specific learning needs.

Nikki's parents made every effort to support his interests and development. They tried to learn how Nikki learned, and shared many insights about him to the teachers and professional who worked with him. He responded well to the organized structure and predictability of his home and his life, and was able to be cooperative and responsive to his parents' expectations. Nikki's parents were strong advocates of securing special services for all children with special needs in the school system. Nikki brought a new dimension to the lives of the Mitchells, and they are devoted to helping him develop a capacity for a meaningful life.

The Mitchells, who are very sensitive to Nikki's feelings, developed a story that he loves to hear—about how he came to be part of their family. Nikki's understanding will expand as he matures. Each time Nikki raises new questions, they add to the story.

How Nikki Came to Be Their Son: An Adoption Story

> *First phase of the story.* There was a family who lived in a big white house with a kitty. This family really wanted a child but could not have a baby of their own. On the other side of the ocean was a little boy who really needed a mommy and daddy. The family that wanted a little boy was told about him and sent for him to come. He flew above the moon and through the stars, and came to be with them. They live in the big white house, with the kitty, and they are now a happy family.
>
> *Second phase: Mrs. Mitchell responded to Nikki's question at 6 years old of whether he grew in his mother's tummy.* Mrs. Mitchell told Nikki, "You did not grow in Mommy's tummy, but you grew in my heart." This response gave Nikki much pleasure and reassurance.
>
> *Third phase.* The Mitchells anticipate that Nikki will want to hear more about his birth parents. They have his original records and his birth certificate, but this part of the story they feel is harder to tell, as it involves actual loss of his birth parents.

Pavao (1998) describes the ways in which a child understands adoption at different phases of development and the Mitchell's story is an example of theier effort to best help Nikki understand.

Loss as a Prelude to New Parental Attachments: Treatment to Help Tanya Recover and Adjust

Ms. Smith, a single professional woman, had been a foster mother for a number of years and yearned to have a family of her own. Although she still cared for Matthew, a foster child whom she hoped to adopt, she applied to an international adoption agency and responded quickly when she was informed that a 2½-year-old girl from a city east of Moscow was available for adoption. Ms. Smith described the arduous journey to the orphanage and the starkness of her first meeting with Tanya: "A little girl was pushed into the bare meeting room by a woman who said, 'Go and kiss your mother.' " Ms. Smith and Tanya sat on the floor together. Ms. Smith recalls, "Tanya was interested in my ability to show her how to play, and in the juice and snacks I brought. Also, she was interested in *anyone who was new and different, as I learned from her subsequent behavior.* There were no toys in the institution except in the director's office. Tanya played for an hour and cried when she was taken away from me, the toys, snacks, and juice I brought." Ms. Smith had noted immediately that Tanya was hungry for food and attention, as are many infants and toddlers who have lived in institutional care (Provence & Lipton, 1962).

When she returned to the orphanage after completing the necessary paperwork, a group of somber caregivers stood on the steps of the orphanage as Tanya was pushed toward Ms. Smith and the waiting car. In the car, Tanya at first seemed passive and did not protest. At her age, she could not understand that she was to abruptly lose contact with her known caregivers, or that her life was taking a dramatic turn. She was interested in the new experience of the car and did not turn back to look at the orphanage as older children are reported to have done.

Later, when asked by the therapist about Tanya's passive acceptance of the departure, Ms. Smith said, "It seemed understandable to me after I read the medical record. She was used to being dragged from pillar to post since birth. She was born 2 months prematurely, and her birth mother left her in the hospital and never returned. She stayed in the hospital, requiring intensive medical care for 6 months, then moved to another placement for a year and finally came to the orphanage. She had pneumonia 11 times and also had hepatitis C. I don't think she understood she was really leaving—she didn't really speak well. It seemed like nonsense syllables. She said 'cat' and 'dog,' and the only other intelligible word was the word for 'myself,' 'Summa.' " The fact that Tanya had a word for "myself" was a positive sign that Tanya was developing a sense of herself.

By the time they reached relatives in Moscow, where Ms. Smith had to apply for an American visa for Tanya, she was worried about her. Tanya ate voraciously, even eating the fluff on her socks, a behavior indicative of pica, a symptom related to deprivation and neglect (DSM IV; American Psychiatric Association, 1994). Equally perplexing was Tanya's interest in everyone and everything, not distinguishing between her adoptive mother and others. She had profound difficulty with transitions, which usually resulted in prolonged tantrums. Transitions were an inevitable part of the trip home, but severe difficulties with transitions and ending activities lasted for many years.

Her tantrums escalated on the long trip to the United States, and Ms. Smith's attempts to comfort Tanya were of no avail. As reported by other adoptive parents, the magnitude of the emotional problems became more apparent on the trip home (Seelye, 1998). For example, on arrival in the United States, the new family stopped briefly at the grandmother's house, and Tanya was drawn to the swimming pool. When her mother tried to take her home, Tanya broke down and had to be carried to the car, sobbing throughout the 2-hour drive. Every separation was a new crisis.

When they arrived home, Tanya met Matthew, Ms. Smith's foster child. Tanya related to Matthew and to other new people in an unusual way. She undressed and waited, as though for inspection. Later on, in therapy, it became clear that Tanya was reenacting experiences in the institution. In treatment, when she played hospital with her dolls, we came to understand that Tanya's undressing was customary in the orphanage when meeting new people.The primary social interaction she received in the orphanage started and ended with a series of caregivers providing bodily care (Castle et al., 1999). In the United States, Tanya benefited from extensive medical attention, but some of it was frightening, as it reminded her of the many procedures in the hospital in Russia. Beyond that, Ms. Smith was overwhelmed by Tanya's poor ability to communicate, her voracious hunger for food and attention, her habit of running away and needing to be caught, and her inability to adapt even to small changes without tantrums. She did not use her adoptive mother as a social reference point, and Ms. Smith often worried because Tanya seemed fearless and was often in danger, for example, when she ran into the road.

How can we understand Tanya's behavior? In the transition to the United States, she lost the context of the orphanage, her known language and food, and the cultural environment to which she was accustomed. However, Tanya's developmental lags were far more pervasive than an adjustment disorder reaction. Her emotional and relational behavior may be explained as attachment disturbances related to the long-term effects of severe neglect, illness, and abandonment. Of concern to her mother was that Tanya seemed to seek the excitement of new things and new people, and her beginning relationship with her mother seemed easily broken. This "indifference" to the importance of her mother was reminiscent of Tanya's experience with a revolving set of caregivers in the orphanage. She had never experienced the deep connection of an attachment with a special caregiver on whom she could depend for continuous care. Many of Tanya's behaviors resulted from past adaptations to her sense that she "was her own caregiver," and her impulsive and precocious behaviors represented primitive self-reliance. As a child without the experience of attachment to a particular caregiver, she did not look to her mother for guidance or indications of safety (Ainsworth et al., 1978).

When a child does not experience the empathy of "the other" in the earliest years, she has little opportunity for imitating and then identifying with the empathetic figure. In this regard, Tanya could not take in her mother's emotional efforts to help her. The lack of synchrony between her mother's wish to help and Tanya's slow response to claiming her as a special person was frustrating. Ms. Smith had the complex task of reaching out to a frightened and often infuriating child.

Ms. Smith sought therapeutic help for Tanya shortly before Tanya's fifth birthday. She had begun to hide her mother's precious belongings, particularly the Christmas lights, but denied doing so. This behavior deeply hurt her mother, who believed that she and Tanya had been forming a closer attachment. She was hurt and puzzled by Tanya's volatile behavior toward her, especially the rapid circular changes from love to rejection to being inconsolable. The therapist accepted the mother's disappointment over the length of time it was taking Tanya to develop a trusting relationship and explained that it would take still more time to understand how Tanya was making sense of everything that had happened to her.

In the first therapy session, Tanya introduced a theme that would remain for a long time: her history in the orphanage and the loss of her birth mother. She drew a picture of a little girl with a Russian hair bow and dictated a story about this little girl who was taken away from her birthplace. The girl returned to try to find her mother, but when she came to the door, only a skeleton answered and did not recognize her. In her story, she tried to convince the skeleton that it was she, Tanya, and she had come to find her mother, but still, no one recognized her.

Thus, Tanya introduced a theme of loss and grief, abandonment and search, that would become part of her play during therapy. Of great importance in the first visit was the feelings of the child in the story, of the loss of her roots, of not being recognized or remembered, and of being stolen and taken away. The Christmas lights were an evoked memory from Russia, and hiding them was perhaps an attempt to retouch the precious things in her past. The child's story of loss mirrored her adoptive mother's reason for having brought Tanya for treatment, her puzzlement and sadness at having lost something of meaning. Like many other children, Tanya found a way to present an important core of her story in the first therapeutic session, linking her own story of loss to her feelings of sorrow and her relationship to both her birth and her adoptive mother.

Through her drawings and play, Tanya dramatically expressed her ambivalence toward her adoptive mother and her conception of what had happened to her. In Tanya's mind, Ms. Smith had taken her away from a memory that she at times recalled as "precious." Despite the actual deprivation and threats to her survival in the hospitals and orphanages, she still longed to return to the fantasy of her idealized "home." Her fantasy of a waiting maternal figure who did not recognize her represented the lost mother and the lost connections to the many caregivers that she had known. Her feelings toward Ms. Smith were filled with ambivalence. In addition to her sense of loss and grief, Tanya's story of her adoption included signs of survivor guilt and feelings that others were suffering, and she had abandoned them.

Over the next 2 years in therapy, Tanya elaborated the following themes in play: abandonment, loss, a parent searching for her, her search for a parent, accidents, hurts, chaos, and being saved. At times, Tanya identified with the kittens in the orphanage and meowed like a frightened animal, skittering away from the approach of the "comforting other." Eventually, the stories and play expressed her situation in extreme terms. She told the therapist, "If God says he loves me, I can live," which also meant that if she could not believe she was loved, she would die.

Gradually, Tanya began to expand her birth narrative to mesh with more age-appropriate developmental tasks. On her seventh birthday, she was given a bead necklace with her name on it, similar to bracelets given to infants for identification purposes. She put it on and asked the therapist to follow her to an outdoor rock pile, where she had played 6 months earlier. She told the therapist not to look, then hid the necklace under a rock. She uncovered it, gravely and triumphantly saying, "*This* is where I was born. See, here is my name. They still remember me there." Tanya then said that when she grew up, she would search for her daughter who lived in another country. This fantasy gave voice to the themes of loss, searching, and reunion, which Tanya repeated in many play constructions as an active attempt to master her experiences. Eventually, Tanya was able to cry and grieve about the possibility of never being able to find her birth mother, although she still wished to return to Russia to make the attempt.

Tanya's relationship with her adoptive mother has become more secure. After therapy sessions, she usually wants to reunite by hugging her. She draws pictures for her and expresses need for her. Sometimes Tanya expresses her fear that when she has done something to upset her mother, she will be left alone again. However, Tanya shows increasing trust in her mother's love and the permanence of their relationship. In her therapist's playroom on Valentine's day, when Tanya was 7, she dictated this poem.

What Makes a Perfect Mother?
By Tanya

6 cups of love
one cup of hugs.
16 cups of patience.
This is what makes a perfect mother.

Tanya hurried to give this to her mother, who was deeply touched. The poem was written with empathy for Ms. Smith; it expressed her awareness of her mother's love and acknowledged the patience that she, Tanya, needed from her mother, to help her grow up.

Transracial and Transcultural Issues for Families

The adoption of transracial children can create special identity problems that parents need to address. Narratives of the cultural and psychological impact of adoption on Chinese girls reveal that when others point out they are "different," they experience challenges to their perception of themselves. Collins (2000) describes how her adopted Chinese daughter was subjected to the remarks of strangers, who "innocently" commented on her facial features and hair coloring, and openly asked difficult questions such as where did you get her, or even how much did she cost. At times people felt free to touch her daughter, as if she were a doll. Chinese American parents sometimes asked intrusive questions which reflected their own ambivalence about transracial adoption. Collins reported that these comments felt like an assault to her young school-age daughter, and raised difficult questions for her which often left her in tears. Collins observed that over time her daughter came to feel her family was different from the "typical" American family as well as the "typical" Asian American family.

Insensitivity, bias, and prejudice combined with the losses that preceded adoption have an impact on the internal life of the child. One young adult said, "I had no idea (as a young child and a teenager) what to do when I was seen as my face" (Griebenow, 2000). Parents of Asian adopted children become painfully aware of some of these unanticipated problems that their children face. Parents have heard them voice their feelings: "Mommy, I want to look like you. Why is our family different? Why do they think I can't speak English? What are we? Are we Chinese Americans or just Americans? Where was I born and where are my parents?"

Parents can use a developmental framework to understand the questions and respond to their children (Pavao, 1998). They need to recognize that this is a family identity problem, not just a problem for the children. It is important to establish links with other transracial families, which provide support for their children and themselves. Recognition of family differences not only cause problems, they can enrich family life and create a sense of pride. Each family must decide how to help the child connect with his/her cultural origin. Researchers find that living in an integrated community in which children can relate to families of similar origin is helpful in supporting identity formation (Feigelman, 2000). It is too early to know the impact of adoption on the self-esteem of Chinese girls, given the reality that the separation from their birth parent(s) was in most cases primarily based on government policy of one child per family, and a bias towards male children.

DISCUSSION

Research literature and clinical reports outline the cumulative developmental risks for infants and children who have lived in institutions without adequate medical and social care. Often, the children continue to experience voracious hunger for food and attention, separation anxiety, hypervigilance, special fears, and difficulty in adapting even to small changes without losing control in prolonged tantrums. The relationships with their adoptive parents can have certain characteristics that represent ambivalence and insecurity in their internal view of human relationships. On the one hand, hiding, running away, avoiding, and testing often persist for a lengthy period of time; on the other hand, extreme clinging and dependence can emerge as well. The children often are physically endangered, since they do not use their parent(s) as social reference points to guide them in the way children do when they have had a family life from the start. For example, Tanya seemed fearless and was often in danger when she ran away from her mother in new situations.

The children are likely to experience early parental loss, social deprivation, a lack of adequate stimulation, and impoverished medical and psychological care. The resulting developmental problems can include postnatal medical trauma; lags in social, cognitive, and emotional development; as well as neuropsychological impairment. The preadoptive histories of these children can include a range of early experiences in various institutions. No two are exactly alike, and practitioners must listen to the unique experiences of each child and family. Some of these adopted children have more difficult beginnings than others, and some are more resilient and emerge more intact than others. The age at adoption is significant, since the longer the experience in institutional care, the greater the potential impact on the neurological, psychological, and emotional well-being of the child.

All children need timely, adequate psychological care and appropriate environmental stimulation to achieve their optimal potential. The cornerstone of a positive holding environment is the provision of individual and responsive care by a primary caregiver who meets the child's early dependency needs. Children who experience early emotional deprivation, pain, hunger, fear, and frustration, and who do not have an adult who can help shield them from the overwhelming stress, attempt to meet their fears with primitive defenses along a fight–flight continuum. These defenses can include self-injurious behavior, hyperactivity and aggression toward others or the self, or withdrawal, passivity, and turning inward. Such behaviors serve as a primitive defense against emotional and physical pain. We can understand Nikki's and Tanya's emotional reactions in the transition to adoption in the light of their previous need to rely on themselves in intolerable situations.

In the vignettes presented here, the adoptive parents offered their children new models of a parental relationship. Unlike adoption at birth, the relationships began after severe deprivation and loss. An uneven symmetry existed between the parents' readiness to attach and the children's bewilderment about the new person. The children, by and large, had little experience with a permanent, stable, and predictable caregiver. It took time for Nikki and Tanya to realize that their parents could provide comfort and fulfill their needs, and that they would not leave them.

Parents who adopt children who have experienced early deprivation and trauma face many challenges. They must help their children develop trust in them and learn to rely on them for comfort and nurture. In addition, parents need to cope with the many developmental problems that remain and seek help, which is costly and time consuming, and for which the outcome for their children is uncertain. They need to deal with their own grief in coming to terms with the emotional turmoil of the children and the difficulties that may lie ahead.

Researchers and interdisciplinary clinicians are attempting to understand the etiology and severity in cognitive, social, and emotional impairment of institutionalized children, and to develop effective treatment protocols for various long-standing medical, developmental, and psychological disorders. Many medical centers now exist for evaluation and treatment (Miller, 1999). The treatment of children with such complex problems requires an interdisciplinary approach. A psychodynamic framework is helpful both in assessment and treatment, and the parents must be an integral part of the process. Long-term treatment is often needed. The therapeutic holding environment must include a recognition of the children's need to develop a new relational experience with an empathetic other. It is still not known how much recovery is possible after such severe early trauma. The age of the child at adoption and the quality of preadoptive care are factors that may account for the more positive adaptation of some children. Other children may need extensive time to develop meaningful, new therapeutic relationships that can help them create rich internal experiences.

Long-term therapeutic intervention can help children identify and integrate suppressed internal feelings, such as fear, longing, grief, and anger, that had been unmanageable in the absence of an empathetic relationship with another. Within a therapeutic relationship, and with the assistance of empathetic caregiving at home, children may be able to create more adaptive defenses against pain and go forward with other aspects of development. As time goes by, new questions emerge in each developmental phase. For example, children will have questions related to their dual heritage and long to know more about their families of origin. Conflicts in identity formation occur in older children, and mourning related to the losses of the past is a theme that continues to emerge over time (Silverman & Feigelman, 1990).

Traumatic early beginnings can never be completely overcome or forgotten but recovery can be significant. Nevertheless, as children reach new phases of development, they remain vulnerable to the early experiences of loss, deprivation, helplessness, and the absence of early intimacy with a significant other. Existential grief related to early loss may be modified but will remain a part of the self. Most parents who have adopted a child from abroad believe that they have given their child a chance for a more fulfilling life. This realization is comforting even when their children have to cope with continuing developmental struggles. We now know more about the dynamics of these early struggles but still require more clinical studies to understand the impact of these difficult early experiences on the long-term ego development and adaptation of children, especially the conflicts that may occur in adolescence and maturity. The study of international adoptions and their ramifications is a work in progress.

6

Skipped-Generation Kinship Care

Grandparents and Their Grandchildren

In the last 25 years, the number of children who have been separated from their parents and placed in foster or adoptive kinship care has increased rapidly. More particularly, since 1970, there has been a 50% increase in the number of children living in skipped-generation families. In 1998, 3.9 million children lived in homes maintained by their grandparents in either informal or formal kinship care (Lugaila, 1998). By the late 1990s, 5.5% of all children under age 18 resided in grandparent-maintained homes. The steepest increases in households maintained by grandparents have been in families where the child's parent(s) are not present (Burnette, 1999).

The circumstances that underlie the increased responsibility of grandparents generally relate to serious breakdowns in the family. Grandparents who unexpectedly become the primary providers for their grandchildren face major lifecycle disruptions as they undertake difficult caregiving responsibilities, especially if they alone maintain the family household (Bryson & Casper, 1998). Indeed, the most vulnerable intergenerational households are the one million families headed by a grandmother alone, or a grandmother living with her grandchildren and a single daughter.

Nationally, these grandmothers carry the sole responsibility for 1,800,000 children (Lugaila, 1998). Over 63% of these single grandmothers have incomes below the poverty line, and 90% are on some form of public assistance. Moreover, their personal health is generally assessed to be more fragile compared to other heads of households (Casper & Bryson, 1998). Among these families, access to health care and social support services is often inadequate to meet the grandmothers' needs, as well as the medical and educational needs of their grandchildren. Overall, children who live in grandparent-maintained households, with or without a parent, are more likely to be without health insurance, living in families below the poverty line, and receiving public assistance (Bryson & Casper, 1998).

The burden of skipped-generation caregiving also falls more heavily on particular ethnic and racial groups in our society. While over 3% of all children in the United States are estimated to live in the care of relatives without a parent present, the growth in such kinship care has been greatest among children of color. Children of color are also more likely to be living in homes maintained by the most stressed of family members, the single grandmother (Harden, Clark, & Maguire, 1997). At the end of the 20th century, 12.6% of African American children were living in a household maintained by a grandparent, as compared to 6.1% of Hispanic children and 3.9% of white children (Lugaila, 1998).

The caregiving burdens of these families are high. In addition to poverty and lack of sufficient social support, many live in impoverished urban communities that offer few community resources (Harden et al., 1997). These sociodemographic factors add stress to the contextual life of the family. Children in these families are also more likely to have experienced loss, trauma, and disruption in their earliest caregiving environments and are therefore often at developmental risk. Thus, the caregiving burdens for these grandmothers, who are sole providers for their grandchildren, are heavy and complex (Burnette, 1999; Minkler & Roe, 1993; Minkler, Roe, & Price, 1992).

In 1922, Mary Richmond, a pioneer in the field of social work, conceptualized a dual paradigm of clinical services as a way to help families who experience multidimensional problems. For grandparents who face both socioeconomic and personal stress, her model suggests that social workers and others providing care and support for these families should consider both direct and indirect action in order to help the family. On the one hand, direct therapeutic action involves the provision of services to support the individual family members. On the other hand, indirect services, such as advocacy and attention to needed social support programs and resources, help to improve the contextual life of the family (Richmond, 1922).

The social services provided to families maintained by grandparents call for an integrated community based approach. This chapter will explore the many complex family and child issues that arise in the intergenerational care of children (Johnson, 1999).

THE GRANDPARENT AS KIN KEEPER AND GUARDIAN OF THE GENERATIONS

Becoming a grandparent is an important step in the lifecycle. As Erikson has suggested, generativity is a significant phase in the lifecycle. Helping to ensure the continuity of the generations of the family often brings a sense of well-being and connection to an aging grandparent and can mitigate against a sense of aloneness and despair (Erikson, 1963). Being a grandparent expands one's sense of identity and life purpose, and brings new hope and pleasure. Across generations and in many different cultures, grandparents have often stepped in to become the primary caregivers for their young grandchildren at moments of crisis in the lives of their children. The natural bonds that exist between generations are evident in the wish of most grandparents to support the well-being of their dependent grandchildren.

Burton (1992), for example, describes the historical roles of black grandparents in kinship care. During the post-Civil War immigration of black families from the South to the North, grandparents often cared for their grandchildren so that their own children could establish themselves in better circumstances. She notes that all three generations benefited from these arrangements. The elderly women gained companionship and in some cases a measure of economic support; their children were free to search for jobs elsewhere; the grandchildren grew up under the watchful eye of a caring relative. Other observers describe the historical involvement of black grandmothers and grandfathers with their grandchildren as a positive cultural adaptation that helped the generations survive the hardships of forced immigration and slavery (Minkler et al., 1992; Stack, 1974). Frazier describes this historical role of black grandparents as kin keepers and guardians of the next generation (Frazier, 1939).

Today, however, grandparents who provide kinship care are often doing so under quite different contextual circumstances. In the past, it was more likely that grandparents were engaged in a shared endeavor with their own children to better the entire family's situation. But during the 1990s, there was a dramatic rise in the number of children from all ethnic groups who *permanently* live in homes maintained by their grandparents, without the involvement of their own parents (Casper & Bryson, 1998).

The dramatic changes reflect the increased incidence of breakdowns in the ability of many families to provide protective care for their children. These breakdowns have been attributed to a wide array of social factors, including displacement of children through split immigration patterns, the growth in drug use among young parents, teen pregnancy, divorce, the rapid rise of single-parent households, the mental and physical illness of the children's birth parents, AIDS, crime, child abuse and neglect, and the incarceration of parents (Minkler et al., 1992).

A complex set of personal and social factors has caused grandparents, particularly grandmothers, to respond to the needs of their grandchildren for a permanent home. Some of the primary factors, can be summarized as follows:

- The number of children in extended foster care has reached a new high, and permanent homes are needed, especially for children of color, older children, and children with special needs, who are hard to place (McKenzie, 1993).
- New adoption guidelines have provided opportunities for grandparents to become formal foster parents of their own grandchildren. Until 1979, willing relatives were not eligible for the government assistance normally available to foster parents. However, the Supreme Court decision in *Miller v. Youakim* (1979) made many Aid to Families with Dependent Children (AFDC) children eligible for federal foster care benefits. And the Adoption Assistance and Child Welfare Act of 1980 (Public Law 96-272), called for placing children in the most family-like setting. These two developments allowed kinship foster parents to receive the same benefits as nonkin foster parents.
- The Adoption and Safe Families Act of 1997 (Public Law 105-89) provides monetary incentives to the states to adopt policies that hasten permanency planning. As a result, some states have begun to recruit grandparents to increase the number of children adopted annually from foster placement.
- Many grandparents wish to keep their grandchildren within their extended family, and within the same ethnic and cultural community as their birth parents. A grandparent may have either a voluntary agreement with the child's parents (informal kinship care) or a legal agreement with the courts (formal kinship care) (Harden et al., 1997).

INTERACTIVE FACTORS IN THE ASSESSMENT OF THE NEEDS OF THE SKIPPED-GENERATION FAMILY

Becoming a primary caregiver and maintaining a family household for grandchildren constitutes a significant interruption in a grandmother's life cycle. While the grandparent may feel satisfaction as she nurtures her vulnerable grandchildren, the assumption of this responsibility may also precipitate new problems. The contextual status of her life situation has changed, and the burden of caring for her grandchildren is influenced by the degree of poverty, and lack of medical and psychological support, the grandmother's own physical and mental health, the developmental status of the grandchild, and depression, guilt, and anxiety about her own child's difficulties. These dynamic factors interrelate and create a new and often unanticipated impact on the psychological and physical health of the grandmother or grandfather (Johnson, 1999).

Traditionally, many of these caregivers have not sought help from professionals, and have tried to resolve family problems within their families and communities. The grandparents face the daunting task of evaluating their new situation and understanding which resources they need to maintain the well-being of the family household. Even when they have identified needs with the help of a child welfare practitioner or social worker, the grandparents may face many barriers in actually finding available support services.

The literature on intergenerational caregiving has considered various ways to conceptualize the most appropriate assessment and intervention strategies for skipped-generation caregiving families. Ecological models that focus on the "person in the situation" are considered the most useful (Aranda & Knight, 1997; Bronfenbrenner, 1977). Studies of caregiver burden focus on interrelated sets of factors that represent various aspects of individual, family, and societal functioning. These three sets of factors are the contextual status of the family, the psychological health of the grandparents, and the developmental status and needs of the child (see Figure 6.1).

An integrated assessment based on the interactive factors presented in Figure 6.1 helps the clinician develop a differential diagnosis that can lead to appropriate social and clinical interventions (Aranda & Knight, 1997). This type of assessment helps address the more global needs of the family as well as the individual needs of the grandparent and children for specific services. The overall objective is to help stabilize and support the household, and to improve the health and well-being of the family members (Burnette, 1999). This assessment model, which integrates the key factors impacting all members of the family, can illuminate the nature of the challenges facing the grandparent, the type of support that could improve the quality and stability of her life, and the experiences of the grandchildren.

For a variety of reasons, developing a working alliance with grandparents may be difficult. Often grandparents feel isolated, and sensitive practi-

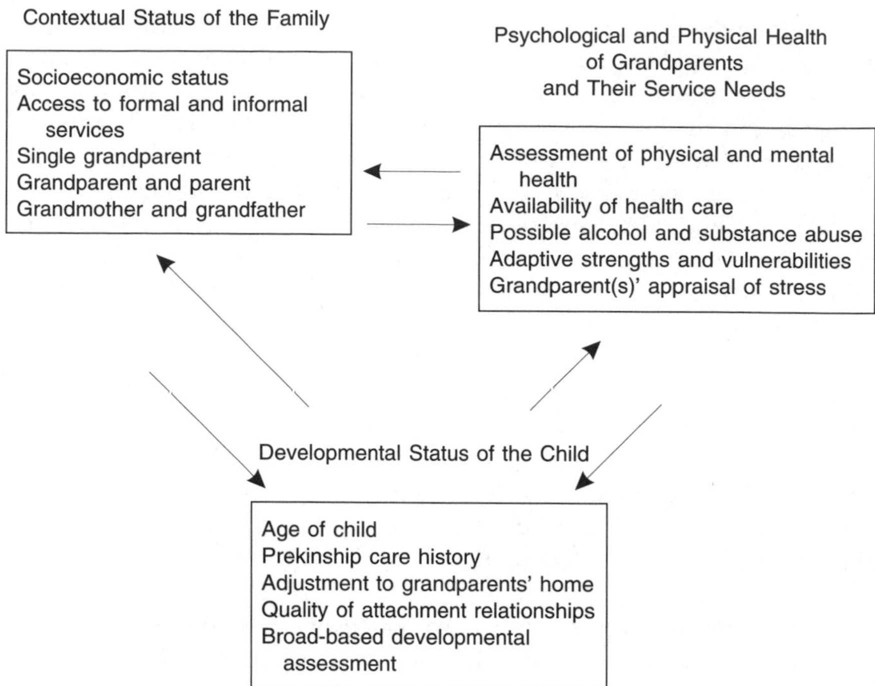

FIGURE 6.1. Interactive factors in the assessment of burden on skipped-generation caregivers.

tioners need to communicate their wish to understand the needs of the family. A practitioner needs to gain the grandparent's trust by becoming aware of grandmother's feelings regarding the loss of her children, understanding her view of her role as a caregiver, listening to the family's particular cultural perspectives on child rearing, clarifying with the grandmother her view of what is the matter, and considering the traditional way in which the family has reached out for help. Only within a helping relationship built on trust and respect for the subjective view of the grandparent, can the grandparent consider possibilities of new avenues for help. Furthermore, the nature of family and community support that is available, and the ties to institutions such as the church, is an important potential resource. Knowing and respecting the important aspects of the fabric of the grandparent's life can convey respect, increase her personal comfort level, and help her join with the practitioner to identify needs and search for solutions.

Institutions and professionals who provide services to the families with multiple levels of need often must develop a network of preventive services to support the strengths that exist. Unfortunately, in communities where a high degree of poverty exists, lack of insurance and difficulty in finding services abound. Even when they are present, however, it is noted that grandmothers often find it difficult to access available resources. Practitioners must often devise significant outreach services to help them (Beleville et al., 1991).

Two recent studies used "the person in the environment" perspective to study the psychological, physical, social, and economic needs of single grandmothers, and found common themes in the lives of Latino grandmothers in New York City and the experiences of African American grandmothers in Oakland, California (Burnette; 1999, Minkler et al., 1992). Most of the grandmothers felt committed to their grandchildren and tried to meet the many responsibilities of maintaining the family, even at the expense of their own health. Keeping the children in the extended family and providing continuity and stability gave many grandmothers a sense of satisfaction and accomplishment (Cox, 1999).

Overall, the studies identified important variables such as poverty, isolation, mental and physical health problems, and high stress related to the degree of caregiving burdens. The strain often resulted in increased illness, depression, and alcoholism. In each study population, the grandmothers said they received neither the help needed for their own chronic health problems nor any relief from stress, fatigue, and loneliness (Johnson, 1999).

The development of outreach services to families is important, as grandmothers overwhelmed by medical problems and stress may not have the energy to seek help and are afraid that if they do, an "outsider" might remove the children. New immigrants, who are neither fluent in English nor used to American mental health and medical practices, may not know about or feel entitled to seek available social services (Gibbs & Huang, 1999).

Some families use informal community ties instead, such as the church or other informal indigenous groups. However, these resources may not be sufficient to address the multilevel problems of the family. The absence of professional services, especially for the elderly in impoverished communities, compounds the problems (Johnson, 1999). Given the focus on Latino and black grandmothers, these researchers also suggest ways in which discrimination and bias may become institutionalized and result in inadequate resources in some communities.

THE DEVELOPMENTAL STATUS OF CHILDREN IN INFORMAL AND FORMAL KINSHIP CARE

The psychological world of children separated from their birth parents and raised by other relatives has been eloquently described in both children's fairy tales (*Hansel and Gretel, Cinderella*) and broader literature (Dickens, 1999; Oates, 1998; Verdelle, 1996). These children's narratives often reveal their sense of abandonment, rejection, and even feelings that they are responsible for their parents leaving them. Over time, as adults, these children often continue to remember the separation from their birth parent with a sense of deep loss and confusion. A poem movingly expresses an adult's remembered feelings regarding her placement following a family crisis (Oates, 1998, p. 282):

> It's a long time ago now, but I remember hiding away to cry.
> When I was a little girl and my mother didn't want me.

The "little girl" in the poem was 6 months old when she was sent to live with an aunt and uncle following the brutal murder of her father and the inability of her mother to cope with poverty as well as the responsibility of caring for eight other children. As she grew up, she came to know her birth family and expressed a wish to live with them. Her yearning for acceptance by her birth mother, however, was rebuffed, and she forever felt herself to be less beloved than others. In the poem, she sadly comes to terms with the reality of poverty and other circumstances that caused her to be separated from her parents (Oates, 1998).

Themes in the Child's Life

Many of the infants and children in kinship care today have been taken in by grandparents because of serious breakdowns in protective parental care. When the separation from parents is precipitated by a traumatic history, the child may have been developmentally "at risk" prior to the separation itself (Paret & Shapiro, 1998). The experience of early trauma can affect both the child's physical health and his/her ability to trust caregiving figures (Hurry, 1998). Despite the caregiver's best efforts, the children may be emotionally volatile and at times unresponsive.

For a new caregiver, it is hard to know if the child is simply responding to the shock of loss, or if the child's behavior represents his/her previous ways of coping in general. It would be difficult to assess correctly the degree of psychological health or pathology based on the child's initial adjustment to the new home. Some important themes are critical to the dynamic relationship that becomes established between grandchildren and their kinship caregivers when adoption follows trauma, loss, and family disruption.

The Experience of Loss

Often, grandparents must cope with a grieving child who may have little or no personal relationship with them. When children begin to live with their grandparents or other relatives, their emotional state and behavior are difficult to cope with and painful to observe. They may experience sleep and eating disorders, and be unable to control their feelings or be soothed. Even when the circumstances that have caused the separation of parent and child are unavoidable, such as the sudden death of a parent, the young child often cannot fully understand or accept the realities of what has occurred. Indeed, young children will process the realities only through the lens of their maturational status. They may become depressed or avoid dealing with feelings of anxiety, sadness, and anger, and act out their underlying feelings (Furman, 1994; Webb, 1999). The children may have many crises throughout development and need therapeutic help to work through the impact of early loss.

The Meaning of Trust

Some of the children who enter kinship care have had the benefit of a secure relationship with a psychological caregiver and have internalized a sense of trust and security. They may be able to retain a degree of robustness and resiliency following the loss of their parent(s). Their experience of having had a meaningful relationship with a parental figure on whom they could depend for the fulfillment of their needs will have been internalized as a template of care. This internalized model of trust in a caregiving other eventually helps them to transfer their affection and trust to their surrogate parent (Hurry, 1998; Stern, 1985).

If the child or infant did not have a primary caregiver upon whom he/she could rely, the capacity to form a relationship with another person may be compromised. When separation occurs, these children often have few internal resources to help them cope. They may not feel that their new caregiver will love them or stay with them. The child who has experienced "broken trust" in relationships may be angry or withdrawn, and this behavior can be as disturbing and frightening to the grandparent or other relatives as to the child.

The Impact of Trauma on Development

The ability of a child to proceed along expected developmental lines in cognitive, social, and emotional development may be impaired by poor health or early neglect and trauma (Freud, 1965). The age at which a child experiences trauma and loss has an effect on his/her overall development. In general, the younger the child, the more vulnerable he/she is to the impact of neglect, abuse, and loss. When a child enters the grandparent's home, he/she may be beset by feelings of inadequacy and unworthiness because of the loss of parent(s), and because of academic and social problems. This sense of inadequacy at school can add to poor self-esteem. The child often needs help in many spheres of development. Progress can be very slow and is often painful and frustrating to the grandparent.

Difficulties in the Capacity to Cope with Feelings

A child's style of regulating strong affects such as fear, anger, and sadness, is also related to the quality of preadoptive experiences. Psychosocial and neurobiological research suggest that chronic exposure to trauma in early childhood may be associated with later behavioral and developmental problems that are difficult to resolve (Cicchetti & Cohen, 1995; Shapiro & Applegate, 2000). Infants and children who have been brought up in chaotic families are known to have great difficulty in the development of normal ego functioning, particularly the capacity to establish a relationship with another and to modulate internal feeling states, such as anger, fear, and anxiety (Anthony, 1983; Tonning, 1999).

Behavioral responses to trauma are organized and described along a "fight or flight" continuum (Selye, 1978). Such behaviors are considered adaptive in the short run as immediate coping responses to stress (Webb, 1999). These patterns are described, in their extremes, as states of hyperarousal and disassociation. The coping literature sometimes refers to these behavioral states with terms such as hypervigilance, withdrawal, and/or "freezing" (Fraiberg, 1987b; Perry et al., 1995).

Grandparents may find it exceedingly difficult to care for a child who is emotionally volatile, and they may feel angry that the child does not recognize the sacrifice that is being made to care for him/her. Diagnostically, it is important to assess whether the child's behavior represents an acute reaction to stress or a more enduring "trait" or adaptation to a prior caretaking environment. An important area of developmental assessment is to track the various levels of functioning a child has achieved within multiple developmental lines (Freud, 1965). It is also helpful to identify at which point development may have slowed. This can reveal the emotional "age" of the child and has implications for the caregiver's expectations and assessment of the child's need. Grandparents or other kinship caregivers often need the counsel and observations of a child development specialist.

Using Language to Bring About New Understanding

When a child is older, however, the grandparents or other kinship caregivers can use expressive language to help him/her understand the changes that have occurred, and the realities of the new family. Children want to know who will live together, for how long, and what contact they will continue to have with their parents. Many older children can understand the context of change and the dimensions of time. The creation of a coherent family narrative is important because the process of constructing the story can help the family master the meaning of the changes they are experiencing. This is essential to the formation of a stronger sense of family identity and the child's development of a more coherent sense of self (Paret & Shapiro, 1998).

Developing Trust in a Caregiver

In her clinical work with children from disturbed or dysfunctional families, Hurry noted that a new empathetic figure, be it a grandparent or another concerned adult, can begin to help the child develop a more trusting relationship (Hurry, 1998). This relationship will take considerable time to mature, but it can be the basis for the beginning of internal emotional growth. A caregiver can enrich the child's milieu by providing an environment characterized by a level of safety, predictability, and empathy that promotes a more coherent sense of the world (Hurry, 1998). Time is needed before the child begins to have a sense that the erratic nature of his/her past world will not reoccur. If the disrupted emotional and behavioral state does not ease over time, then a more complete dynamic and neuropsychological assessment of the child's developmental status is needed.This assessment may indicate the need for more specific and intensive treatment (Chethick, 2000; James, 1994; Webb, 1999).

In summary, grandparents often need professional assistance to help them respond most effectively to their grandchild's emotional needs. Guidance may be needed to help grandparents find the words to validate the child's sense of loss and disappointment, as well as to help assuage any guilt that he/she may have in feeling responsible for a parent's illness or other difficulties. Grandparents, who are themselves grieving the losses involved with the parental crisis, often may find it difficult to tolerate the tears of their child or grandchild. The interruption in their own lifecycle has caused a rupture of the sense of self, and they must find supportive or therapeutic help for themselves as a prelude to being able to empathize with the dependent needs of a child in a state of anxiety and fear (Fraiberg et al., 1975).

A complicating factor in skipped-generation adoption is the manner in which the relationship between the child and birth parents continues. The grandparent may feel shame, guilt, and a sense of failure about what has happened to the family. These feelings may be important factors in the grandmother's willingness to take care of the children. However, she may also feel despair about the poor outcome for the children, and these feelings can affect the ways she relates to her grandchildren. In some cases, fearing the disruptions that often occur when the birth parent(s) visit, grandparents may discourage the parents from coming. What does it mean to the birth father and/or mother when contact is broken with the child in this way? Clearly, the grandmother's feelings and actions can add to the grief of the birth parents and the child. If the father or mother withdraws further, this new abandonment can be hurtful to the child. Therapists and family counselors have to identify the primary patient they are serving in the family, and also to consider the intergenerational needs of family members.

CASE ILLUSTRATIONS

We first consider two vignettes that illustrate how two preschoolers, Neesey and Linda, used their early attachment experiences with their mothers and with their grandmothers to help them overcome the shock of being suddenly left in their grandmother's care. Neesey and Linda were each abruptly left by their mothers in the care of their healthy grandparents at a time of crisis. Although both children suffered a significant psychological setback at the time of separation, with the care of their grandparents, they eventually recovered their previous level of ego functioning. Nevertheless, the crisis had a long-term impact on their psychological development.

Neesey and Granma'am

The important role of the grandparent as kin keeper and guardian of the generations was eloquently described in the novel *The Good Negress* (Verdelle, 1996). A tragedy occurred in the family of a 5-year-old girl,

Neesey, when her father died very suddenly. Her grief-stricken mother, Margarete, brought Neesey south to be left in the care of her grandmother, whom Neesey called Granma'am. Margarete returned to Detroit, with Neesey's brothers, to try and rebuild her life.

Neesey's grandmother was a strong and able woman. Although poor, Granma'am supported herself and Neesey through hard work, self-sufficiency, and a spiritual sense of purpose. Meaningful relationships existed among siblings, parents, the community, and the church. Suddenly, when the crisis surrounding Neesey's care arose, Granma'am used all of her own resiliency to cope.

Neesey experienced the abrupt separation from her mother as a betrayal, which left her in temporary shock. Verdelle (1996) describes the little girl's feelings upon waking up on the morning she realized that her mother had gone.

> When she awoke, the sudden absence of her mother had shattered her world. "Where's Mama?" I was screaming; my voice was quavering, wild, quick. I jumped up. The chair legs scraped against the kitchen floor. I stood as tall as I could on the floor. I looked directly at a face and mouth that did not move, (grandmother) eyes that looked surprised but ready too, somehow. The whole situation answered, with a shudder, and a sucking sound: "*she's gone.*" I tore away from the table, my arms heavy like they was wet and wrung out. They swung very late behind my hurly-burly hurt. I upset the neat breakfast plate with my wet rags for arms. Off the plate and the table went the *swiped* boiled egg, it landed in the chair, it rolled off onto the floor. The shell crumpled at the compact hit, and the egg rested there, *displaced,* and on its side. The *cracked pieces of shell hung together*; it was that tough-but-thin inside skin. One boiled breakfast egg preserved through the fall.
>
> *Disbelief is an emotion*, you know. Like an ocean and its major pulse, *it can overtake you. It can blind your eyes and block your ear canals. It can knock you to a depth. Both my hopefulness and my faith in my mother went flat. I felt so completely betrayed.*" (pp. 2–3)

In reading these words, we see that Neesey was frightened to the point of being unable to function. Her senses were overcome by profound terror and the feeling that her internal sense of security was "ripped" out of her. The novel continues to describe the way in which Grandma'am helped Neesey to overcome her grief and to continue to have hope for the future. Accustomed to hardship, the grandmother acknowledged the child's grief in words but she did not dwell on it. She kept the child close to her, engaging her in the work of the household. She spent endless hours talking to her, teaching her how to cook, to plant in the garden, and to create family connections and ties. Neesey came to feel that she belonged and was highly valued.

Neesey experienced a solid, emotionally satisfying relationship with her grandmother, who offered her empathy but sternness regarding her feelings and thoughts. Grandma'am gave her time to recover and was patient with Neesey when she was sad or angry, and encouraged her to go forward and learn. It was this relationship that made it possible for Neesey to become excited about new learning and new friends, and to master the many transitions and conflicts that arose as she grew up.

Neesey identified with her grandmother, and took on many of her ways, particularly caring for others. While these abilities gave her a sense of mastery and calmed her fears, she took on responsibility far beyond her years, and did not easily express her own internal thoughts and feelings. Like her grandmother, Neesey never outwardly complained.

Nearing adolescence, Neesey was taken to Detroit and reunited with her mother, her mother's new husband, and her older brothers. The relationship with her mother was not the same as it had been, and Neesey felt distant from her, neither expecting nor asking for understanding or care. Neesey helped her mother with the housework and the new baby but she no longer saw her mother as a parent and refused to call her Mommy, calling her by her first name, Margarete.

Her grandmother had become the psychological parent who had given Neesey the inner strength and security to survive. She identified with her grandmother and relied on this internal image when she encountered new problems. It was the relationship with her grandmother that allowed Neesey to respond to the help of a classroom teacher who recognized her ability and supported her development at school. She was able to grab onto the rope offered by a teacher who acknowledged her exceptional intellect and the satisfaction that could come from the study of expressive language. Hurry (1998) stresses that a secure relationship with even *one* person, even for only a short time, may provide the foundation for a mode of relating that can later be utilized when an appropriate attachment figure is found. The presence of her grandmother as a "knowing witness" made a decisive difference in Neesey's development. As she reached young adulthood, Neesey continued to evaluate her choices and feelings in terms of her past experiences.

Linda and Her Grandparents: A Case Vignette

Linda was already a preschooler when she went to live with her grandparents in the Midwest because of her mother's drug addiction. The grandparents, Mr. and Mrs. Knight, a middle-class family, made a full-time commitment to nurture and be responsible for Linda. Following the permanent separation, Linda was in a state of shock and developed many difficulties. Despite the fact that her mother, Emma, used drugs and was often neglectful, Linda and Emma were attached to each other. Linda's sleep was disrupted by nightmares, and her days were often filled with sadness. She longed for her mother to come back. She had fantasies that this would happen and was repeatedly heartbroken when the wish did not come true. Her grandmother accepted Linda's longings for her mother, and her expressions of grief, and tried to comfort her.

Eventually, Linda began to accept her grandmother's love and to become more attached, turning to her when she felt ill or sad. Her behavior and actions gradually became more typical of a child her age, and she progressed, playing with friends and doing well at school. Linda received help from a school social worker, and her grandmother became more attuned to her needs and could recognize when she was anxious and needed reassurance. The social worker, Mrs. Kahn, tried to help Linda put her thoughts into words and talk about her hopes and wishes. As Linda began to rely on her grandmother, she began to form a stable internal representation of her as a primary parental figure. The quality of the attachment relationship between Linda and her grandmother was built on trust and an expectation of empathy. As this relationship deepened, Linda became confused about whom to call Mommy, her grandmother or her mother, but she thought of her grandmother as her mother.

As with many adopted children, Linda reexperienced the narcissistic wound of early rejection in adolescence (Brodzinsky & Schechter, 1990). When she became an adolescent and met new friends at school, the reality of her unique family situation became more painful. When friends would ask her to tell about her family, Linda was embarrassed about her situation. Her feelings toward her mother and grandmother became more intense and confusing. She felt anger toward her mother for leaving but also wanted her to come back and be there with her. The increased longing for her mother that returned, along with a renewed sense of loss and discomfort regarding loyalty conflicts, was hurtful to her grandmother.

Linda's grandmother and her birth mother had both been important attachment figures, but each of her "mothers" had very different symbolic meaning. In some way, Linda blamed her grandmother for the loss of her mother. Whether the behavior was warranted or not, Linda's grandmother became the recipient of anger that may have belonged to the mother. Linda's self-esteem at this point was fragile. With the help of a therapist, Linda began to come to terms with her conflicted feelings and was able to proceed in her search for her own identity. As a young adult, she was able to express deep love for her grandmother.

It is suggested that feelings of early loss at one stage are often reevoked at a later stage of development (Balint, 1968). During adolescence, the time when children begin to consider a new level of separation and autonomy, they need to have confidence that the parental attachment figure will be there. This sense of security helps them as they risk taking new steps away from the family (Blos, 1967). Unlike most children in skipped generation families, Linda was fortunate in having both an emotionally solid grandmother and grandfather. The availability of two grandparents gave her the opportunity to internalize a model of dynamic interactions between multiple family members.

SUBSTANCE ABUSE AND THE ADAPTATION OF CHILDREN TO ADOPTION

One of the most difficult prekinship care experiences is that of children of drug addicted parents, especially when cocaine has been the source of the addiction. In such families, children may be exposed to high-risk medical conditions *in utero*, as well as high-risk psychological conditions in the postnatal environment. We know that if a child has suffered from drug exposure, poor nutrition, or inadequate health care in the neonatal period, he/she is at risk for atypical neurological development, prematurity, low birthweight, and general problems in state regulation at birth. Some children continue to show signs of atypical development in the cognitive, social, and emotional spheres throughout childhood (Chasnoff et al., 1998).

Approximately 11% of children born in the United States in 1998 were exposed prenatally to drugs, most often cocaine (Chasnoff et al., 1998). Many of these children are now in the care of their grandparents (Minkler et al., 1992). The grandparents who care for these children in either informal or formal kinship care face a difficult caregiving challenge because the impact of drugs and/or an early chaotic environment carries long-term developmental consequences.

An infant exposed to drugs *in utero* is likely to have unusual symptoms that require special caregiving. Excessive irritability, frequent tremors and startles, poor eating and sleeping patterns, and poor muscle tone are frequently observed. Abnormal sensorimotor, cognitive, and social interaction response patterns may be observed throughout infancy (Chasnoff et al., 1998). These infants require special care in which caregivers need to be attuned to their extreme sensitivity to external stimuli. Given these medical conditions, ongoing assessments and frequent doctor or hospital visits may be required and constitute a great effort for the grandparent.

Furthermore, many of these children continue to have developmental difficulties as they become preschoolers and enter kindergarten. Teachers have reported seeing short attention spans, inconsistent behaviors and abilities, poor motor coordination, uncontrollable mood swings, language delays, and other problems (Norris, 1991). However, it is difficult to assess how much the developmental delays and psychological impairment are due to the exposure to drugs *in utero* and their postnatal aftereffects, and how much is related to early abuse and neglect (Chasnoff et al., 1998).

Whatever the etiology of the developmental difficulties, these children require assistance in many developmental areas: special help in the classroom, evaluation of special learning problems, and therapeutic intervention for emotional trauma. At the same time, it is important that children not be labeled as "crack babies," since this carries a symbolic meaning of hopelessness and interferes with the development of responsive educational strategies. The label "crack baby" can create powerful expectations of failure, and therapeutic efforts should not be curtailed prematurely (Barth, 1991, p. 130).

The Burden of Care for Children from Drug-Addicted Parents

A study of the burdens to grandparents who provide a home for the children of their cocaine-addicted daughters reveals the extensiveness of the children's psychological and physical needs and the complex caregiving required (Minkler, Roe, & Price, 1992). Intensive medical care for the child may disrupt the grandmother's ability to work. The following brief vignettes reveal the multiple burdens for grandparents as they try to nurture their grandchildren in crisis.

A 62-year-old grandmother described her experiences in soothing and reassuring the two grandchildren who had recently come to live with her: "They feel like they don't trust you. They have their eyes on you at all times, the minute they hear you walk. . . . I guess they lived in fear so long. . . . I guess this is what they had to live with, with all the drug people in the house. They didn't know what to expect. It is this fear—fear. But they seem to be coming out of it" (in Minkler & Roe, 1993, p. 163).

Another grandmother in the study described her 3-year-old grandson: "He used to just scream. Every time I'd start getting dressed, he'd think I was going to leave him. He'd say, 'Don't leave me!' . . . He'd stand in the door till I got back when I went to the washroom" (in Minkler & Roe, 1993, p. 163).

How do we explain these behaviors? These children endured early drug-related trauma, including the absence of a stable relationship with their parent. Lack of trust in the permanence of their caregivers and expectation of abandonment led to constant vigilance to protect themselves from the terror of being left alone. Their behavior was related to their primitive ways of dealing with anxiety as they had been left alone to cope with trauma and fear in their earliest years. Even with the grandmother's help, it may take a very long time for these symptoms to abate. The children may be able to develop new and more mature adaptive capacities if their lives become less chaotic and they can rely on a long-term, stable relationship with their grandmother. The grandparents interviewed in the study seemed to understand that the children had special needs and that their fears and behaviors were related to the trauma they had experienced. While some grandparents had the health and resilience to respond to the needs of these children, others required extensive professional help to cope with the children's anxiety and help them establish a more secure relationship.

The grandmothers in the Minkler and Roe's study (1993) also identified another problem. Conflicts of loyalty arose over the grandparent's concern for the protection of the grandchildren and the termination of parental visits because of the emotional chaos these visits often caused. While some parents became more stable, many did not, and the erratic visits often disturbed the children (Tonning, 1999). Their emotional reactions to frightening visits emerged in behaviors such as mood changes, hiding, tantrums, refusal to eat, or aggressive behavior. The disturbances resemble the reunion patterns of children classified as having an insecure or disorganized attachment to their parents (Ainsworth, 1979b; Cassidy & Shaver, 1999). The grandmothers were aware of having to walk a fine line between helping to promote a bond between parent and child, and protecting the child from repeated disappointment and anxiety. Many grandparents wanted to keep the doors open to their children, but when conditions become too intolerable, some chose to protect their grandchildren, even at the expense of prohibiting parental visits (Minkler & Roe, 1993; Burton, 1992, 1999).

Nevertheless, as in other studies, the grandmothers who were able to cope expressed a personal sense of pride in keeping their families together and relief in knowing that their grandchildren were finally cared for and safe. Their role as guardians of the next generation gave them a sense of satisfaction in doing an important job and a heightened sense of self-worth and purpose (Johnson, 1999).

An example of the plight of grandmothers who must concern themselves with both their children's needs and those of their grandchildren was recently reported in an article in the *New York Times* (De Parle, 1999).

Case Vignette: Mickey, Max, and Jessielean

Two young toddlers, Mickey, age 2, and Max, aged 3, had been living with their single mother, Jessielean, in Milwaukee, Wisconsin. Jessielean, had a turbulent personal history. The transition to kinship care occurred after Jessielean was sentenced to jail for 4 years, following her conviction for theft. The children's 43-year-old grandmother, Ms. James lived alone, and was hardworking, poor, and had many physical ailments, including obesity, high blood pressure, and arthritis. She also suffered from emotional depression and physical exhaustion.

When her daughter went to jail, Ms. James was overwhelmed by the two frantic toddlers, who were often out of control. In addition, they were unresponsive to her efforts to soothe them or set limits on their behavior. Ms. James struggled to feed, clothe, diaper, and bathe the children who resisted her care. Mickey and Max engaged in dangerous play and required even closer supervision than most toddlers. They clogged Ms. James's toilet, colored her walls, and reduced the wood panel of her dresser drawers to a pile of splinters. At times, the children flew into hour-long rages, and Max sometimes rammed his head against the wall. Ms. James soon sought psychiatric assistance from the local child welfare agency for this little boy, as she was at her wits' end (De Parle, 1999).

The early prekinship care history of these children contained many high-risk factors. Their young mother, Jessielean, had a history of drug addiction, and the contextual life of her home was unstable, violent, and fragile. The children had been known to protective services and their case histories included evidence of neglect, lack of adequate nutrition, abuse, and chaotic circumstances, with repeated episodes of violence. Jessielean had recently lost her welfare status when the new "welfare to work laws" reduced the welfare rolls. Soon thereafter, she was arrested for stealing some goods at a local store.

The children's emotional and behavioral difficulties preceded their entry into their grandmother's home. Their emotional and developmental status was fragile, and they showed signs of only meager connections with available attachment figures. Left to their own resources at an early age, their attempts to cope with hunger and anxiety were primitive. Their behavioral symptoms of hyperactive running, hitting, hurting themselves, and head banging are seen in many neglected children. They had not experienced the human comfort that could have helped them mediate strong feelings of anxiety, anger, or sadness (Freud & Burlingham, 1944; Shapiro & Applegate, 2000).

The children's adaptive behavior was far behind what one might expect of their age group. In addition to limited evidence of beginning structure in the cognitive, emotional, and social sphere, there were deficits in comprehensive and expressive language, such as listening and responding, and evidence of poor capacity to mediate feelings, with a low threshold of frustration tolerance. They were also unable to use words to communicate feelings and needs. Ms. James would need a great deal of assistance, not only in terms of economic and social support to help her stabilize her own household, but also to obtain health care and support for herself. Furthermore, she needed professional guidance to evaluate the treatment needs of the children.

At the same time, the children's mother, Jessielean, was deeply depressed and needed comfort from her mother. Although Ms. James cared about her daughter, she was also very angry about what had happened to the grandchildren and the burden she was facing. When she visited her daughter in jail, Jessielean broke down in tears. Her mother lost control and yelled at her, "Don't you cry—I'm the one crying. I don't want to hear you're depressed—I'm depressed" (De Parle, 1999, p. 24).

The plight of Ms. James's family illustrates an extreme case of the burden on a single grandparent when there are significant intergenerational needs. She needed assistance to cope with poverty, illness, isolation, and the needs of two very disturbed toddlers. Overwhelmed and depressed, she was concerned for her daughter as well.

A therapist seeing this family would need to develop short-term treatment plans emphasizing the immediate psychological and physical safety of the children and the health of the grandmother. The longer-term interventions would need to focus on the recovery of the children and the extensive support needed by the grandmother, so that she could provide stable and empathetic care during the next critical years. The development of a working alliance that attends to the grandmother's own needs and her concern for her grandchildren is important.

Jessielean was in dire circumstances. Alone, and depressed, she desired to continue a relationship with her children and her mother. For Mickey and Max, it was important to maintain some relationship with their mother. That family attachment relationships existed is evident, but they were fraught with conflict and despair. A combination of individual and family therapy was critical in maintaining the significant relationships between the members of the family.

DISCUSSION

Informal and formal kinship care are clearly complex forms of family life that pose many economic, psychological, and health challenges for each of the generations involved. Mary Richmond has emphasized that practitioners should be cognizant of the importance of providing both direct and indirect services to families with multiple needs (Richmond, 1922). This is especially relevant when dealing with the distinct problems faced by grandparent-maintained households. The burden of grandparental care has fallen disproportionately on families in poverty, families of color, and grandmothers who maintain the family household alone, without the presence of their own children (Casper & Bryson, 1998).

At the time of adoption or foster placement each person in the strained skipped-generation household has particular needs related to his/her own emotional status and particular phase in the lifecycle. The child is likely to be in a state of confusion and loss. The parent(s) have lost the care of their child and may be suffering from physical or mental illness and/or addiction. The grandmother is experiencing a major disruption in her lifecycle and needs to adjust to the burden of caregiving a second time. Often lack of financial resources, poor health, and isolation compound the family's dire situation.

The case vignettes presented here illustrate the impact of early experiences on the adaptation of children to grandparental care. Neesey and Linda, for example, had the opportunity to develop meaningful relationships with their grandparents before the separation from their mothers. They had a certain degree of internal robustness and resilience, and a capacity to trust in the "other" that helped them establish meaningful relationships with their grandmothers. While they still experienced deeply the impact of the loss of their parent(s), their earlier strengths allowed them to utilize the "love" of grandparents who wished to care for them.

On the other hand, two toddlers, Mickey and Max, in a chaotic situation since birth, as their mother was heavily addicted to cocaine, came into their grandmother's care when their mother was imprisoned for petty theft. The years of early neglect gravely affected their ability to trust and to establish a reciprocally satisfying relationship with another person (Tonning, 1999). The relationship between the boys and their grandmother, Ms. James, was fraught with ambivalence and conflict, in circumstances compounded by the imprisonment of the boys' mother and the grief of all family members. The children's emotional needs made it even more difficult for their grandmother to provide the care they desperately required (Johnson, 1999).

Models of assessment that consider the "person in the environment" situation are helpful in addressing the contextual, social, and economic status of the family, as well as the psychosocial status of the child and the grandparent (Johnson, 1999). Often, the family is in crisis. Short-term intervention plans are needed to help the family reach a level of stability. Timely provision of adequate resources and services is critical to sustain the family. The long-term treatment needs of the family may take some time, while the practitioner evaluates the needs of the child and establishes a working alliance with the grandparent. This alliance can enable the grandparent to join with the practitioner in establishing long-term treatment goals with which they both feel comfortable. Often, grandmothers are reassured when they know that a long-term plan is in place to help their grandchildren (Minkler & Roe, 1993).

Where poverty, lack of social support, and unmet medical and treatment needs exist, the professional must reach out and work with institutions and agencies that can help shore up the economic, health, and social requirements of the family. Often, this involves efforts to improve the general resources that help to reduce poverty and coordinate care among various community resources, such as child welfare and child care programs (Johnson, 1999).

Interventions to assist grandparent-maintained households need to include primary prevention outreach programs as well as accessible tertiary care treatment services. Informed outreach programs are especially important for grandmothers who may not be fluent in English and do not have information about resources that are available for them (Johnson, 1999). Such a program is being developed at the University of Medicine and Dentistry in New Brunswick, New Jersey. This prevention program, known as the Children at Risk Resources and Intervention Program (CARRI), includes direct services through home visits, the provision of access to hospital based guidance and education, and social support for foster care and adoptive grandmothers whose families have been splintered due to immigration patterns.

Finally, this chapter has described the strengths and vulnerabilities of skipped-generation families and the important contribution that grandparents are making to the well-being of their grandchildren. A lack of social, economic, and therapeutic support often impairs the willing grandparents' ability to fulfill their valued role as kin keepers of the next generation. Social work practitioners and others involved in child welfare need to advocate for public support to sustain these vulnerable skipped-generation households (Hegar & Scannapieco, 1999). As Maslow (1954) has indicated, it is hard for anyone to address internal issues when basic external needs are paramount.

Dr. Arthur Kornhaber, president of the Foundation for Grandparenting, comments: "When we are pushed together because of parental fatigue or marital failure, we've got to sit down and look at what is best for all of us, especially the children. Grandparents and grandchildren have a magical bond" (Sharp, 1999, p. D-2). As a society and as professionals concerned for families and the well-being of vulnerable children, we must help to sustain the skipped-generation caregiving family as a significant societal and family resource.

7

Open Adoption

Family Attachments and Identity Formation

A quiet revolution is taking place in the practice of adopting children at birth. Since 1917, most nonkinship adoptions of infants at birth have been based on a presumption of closed relationships between the birth parents and the adoptive family (Cole & Donley, 1990). The premise of these *closed adoptions* was the belief that it was best for all members of the adoption triad to have closure on the past in order to help everyone adjust to the new family realities. The enactment in 1917 of the first *sealed records law* in Minnesota meant that information identifying the birth family was to be kept permanently sealed in the custody of the court or the placement agency (Baran & Pannor, 1990; Sorosky et al., 1989). These laws eventually became associated with the closed model of adoption practices that became "the best interest adoption standard" (Foster, 1973). This model assumed that closure on the past would help the birth mother close this chapter of her life and help the adoptive family develop a strong family structure that would benefit the healthy development of the child (Baumann, 1997; Wegar, 1997). This approach, which has defined standard adoption practice in the United States, is being transformed.

At the turn of the 21st century, many families, as well as researchers and practitioners in the field of adoption, are challenging these ideas and advocating new forms of adoption, called "open adoptions," in which the identities of both the birth and the adoptive families are known to each other and lines of communication remain open between them. Sometimes the birth parent has a voice in choosing the adoptive parent; and both the birth parent(s) and the adoptive parent(s) agree on the nature of further contacts between them. Although there are various models of open adoption, a basic aspect of these approaches represents a fundamental change in the nature of the relationship between the members of the adoption triad—the birth parents, the adoptive parents, and the child (Ryburn, 1994; Wegar, 1997).

Much debate continues as to the potential costs and benefits of open rather than closed adoptions for the psychological well-being of the adopted child and the ability of the adoptive family to form strong identity boundaries (Baumann, 1997; Ryburn, 1994; Wegar, 1997). The model of open adoption brings new perspectives to the consideration of issues often seen in clinical practice: the symbolic meaning of adoption for parent(s) and children; the child's lifelong effort to resolve the losses inherent in adoption; and the child's search for identity over time, particularly in adolescence. In all adoptions, abandonment and loss of love become part of the child's attachment history and are often linked together as the child tries to integrate his/her dual parental heritage. These themes often emerge in the clinical narratives of children who have sought therapeutic help at specific phases of their lives (Brodzinsky & Schechter, 1990).

Open and closed adoption models are inherently different in their approaches to the ethical, moral, and psychological questions that affect all members of the adoption triangle. Each model presents a different perspective on the dynamic interaction among the members of the adoption triad. In open adoption, both the birth parent(s) and the adoptive parent(s) develop a special relationship with their child. The adoptive parents have the difficult task of forming a secure attachment relationship with their child while maintaining a degree of openness with the birth parent(s). The birth parent(s) retain a connection with their child but must adapt to the reality that they are not the primary attachment figures. The dynamic interactions between the two families may create pain and stress at different moments in time. On the one hand, recent studies suggest that the opportunity to work through the complex family dynamics may benefit all members of the adoption triad. On the other hand, the emotional health of the birth and adoptive parent(s) is critical to establishing and maintaining a viable open relationship between themselves and their child (Berry, 1993; Gritter, 1989; Ryburn, 1994). Often counseling, education, and guidance are needed to help sustain this complex family structure.

We hope this chapter will further understanding of the "shared fate" of all members of the adoption triad (Kirk, 1964). These insights have significant implications for clinical practice. Open adoption expands the nature of the experiences of all members of the adoption triad and enables us to explore the dynamics of adoption through the lens of the experiences of the birth parent(s), the adoptive parent(s), and the child.

THE LEGAL AND SOCIAL TRANSFORMATION OF ADOPTION PRACTICE

From Sealed Records to Open Adoption Practice

The following quotations represent important aspects in the debate over whether adoption records should be sealed and/or the circumstances in which they should become open.

> *From a speech by William Pierce defending the importance of keeping records sealed:*
>
> "Our society says that privacy is a really important thing, that people have a right to privacy . . . it is not a presumption, it's what the United States Supreme Court says—It says that a person does have a right to privacy. And another person's need for information doesn't destroy your right to privacy." (in Wegar, 1997, p. 17)

> *From Lifton (1976) supporting the opening of sealed records:*
>
> "Adoptees view the policy of confidentiality as a euphemism for putting everyone's rights over their own, although as babies they had no say in the transaction." (in Wegar, 1997, p. 17)

These quotes represent two diametrically different reactions to efforts to modify sealed records adoption laws. The questions being debated are whether existing sealed records practices should be changed to allow adoptees and birth parents to search for each other more easily, or whether confidentiality should be continued as in the initial agreement of the adoption. As Kirk (1981) stated, adoption is a kind of family formation that entails a pattern of social relationships among the members of the adoption triad as well as a legally established social institution. These laws and social relationships are transformed through time as our understanding of the needs of families and children changes.

It is not surprising that the history of adoption law in our society mirrors our changing cultural norms and values. In the earliest centuries of American history, there was no legal framework for adoption (Baran & Pannor, 1990; Cole & Donley, 1990; Sorosky et al., 1989). The pragmatic needs of families for assistance and the needs of orphaned and homeless children for nurturant families came together on an informal basis, without the legal framework of formal adoption laws that developed later. There was no concept of secrecy surrounding adoptions or of a need to preserve the birth parents' anonymity. In fact, a suggestion that the child should be permanently separated from his/her known family history was considered to be morally wrong in the early decades of the 20th century (Foster, 1973). On the other hand, without guidelines and laws for adequate care of nonbiologically related children, many abuses occurred (Baumann, 1997; Wegar, 1997).

In 1917, Minnesota passed the first laws prohibiting the release of identifying information about the birth parents' identity. By 1929, in every state, adoption laws were designed to prevent abuses and to meet the current "best interest standards," including sealed records provisions. The presumptions underlying these sealed records laws was that this was the best way to protect the welfare of the "parentless child" and the privacy of both the adoptive family and the birth parent (Baran & Pannor, 1990; Cole & Donley, 1990; Sorosky et al., 1989).

These laws reflected the social attitude of the time that the child needed to be protected from the stigma of a connection to the unwed birth mother and the stigma and status of being illegitimate. In addition, the adoptive family needed to be protected from the intrusion and potential conflict of a relationship with the birth parents and negative perceptions about the worth of an adopted child. Finally, the birth mother needed privacy to have a second chance to forge a new life. These adoption laws and practices reflected the view that all members of the birth triangle would be better off if they could "forget" the past and deny the unspoken reality of their shared fate (Baumann, 1997; Kirk, 1964; Wegar, 1997).

In the 1930s and 1940s, private adoption agencies, primarily staffed by social workers, developed policies and procedures that enforced the sealed records practice (Baran & Pannor, 1990). The actual impact of closed adoptions on persons in the adoption triad was not evaluated during these decades. The issues of grief and loss were not fully understood, and change in social policy or adoption practices was not seriously considered (Baumann, 1997). In fact, after World War II, new laws required that birth records be sealed and new birth certificates be issued in the names of the adoptive parents (Baran & Pannor, 1990). This increased confidentiality resulted in the total severance of the biological parents from the adoptive family.

Legal decisions were in tune with the dominant cultural belief that it was the experiences in the adoptive family that counted, not the biological inheritance of the child. The shaping of social and cultural beliefs was supported by new studies in psychology that focused on the relationship between infants and parental caregivers as the most important predictor of future development (Ainsworth, 1979b; Freud, 1966; Freud & Burlingham, 1944; Winnicott, 1956). At the time, it did not seem critical to know about the birth family's medical or psychological history. More recent research, however, has demonstrated how much genetic history can affect the developmental pathways of the child in the spheres of physical and mental health, temperament, aptitudes, cognition, and talents (Cadoret, 1990).

Closed adoptions and sealed records were believed to benefit the psychological adaptation of the birth mother, the adoptive parents, and the child. It was thought that without contact with the birth parent, all members of the birth triad could put aside their losses. The adoptive parents wanted closure to help the family mirror biological parentage, so that their pain of infertility loss could be forgotten. The birth mothers needed to forget or overcome the loss of their infants more quickly, and the children needed to claim their new parents as truly theirs, without suffering the thoughts of rejection and loss of their biological parents and roots. We now know, through the narratives of many persons and the work of clinicians and researchers in adoption, that *all* members of the adoption triad deal with the reality of adoption in different ways, at different moments in their lives. The door to the identities of the members of the adoption triad may have been sealed in law, but not in the internal worlds of emotions, fantasies, and thoughts of all those involved (A. Brodzinsky, 1990; Wegar, 1997).

New Ideas and Social Change

In the late 1960s and early 1970s, the Civil Rights and feminist movements questioned many of the accepted cultural norms and values in our society. In general, there was a reevaluation of the pervasive discrimination that existed for minority and marginalized groups in our society (Lamb, 1999; Mintz & Kellogg, 1988). Great interest developed in discovering one's roots and building pride in the survival of those who had overcome great hardship resulting from discrimination, poverty, sexism, and racism.

These ideas also led to questioning the sealed records laws that affected adoption practice. For example, the harshness of the social stigmatization of single parenthood and the plight of unwed birth mothers was questioned anew (Cole & Donley, 1990). Advocates for change referred to the human costs to birth parents of the sealed records policies and to the negative public attitudes toward birth parents who placed their children for adoption (Baumann, 1997; Sorosky et al., 1989). Were not these birth mothers forced to give up their babies because of lack of financial and social support? Was it right to prevent them from knowing where their children were, or to prevent the adult adoptees who wished to know their roots from finding their parents? In the 1970s, unmarried birth fathers were recognized as having legal status, and they also began to express their desire to be heard. Their voices contributed to the beginnings of change as they asked for a role in decision making regarding their children (Baumann, 1997).

As a result of these developments in the 1970s, multilevel challenges to the sealed records practice were launched (Lifton, 1977). The opening of sealed records became the focus of debates between private adoption agencies that generally supported keeping the status quo and the vocal advocacy of many grassroots groups and individuals who demanded change. Some advocates believed that those who had agreed to adoption on the basis of full confidentiality had a right to their privacy and should not have to fear intrusion into a developed life (Pierce, 1990). On the other hand, advocates for the right to find a parent argued that each child had a basic right to know about his/her birth heritage and lost kinship connections (Lifton, 1976). In Lifton's thinking, the importance of search to the adoptee was related to the need to know about one's past in order to achieve an integrated sense of self and a meaningful individual identity (Lifton, 1977, 1988, 1994; Saffian, 1998).

Clinicians began to take more seriously the impact of closed adoption on children. They recognized that the adaptation to adoption is a lifelong process, often intensified in adolescence, when youngsters struggle with identity formation issues (Schechter & Bertocci, 1990). Mental health literature presumed that the adoptees would never know the true facts regarding the identity of their birth parents and would work out their need to integrate their dual heritage through fantasy (Stone, 1972). There was, however, increasing clinical evidence that many adolescent adoptees became preoccupied with their birth heritage. The sealed records laws that were intended to protect the confidentiality of adoptees actually created significant hardships for young adults who were having great difficulty in forming an integrated sense of identity. Rather than feeling protected, secrecy and cutoffs from their birth parents increased their sense of abandonment and difference (Schechter & Bertocci, 1990).

The ongoing debate precipitated new legal approaches to the question of sealed records. Eventually, some states began to develop procedures wherein children and birth parents could have some access to parental medical records. Also, special registries were established to enable parents and children to locate each other if both expressed this wish. Many agencies adopted a more liberal practice of releasing medical information, and states began to debate new laws that would make the search process easier.

Despite all of these efforts, by the mid-1990s, only three states—Alaska, Kansas, and Tennessee—had laws permitting adult adoptees the right to obtain genealogical information without a court order or the consent of the birth parents (Wegar, 1997).

The Evolution of Open Adoption Models

Although the efforts of the search movement raised the consciousness of many people regarding the social attitudes that shaped adoption practices, these insights alone would not have led to the present transition from closed to open adoption models. However, changing social and cultural attitudes, and the small number of infants available for adoption, combined to create new adoption practices. Prominent among these are open adoption models. The following events have been of great importance:

- Fewer healthy newborns are available for traditional adoptions, and many intentional parents are seeking a child. The rate of white women who release their infants for adoption decreased from 19% in 1965 to 3% in 1988, while the analogous rate for families of color, which has always been low (approximately 2–3%), remained constant. As of the mid-1990s the estimated wait for a healthy infant is from 1 to 7 years (Evan B. Donaldson Adoption Institute, 2000).
- There are multiple reasons for these changes. Availability of contraceptives and legal abortion gives women more control over their reproductive lives, and fewer infants are born whom parents place for adoption. Older children with special needs, however, continue to await adoptive families.
- Freed by decreasing stigmatization of single parenthood, single parents are more willing to keep their children. They are more aware that giving up a baby may leave lifelong scars for parents and children.
- The Civil Rights movement and the resulting Freedom of Information Acts also advanced the ideas of openness in adoption (Sorosky et al., 1989).
- Birth parents who wish to place their children for adoption feel more empowered to make choices for their infants and to express their wish not to lose all contact with them. Eager adoptive parents are more willing to consider new types of relationships with the birth parents (Fein, 1998).
- Family diversity is increasing in our society, now including families of divorce, stepparent families, blended families, and reconstructed families (Lamb, 1999). Many children have adjusted to relationships with different

parental figures in extended family systems. *The relationships in families involved in open adoption are seen as somewhat akin to complex extended kinship families.*

• In closed and open adoption state laws protect the right of birth mothers to change their minds about adoption and protect the legal status of adoptive families. In both closed and open adoptions, the adoptive parents have legal custody and responsibility for their child, and the child has the same legal relationship to the adoptive parents as a birth child (Gritter, 1997).

• Independent, private, and not-for-profit adoption agencies are changing their policies regarding open adoption to accommodate the wishes of birth parents.

• The psychological benefits of open adoptions and the need to rethink adoption practice is supported by many clinicians who are increasingly aware of the psychological cost of closed adoptions to child and family well-being (A. Brodzinsky, 1990; Kirk, 1981).

• Both the National Committee for Adoption and the Child Welfare League of America have acknowledged positive aspects of openness in adoption but have stopped short of support for opening previously sealed records. Thus, while respecting the rights of privacy of those families who made decisions based on one model of adoption, they are supporting the idea that change in adoption procedures may be helpful (Amadio, 1991).

THE ADOPTION TRIAD: PSYCHOLOGICAL ISSUES IN CLOSED AND OPEN ADOPTION

The Narratives of Birth Parents

Practitioners have seen firsthand the grief of birth mothers in placing their children for adoption. Recent research on the postadoption experience of birth mothers demonstrates that relinquishment and adoptive placement is a traumatic experience; often guilt and remorse remain with them throughout their lives. For many women, "the experience of surrendering an infant for adoption is nearly an intolerable loss" (A. Brodzinsky, 1990, p. 304). Until recently, unmarried birth fathers had no legal status in relation to their child and no say in the birth mother's decision. The experiences of birth fathers who have given up a child has not received sufficient clinical attention.There is clinical evidence, however, that fathers also experience deep grief and sometimes great anger over the loss of a child, particularly if they have not been consulted. Often, they try to reclaim their children later (Carbone & Decker, 1999).

If the biological parents consult an agency regarding adoption decisions, they may be helped to explore their feelings and the complexity of their decision. It is advisable that birth parents become aware of the difficult issues that may develop, so that they can make more informed choices and be prepared for dealing with the future conflicts and ambivalence that may occur. The adoption counselor has the sensitive task of developing a working alliance with parents who may have disparate feelings and views regarding their own needs and wishes. The role of the father in adoption decisions can be supportive for the birth mother or create great, additional stress, depending on a number of factors: the circumstances of the pregnancy; the relationship between them; their capacity to care for their child; and their commitment to each other and/or to their child. Even when conflict exists, each person faces the grief of giving up his/her biological child. The counselor has three clients—the birth mother, the birth father, and the unborn child. Crisis intervention is helpful in clarifying and exploring the issues. In relation to adoption planning, the therapist's knowledge of potential benefits and difficulties, and his/her clinical empathy and objectivity can help maintain an alliance with the parents in a potentially conflicted relationship.

Researchers have found that birth mothers have different emotional reactions to closed or open adoption models depending on their defensive adaptation in coping with loss and grief. For some, closure is helpful in the immediate crisis (Blanton & Deschner, 1990). This defense may continue for many years; even at a later point in life, some birth parents cannot express feelings about the adoption and do not wish to deal with the subject. This resistance may continue even when they seek therapeutic help for ostensibly unrelated reasons. The denial and secrecy can come at a great emotional cost to future recovery. On the other hand, birth mothers who choose open adoption may be better able to tolerate feelings of loss and ambivalence. A mother can take great comfort in knowing her child as he or she grows up, while accepting that she cannot be the primary parent (Berry, 1993). Open adoption enables some birth parents to internalize a less negative sense of themselves because they have chosen the adoptive parents whom they feel will value and treasure their child. The separation from the baby can be less traumatic, relieving guilt and allowing the birth mother to move on more easily with her own development (Gritter, 1989; Ryburn, 1994).

Some open adoption allows birth parents to choose different levels and patterns of relationship with their children and their adoptive families. This choice depends on their own comfort with the complexity of the situation and the wishes of the adoptive parents (Gritter, 1997). Birth parents and adoptive parents must negotiate the continuing relationship between them and the nature of ongoing contact with their child. At times, the children themselves may find the contact with the birth parent very difficult, especially during the latency years, when they understand the meaning of adoption more fully (Brodzinsky & Schechter, 1990). This may be a painful conflict that birth parent(s) and adoptive parent(s) need to resolve with the "best interests of the child" in mind.

At the time of adoption, the relationship between the birth parent and the chosen adoptive parent can be one of hope and idealization. The birth parents may see the adoption as a chance for upward mobility of their child. Over time, however, the birth parent(s) may unconsciously wish that they could also be surrounded by the love of the adoptive parents who are nurturing their child. The reality that the adoptive parent is not also adopting them can be difficult. Therapeutic help may be needed to sort out the disappointed fantasies and wishes they have had for themselves and to work toward a more realistic expectation of their "kinship role" in the family. In some cases, the sense of limited "love" and acceptance for themselves may reevoke feelings of rejection from their past, and threaten a positive relationship with the adoptive parents and the child (Fraiberg et al., 1975).

Often, in order to sustain a relationship with each other, both the birth parents and the adoptive parents need professional help in working through these issues. In many cases, community based, nonprofit, private agencies have more experience and capacity to provide a range of services to families than do independent, for-profit placement agencies. These agencies may operate nationally and usually have neither the resources nor the commitment to provide continuing contact with families (Emery, 1993).

The working alliance with the birth parents is very complicated, and case workers must become aware of their own inner attitudes and biases. When issues of separation and loss are dominant, strong feelings may emerge for the professional as well as the parents. Another value-laden and emotional issue is the consideration of benefits or difficulties of cross-racial adoption. At one and the same time, the caseworker may wish to help the birth parent(s) come to their own decision about adoption planning but may also have an opinion as to their capacity to handle the complexities of open adoption. Furthermore, if the birth parent(s) are emotionally disturbed, the clinician may have serious concern about the effects of open adoption on the child. Ethically, the clinician has the obligation to convey all sides of the issues while maintaining empathy with the birth parent(s).

The Adoptive Parents

Clinical experience with open adoption suggests that adoptive parents should be prepared for the unique aspects involved in open adoption practices. They are undertaking a process of family building in which the usual family boundaries are not present but must be created carefully. At each phase of the process, new questions emerge. Families who consider an open adoption come to this crossroad for many reasons: Some parents experience years of infertility treatment and loss before giving up the dream of a biological child, and are reluctant to wait the typical 5–7 years to adopt an infant at birth; single, gay, or lesbian intentional parents may face discrimination in traditional adoption agencies; and members of a specific ethnic, religious, or racial background may face barriers in traditional adoption agencies (Bartholet, 1993).

To some degree, parents considering open adoption are aware that it has some risks. They worry about the possibility of maintaining the integrity of family boundaries and the ability to raise their children without undue pressure or interference from the birth parents. They realize the emotional risk they may experience if they are rejected by birth parents (Gritter, 1997). For intentional parents who have already experienced loss of self-esteem because of infertility or other barriers, the search for acceptance is fraught with anxiety.

Once accepted as adoptive parents, they are involved in a new relationship with the birth parents, often supporting them during pregnancy. All adoptive parents need to work through the sadness they feel for the birth parents' loss and their own guilt about becoming the caregiving/primary parents. In open adoption, when the birth parents are actually known, these feelings may be intensified. Many clinicians have found, however, that the fact that they were chosen by the birth parents helps adoptive parents to feel worthy and special (Ryburn, 1994). The birth parents' acceptance helps them more easily develop a sense of parental entitlement to claim their children (A. Brodzinsky, 1990).

Once adoption occurs, open adoption mirrors traditional adoption in that the adoptive parents can begin to form an attachment to their infant almost at birth by fulfilling the infant's earliest physical and emotional needs. This opportunity to care for and comfort their infant during its earliest days can help the parents establish a strong emotional connection to their child, strengthening the bond between them. Moreover, the child will have the benefit of continuity and stability in starting life within the circle of a permanent family. Children who are securely attached to their adoptive parents develop an internal representation of this relationship upon which to rely. The quality of this attachment is unique to the psychological parents (adoptive parents) and is not easily transferrable to others, including the birth parents.

In all adoptions, the parents have a dual task; they are expected to make the child their own, yet find a way to explain to the child that he or she has been adopted (Kirk, 1964). Clinical experience reveals that even very young children can differentiate the nature of relationships with their primary attachment figures from other relationships with extended family members. The adoptive parents can be reassured that they will always be the primary attachment figures for their children. As we shall see in the case vignettes, young children respond to their primary parents in a very different way than to members of the extended family, including their birth parents.

The adoptive parents need to find appropriate words to talk about the open adoption and to introduce the birth parents to the child. Talking about this sensitive issue is very difficult. The parents must keep in mind the developmental age of their child and his/her capacity to understand the meaning of the adoption. Over time, the narrative will deepen in response to new questions that emerge. A 4-year-old, for example, can understand the words, "This is the lady in whose tummy you grew, and Daddy and Mommy are the ones who will care for you forever." Children, even at this age, will ask many questions, seeking reassurance that their families will be there forever. Later on, the child may begin to have a more complex set of fantasies and expectations about how he/she is related to both sets of parental figures. These new questions about identity and identifications can be a challenge to parents, reevoking painful feelings about earlier losses.

A key issue in the success of open adoption is the quality of communication in the adoption triad (Baumann, 1997; Ryburn, 1994). In a recent study that evaluated the ways in which parents speak to their adopted children about their heritage, no perfect model emerged (A. Brodzinsky, 1990). Rather, the most important factor was the readiness of the parents to respond empathetically to the child's questions, which become more complex and abstract over time. The sensitivity of the communication is paramount to enhancing the positive feelings children have about themselves and their birth parents, as well as their relationship with the adoptive parents. In open adoptions, the communications between child and birth parents directly address the invisible reality of adoption. Otherwise, the child is left to deal with his/her fantasies of the "not said."

Finally, many adoptive parents report that knowing their child's birth parents helps them recognize that their child reflects both the genetic endowment of the birth parents and the heritage of the adoptive family. In closed adoption, for example, many adoptive parents subconsciously fear that their child will identify with a fantasy of the unknown parent. Many adoptive parents fear signs of aggression or sexuality in their children and may become overly anxious because of fantasies regarding their child's family history. For the parent who is fearful of the unknown, the child's normal aggressive play may evoke the ghost of the unknown birth parents. When the birth parents are known, adoptive parents are better able to assess their child's needs and attributes more accurately (Ryburn, 1994). The imprint of the child's biological heritage in terms of health, physical appearance, temperament, strengths, passions, talents, and resilience becomes clearer. As in all families, the parents may not find it easy to accept and encourage the child's attributes and proclivities. But this acceptance and encouragement is critical to the child's psychological and overall development.

Practitioners who work in open adoption need to support the adoptive parents' role as the primary parents while acknowledging that the problems that arise are intricate. There are no simple solutions. The guiding principle of keeping the developmental needs of the child in mind can assist the parents in working through the complex extended family dynamics.

Special Issues for Children Raised in Open Adoption Families

The child's understanding of the meaning of adoption changes across developmental phases. For example, at the age of 4, children may initially feel happy about being "chosen" by their adoptive parents and accept that their birth parents could not take care of them. By the early elementary school years, as cognitive development proceeds, children become more aware of the loss involved in adoption and the reality of their dual heritage. In school, for example, a child is likely to be asked to talk about his/her birth story, and the realization of being different from other children can be experienced with some degree of shock. This new awareness can be the beginning of a heightened self-consciousness and can precipitate developmental disruption, self-doubt, and feelings of loss (Brodzinsky & Schechter, 1990).

For children in closed adoptions, bewilderment about their origins can contribute to increased levels of identity confusion and lead to a sense of shame, embarrassment, and lowered self-esteem. Often, children develop fantasies about their birth parents and imagine reasons for the parents' decision to let them go. Most children tend to blame themselves for the abandonment and this perceived rejection may be internalized as a sense of being undeserving and unworthy.

Open adoption can provide a greater degree of reality that reframes the adoption problem. For children, ongoing contact with birth parents can be experienced as a confirmation of self-worth, as they can take comfort from the fact that their birth parents still care about them. This interest can bolster their self-esteem (Ryburn, 1994). As children get older, there may be a clearer grasp of the reasons for adoption.

However, the child's relationship with his/her birth parents can be fragile and change over time. Without a strong psychological bond, ambivalent feelings may emerge as the child realizes that the birth parents' "love" may be limited and disappointing. In some cases, when the birth parents' feelings change and they withdraw from contact, the adoptive parents cannot easily shield their child from the disappointments that may occur. For example, a child who had not wished to see his birth mother for many years was nevertheless devastated when she did not send a birthday card. At other times, the child may experience loyalty conflicts and survivor guilt if the birth parents are in difficult circumstances and their lives are much more unhappy and distressed than that of the child's adoptive family.

All children are vulnerable to identity conflicts during adolescence; for adopted children, this may be more difficult (Brinich, 1990; Hoopes, 1990). Adolescents may project their struggles for independence onto the adoptive parents and preserve the fantasy of the birth parent as the good parent, or, alternatively, have conflict with the birth parent and reject that relationship temporarily. The presence of dual sets of parents may lead to identity confusion. The child needs the adoptive parents to be patient and understanding in order to resolve the complex process of identity formation and the development of mature independence (Brinich, 1990).

Children in closed adoption often experience a deep need to know more about their birth heritage and often fantasize about who they are. A seventh grader, when asked to write an essay about her family, chose to write about her fantasies of her birth mother, who was of a different racial and ethnic origin, rather than write about her adoptive parents. This brought great anguish to her mother and father, who felt rejected. They also felt angry that after all they had done for her, she preferred to talk about her unknown mother. It was difficult for them to empathize with their daughter's effort to resolve her confusion about adoption and her own self-worth. This idealization of the birth mother was a problem that the family brought to therapy. Children in open adoption may be better able to work through a search for their own identity. The birth parents may have positive and/or negative attributes as identificatory figures. Children may identify with some aspects of the birth parents that conflict with the values of the adoptive family. In both instances, children can use the reality or the fantasy of birth parent(s) to work out adolescent conflicts with their adoptive parents.

Thus, despite many advantages for the child, open adoption is not a panacea (Berry, 1993). The reality of the involvement of birth parents in the developing life of the adopted child poses some hazards. If the birth parents are unable to accept the adopted parents' role as primary, their intrusion may threaten the child's sense of security (Berry, 1993). In some cases, the adoptive parents have to shield their child from involvement with birth parents who are psychologically disturbed (Ryburn, 1994). In other cases, when adoptive parents have not kept to the agreements they made about access and sharing of information, the birth parents can often feel, and be, helpless in influencing such decisions. These stresses can be compared to other nontraditional families, such as stepfamilies and blended families in which the psychological parents need to help the child deal with complex sets of relationships (Lamb, 1999).

Clinical work with children in open adoptions can borrow from the work with children in traditional adoption, in families of divorce, and in blended families. In all these situations, the children have had to deal with attachment losses and attachment gains. The therapist can become a new object, providing a relationship based on trust, stability, empathy, and neutrality. Within this relationship, the child can find a safe place to express his/her anger, pain, and confusion. The transference relationship, however, may be fraught with feelings of both anticipated loss and rejection that may keep the child at a distance even though he/she may long for closeness, reassurance, and acceptance.

THREE OPEN ADOPTION MODELS

Model I. Independent Open Adoptions: Searching for the Right Match

Independent adoptions are brokered through independent adoption centers, lawyers, or others in a position to bring together intentional families and birth parents. Often, the birth parents and adoptive parents live at a distance from each other, in different states or even different countries. Today, web sites are available in which parents can contact private individuals or agencies seeking adoptive parents. What distinguishes for-profit, independent adoptions from traditional agency adoptions is that most traditional agencies have long-standing practices and specified criteria for the selection of adoptive parents. In addition, traditional agencies often provide counseling services intended to protect the future well-being of the child, the birth parents, and the adoptive parents (Emery, 1993).

In independent open adoptions, a preadoption courtship may develop between the birth mother and the intentional parents, who often are desperate to find an infant. The adoptive parents may prepare albums, letters, and biographies of themselves to demonstrate their ability to provide good care to their child. In this early search period, the intentional parents are at risk for disappointment and loss, since they are either competing with other intentional adoptive parents and may be rejected or, if accepted, may face the possibility that the birth mother will later change her mind. Even if a birth mother has accepted financial help during her pregnancy, by state law, she has a specified time period in which she and/or the baby's father may change their minds. The prospective parents may become personally involved with the birth parent(s), and if the process then breaks down, disappointment is intense. Two brief examples illustrate the poignancy of the dramatic issues that may arise in open independent adoptions.

A Completed Open Adoption (Fein, 1998)

Mr. Rosario and Ms. Elniskey chose Mr. and Mrs. Weilacker to be the parents of their baby. Mrs. Weilacker lived in a western state and received the name of the family from an independent agency. Ms. Elniskey and her boyfriend, Mr. Rosario, decided to place their unborn child in an open adoption. Mr. and Mrs. Weilacker, both 39, had endured several unsuccessful years of infertility treatment. Ms. Elniskey already had given birth to three children who were all under age 5 and, given the family's difficult circumstances, she and the birth father agreed to give the baby up for adoption. As an adolescent, Ms. Elniskey had given up a baby in a closed adoption and still grieved over this loss. She did not want to lose track of this baby but, for various reasons, including poverty, was too overwhelmed to keep the child and did not believe she could care for all of her children.

Mrs. Weilacker had been working with an independent placement agency and, at the suggestion of agency personnel, wrote a "Dear Birth Mother" letter to Ms. Elniskey to demonstrate that she and her husband would have the ability to provide good and loving care to her unborn child. After being contacted by Ms. Elniskey, Mrs. Weilacker went to see her and was accepted as an adoptive parent. She provided emotional and financial support throughout the pregnancy. When the baby was born, Mrs. Weilacker returned to help Ms. Elniskey take care of her son, Nicholas, and each mother supported the other. Nicholas's birth mother was emotional in the hospital but once home with her other children, she was overcome by their needs and thought she had made the right decision.

Ms. Elniskey wrote a note to be given to Nicholas when he was older. She explained that as parents, she and his father wanted him to be safe and loved, and had found the right family who could care for him. Mrs. Weilacker brought the baby and his birth mother and father to her home to show them the baby's new home and to meet the adoptive father. Both families agreed to keep in touch in the future through letters, photographs, and visits.

While both families had good intentions for Nicholas, they had a very special situation to deal with; one that would take on different meanings over time. Ms. Elniskey commented on the meaning of the open adoption to her: "Nicholas has to get on with his life and we have to move on with ours. At least our lives won't be entirely separate, but I can't really imagine how it will all be in a month or a year from now" (in Fein, 1998, p. A-30).

What can we expect Nicholas to understand as he grows up, and how can we foresee the relationship between the two sets of parents? We can expect that as an infant and toddler, Nicholas will develop an attachment to his adoptive caregiving parents. He may know the names of his birth mother and father, but he will not fully understand their relationship to him for a long time. When Nicholas begins to ask questions about his birth parents, his adoptive parents will need to reassure him that they will always care for him and that he will never lose them. It will be important to convey to Nicholas that he is their son, whom they love, and that he will forever be a part of the Weilacker family.

As Nicholas gets older, he may wonder about the reasons his birth parents placed him for adoption. The responses to his questions will need sensitive consideration by his adoptive parents. His birth parents will always be part of his life narrative, and this knowledge may mollify a sense of rejection and loss. However, his birth mother was able to care for the other children, and he may question their decision not to care for him. He may also have feelings of remorse or guilt that his needs were too overwhelming to merit their care.

In knowing his birth parents, he is likely to become aware of the differences between them and his adoptive parents, and the ways in which he resembles or is different from each of them. He will need the strong affirmation of his adoptive parents to accept him as he is, including his ethnicity, temperament, racial heritage, and attributes. He will know about his birth parents and his genealogical roots, and will have a different set of relationships with each parent. He will need to work through the potential conflicts of identification and differentiation in the process of identity formation and will benefit from his parents' capacity to support him.

Living at a distance from Nicholas's birth parents, the Weilackers are likely to build strong family boundaries. The adoptive parents are legally

Nicholas's parents, and the decisions about his health care, discipline, nurturance, caregiving, and education are entirely in their hands. It is difficult to know how close or distant the families will become and what points of difference may arise. In many cases, the adoptive family takes strength from the knowledge that the birth mother and father know their child is being taken care of properly (Ryburn, 1994).

An Independent Open Adoption That Did Not Reach Completion

In their beautiful and descriptive memoir, Linda Carbone and Ed Decker describe their difficult, 9-year journey in the attempt to have a biological child through new forms of assisted reproductive technologies (Carbone & Decker, 1999). They narrate the emotional and physical hardships that Linda encountered in undertaking extensive fertility treatment and the toll this took on them as a couple. After three miscarriages, they decided to try to adopt a child in an open adoption, with the assistance of an independent lawyer. In response to newspaper ads, they were contacted by a young high school student in late pregnancy. As soon as the infant was born, they flew to the hospital to meet the birth mother and the baby, whom they already considered their son. Linda and Ed were still recovering from their decision to forego further fertility treatment and were making the transition to the challenge of "loving" an adopted child. When they met the extended family and the birth mother, they were allowed to hold the baby and to begin mentally to claim him as their own. But within a short period of time, during which they relaxed their anxieties about the potential loss of yet another baby, the birth mother changed her mind. The adoptive parents could understand her decision, yet the loss was deeply felt. The heartbroken adoptive father wrote about his feelings when he heard that the adoption would not be completed: "It was like someone had died, although I knew the child was alive and well. But *our* child had died" (Carbone & Decker, 1999, p. 205).

In open adoption the adoptive parents can begin to create a psychological tie with the birth family and the baby before the adoption has been fully decided upon by the birth parent. For those parents who have already experienced the disappointment of infertility or miscarriages, the birth mother changing her mind is yet another blow for which the parents have had little preparation. Some intentional parents continue their search for a child, seeking new directions such as post-foster placement adoption or international adoption. Others benefit from counseling in which they attempt to deal with their grief.

Model II. A Community Adoption Agency and Modified Open Adoption Program

The Children's Home Society in Trenton, New Jersey, has a long history of serving its community. It began as an institution concerned with adoption and the needs of homeless children. Recently, the agency developed a more expansive and open approach to adoption, including a modified and flexible version of open adoption. When birth mothers and fathers seek help, the agency caseworkers describe the various models of open, closed, or modified adoptions and seek the birth parents' opinions as to their preferences and wishes for their child and themselves. Some birth families wish for closure; others wish to be able to have some continuing knowledge about their children. Similarly, the intentional adoptive parents who apply to the agency are interviewed about their interest in participating in open adoption models.

The agency tries to match the wishes of the birth parents with the attitudes and willingness of adoptive parents regarding the nature of the relationship agreed upon between them. The flexible adoption models the agency offers help the birth parents and adoptive parents to choose a plan that is in the best interests of all members of the adoption triad. The agency provides counseling to the young mothers who seek their help. Many of the pregnant young women who approach the Children's Home Society are coping with the adverse effects of poverty, as well as emotional and medical difficulties, including drug addiction. Making a decision about adoption is difficult, but many birth parent(s) feel empowered by having a role in choosing the adoptive parents and being able to know about their child's development. The Children's Home Society has thus constructed a flexible approach to helping birth parent(s) and adoptive parents make plans for adoption. Their policy of lifelong service acknowledges that adoption is a lifetime process, with new questions emerging over time.

The Children's Home Society tries to assess the ability of the dual sets of parents to establish a workable relationship. This process considers many psychological attributes, such as the capacity for empathy and reality testing, the capacity to modulate strong feelings and establish clear role boundaries, and the ability to consider the emotional needs of the growing child. Although the Children's Home Society tries to evaluate the best model for each parent, at times the families cannot continue to live up to their commitments and relationships break down. This is difficult, and the agency is often called upon to provide guidance, information, support, and therapy to either/both the birth parent(s) and/or the adoptive families. If conflict and instability is not resolved, the child can become confused and fearful, and consequently experience waves of turmoil about his/her security and identity (Baumann, 1997; Ryburn, 1994).

Model III. A Full Open Adoption Model in a Family Agency in Northern Michigan

In the last 20 years, a group of adoption agencies in Northern Michigan has created a totally new approach to adoption practice. One such agency, Catholic Human Services in Traverse City, was a leader in the transition from closed to open adoptions. The guiding spirit of this program is the Director of Adoption Services, Jim Gritter, MSW. The grief of birth mothers caused Mr. Gritter to rethink the premises that underlie closed adoption practices. In his books, *Adoption Without Fear* (1989) and *The Spirit of Open Adoption* (1997), Mr. Gritter suggests that the practice of open adoption has profound benefits not only for the birth mother but also for the psychological well-being of all members of the birth triad—the birth parents, the adoptive parents, and the child.

In *The Spirit of Open Adoption*, Gritter (1997, p. 20) describes key aspects of the full open adoption model:

- The birth family selects the adoptive family.
- The families meet each other face-to-face.
- They exchange full identifying information.
- They establish some framework for an ongoing relationship (letters, phone calls, and/or arranged visits).
- The adoptive family has full legal authority as the child's parents and full decision-making power over the best interests of the child.
- Because of the complexity of open adoption, the adoptive parents are asked to participate in intensive group programs to help them understand fully the processes of open adoption. Many services are provided to the adoptive parents during the pre- and postadoptive phases.

Sarah and Her Family

Mr. and Mrs. Van der Haagen became part of the agency's open adoption program with some apprehension and uncertainty. They experienced the anxiety of not being chosen a number of times and often became frustrated and discouraged with the length of time it was taking to adopt a child. After a year, they were told of the possibility of adopting a baby from a young unwed mother named Phoebe, who was in her eighth month of pregnancy.

They met the birth mother and soon overcame their nervousness. The parents eloquently recall the first meeting: "The impact of the meeting was dramatic. We did not realize it at that time, but that meeting linked us forever as family. Our worlds had grown in a profound manner" (in Gritter, 1989, pp. 11–12). The parents met again at the hospital when Sarah was born. Although letters and photographs were exchanged after the adoption, the families did not meet again until Sarah was 3 years old.

Phoebe had made significant progress in her life and wished to see Sarah. The family had shared with Sarah the birth narrative. A precocious and secure little girl, Sarah opened the door when her birth mother arrived and said, "Hi, I'm Sarah. You must be Phoebe. Come on in. This is my Mom. Her name is Julie . . . This is my Dad. His name is Ric. And here is my baby sister, Laura. She's adopted too. . . . " Later on, Sarah turned to her adoptive mother and said, "Mom, did you know that I started in Phoebe's tummy?" (in Gritter, 1989, p.12).

This anecdote reveals that at age 3, Sarah had a strong sense of family identity and a firm sense of connectedness to her adoptive mother and father. She also had already begun to incorporate her birth narrative into the telling of her "life story" and had a positive sense of self within the special nature of her family history. Yet the full meaning of the adoption remained concrete, and only later would she begin to understand the more complex issues involved. As Sarah grew, she wondered which characteristics she had inherited from which parent, noting that she probably got her patience from Pheobe but her "silliness" from her dad. The adoptive parents were able to respond to Sarah's increasingly complex questions about her dual heritage, including some challenges relating to their parental authority. The Van der Haagens were confident in their role as parents for Sarah and her sister. Mrs. Van der Haagen commented on her feelings about being Sarah's mother and the efforts she and her husband made to clarify their role:

> "We sense a concern that if our daughters have two sets of parents there is confusion of parental authority. But we are confident in our roles as nurturing parents and know that Phoebe would never undercut our authority with Sarah. We also sense that people fear there must be competition for Sarah's and Laura's love between the two families. But this simply has not happened. In the beginning of Sarah's relationship with Phoebe, Sarah questioned me. 'Are you always going to be my mom?' And 'Could I ever live with Phoebe?' With reassurances and explanations that I was her mom but that Phoebe would always be a special person in her life, she settled it in her mind that she was, in her words, 'lucky to have two moms to love.' " (in Gritter, 1989, p. 14)

Not all parents have the inner security to approach open adoption relationships with the same assurance and good sense as occurred in Sarah's family. Sarah was also a resilient and thoughtful child, and able to cope, with her parent's help, in understanding her dual heritage, and to differentiate between the roles of her two mothers. She grew up to be a talented and accomplished young person, with a coherent sense of her dual heritage that combined her distinctive relationships with both her biological and adoptive parents.

DISCUSSION

The practice of open adoptions constitutes a major change in our society's way of thinking about the relationships among all members of the adoption triad. While there are many potential difficulties in this new form of adoption, the different models of open adoption allow birth parents and adoptive parents to choose the pathway that is most appropriate for themselves. At the same time, the open adoption model may not be suitable or best for all birth parents or adoptive families (Berry, 1993). For example, a closed adoption may help some birth parents cope more effectively with their grief, while others are comforted by the opportunity to have knowledge of, or contact with, their child over time (Berry, 1993; A. Brodzinsky, 1990).

While some adoptive parents may fear that open adoption may bring intrusion into their lives and create conflict and confusion for their children, others feel that knowing the birth parents may help them understand their child more empathetically and be of more assistance to their child. Advocates of open adoption suggest that the great potential advantage is that children sense their roots as expansive rather than constricted. The sense of abandonment may not be so profound if the child has a more "knowing" sense of his/her birth parents (Baran & Pannor, 1990).

In open adoptions, parents find they can communicate more openly with their children about their feelings and questions regarding their birth history and the meaning of adoption (Baumann, 1997). Practitioners state that the continued relationship with birth parent(s) contributes to children's developmental well-being. In this regard, children may achieve a greater sense of self-worth and self-esteem, an improved capacity to integrate their dual heritage, a greater ability to complete their search for identity, and a more coherent view of themselves as young adults (Baumann, 1997).

The glue that holds this new set of relationships together in open adoption is the ability of the adoptive parents and the birth parents to form a relationship that addresses the reality of their roles and is built on a shared concern for the well-being of their child. Clearly, a modicum of goodwill between the birth parents and the adoptive parents is necessary. As the child matures, he/she may express a new range of ambivalent feelings about his/her complex family world. Sensitivity and common sense are required on the part of birth and adoptive parents to understand the changing emotional issues confronting the child. Psychotherapy, guidance, and support can address the needs of the child and/or the parents at moments of maturational crises (A. Brodzinsky, 1990).

In their book, *Adoption and the Family System: Strategies for Treatment*, Reitz and Watson (1992) conclude that the three most critical issues of closed adoptions are unresolved losses by both adoptees and birth parents, denial by the child and his/her family of the dual family ties, and diminished self-esteem of the adoptees and birthparents. Open adoption is thought to decrease the negative effects of each of these identified processes. While many problems need to be resolved, each member of the triad, while struggling with deep human issues, has the opportunity to develop a compassionate understanding of the others (Baumann, 1997).

Finally, there is the matter of the rights of individuals to have access to their genealogical history. Randolph Severson has addressed this topic in the following words: "With regard to open records and open adoptions, it does not matter whether adoption harms or helps, whether it wounds or cures, whether it solves problems or creates them. The essential point is that every human being on the face of the earth has the right to look into the eyes of those from whom they drew life and to whom they gave life and to know their names and stories; . . . no human law or convention has the right to deny them this inalienable human right" (Severson, 1994, p. 112).

Kirk has described the nature of the relationship between adopted children, their birth parents, and their adoptive parents as being a shared fate (Kirk, 1964). In adoption, the parental families have shared a common human effort to provide care that is in the best interests of their child. Open adoption may more easily allow for the creation of empathetic bonds between members of the adoption triad in the face of loss and difficult human decisions. Furthermore, in the minds of adopted children, the relationship between their two sets of parents represents a symbolic acceptance of their birth history, their dual heritage, and, by implication, themselves.

III

Assisted Reproductive Technology and Family Formation

8

Social and Scientific Changes in the Formation of Families

In 1978, dramatic changes occurred in the science of human reproduction. Louise Brown became the first infant born as a result of a new clinical application of assisted reproductive technology (ART) known as *in vitro fertilization* (IVF). She was the first "test tube" baby, and her birth transformed the way we think about conception, birth, and the meaning of family. Since that time, ART has flourished and many new clinical procedures have been developed. At the current time, these procedures are used by approximately 15% of infertile couples in the United States and by many single women and gay and lesbian families. The growth of the clinical practice of ART in the United States since the birth of Louise Brown is evident in the following statistics (Institute for Science, Law, and Technology Working Group, 1998).

- Approximately 75,000 babies are born annually through the use of ART.
- Approximately 60,000 of these births result from donor insemination.
- Fifteen thousand of these births result from the use of IVF in the laboratory.
- At least one thousand births per year occur through surrogate or gestational parenthood, and this number is increasing each year.

The numbers of infants born through ART is now twice the number of infants available for adoption at birth. National data reveal that during the late 1990s, only 30,000 healthy infants were available for adoption at birth each year, and this number could not meet the demand of parents eager to adopt a healthy infant. More infertile couples are using ART in their efforts to have a child, although the rates of success are modest, and vary a good deal from clinic to clinic, and from individual to individual (Institute for Science, Law, and Technology Working Group, 1998).

The new advances in our understanding of the biological mechanisms of human reproduction and associated clinical interventions have broadened the opportunity of many families to consider having a child. The separation of conception from intimate sexuality and the possibility of collaborative parenthood, however, have raised many important psychological, legal, and ethical questions about the concept of the family. Furthermore, for parenthood, the clinical possibilities now available through ART have changed the long-standing norm that marriage and biological parenthood provide the basic definition of the family. In addition, because of the social and scientific changes in our society, single parents, lesbian and gay families, heterosexual couples with infertility problems, and those families with medical or genetic diseases may now consider having a much-wanted child. In this context, the legal and ethical issues that have arisen underscore the importance of reproductive rights and acknowledge that family life is a major aspect of self-fulfillment and self-identity.

This chapter provides an overview of the medical and psychological issues that occur in the formation of families through new forms of parentage made possible through ART practices. The evolving development of these new clinical practices in human reproduction has significantly transformed how we think about the formation of families and the meaning of parenthood. The rapid revolution that has taken place in the last generation is still in the process of change. As a result, clinical knowledge is still accumulating, even as new scientific possibilities emerge. As yet, there is scant study and less than full understanding of the psychological implications of ART for parents and children (Macklin, 1994b).

The new pathways to parenthood made possible by ART offer hope to many intentional parents. However, the process of becoming a parent using ART can qualitatively change the traditional phases of conception, pregnancy, and birth. Because of these new experiences, many families confront unique questions about the construction of parenthood and the formation of a family identity. Families face difficult medical experiences and often have spent years working through the painful problems of infertility and other barriers to their parenthood prior to their decision to use ART. Subsequently, they may experience *years* of uncertainty, and the hopeful birth mother may also undergo painful and time-consuming medical treatment that can result in stressful, dynamic reactions within the family (Domar, 1997; Hodder, 1997). Couples frequently seek the guidance and support of family therapists, medical social workers, or other clinicians during their efforts to become parents. They do so to help them explore the sometimes difficult medical and personal choices they face, including the decision to forego further treatment and consider other alternatives (Leiblum, 1997).

Intentional parents who take advantage of ART generally receive good medical care from their physicians. However, less attention is given to the psychological issues and family problems that can occur during the "trying" years of treatment. Furthermore, while the joy of the arrival of a healthy baby after years of committed effort is genuine, parents are often beset by the emotional aftereffects of the long quest. In addition, new and unanticipated questions can emerge regarding the ways in which the complex birth history of their child has affected their perception of themselves as parents. Furthermore, the children may eventually need help in understanding particular facets of their complex birth history (Burns & Covington, 1999).

In a wider social sense, new forms of ART have led to the need for a broader definition of the family itself, since these techniques can be used by infertile couples, single parents, and gay and lesbian couples, as well as couples who wish to circumvent family genetic disorders. Thus, these technologies have allowed for new social configurations of parenthood and family. For example, IVF has made it possible to approach the formation of a family by recruiting egg and or sperm donors and/or a surrogate gestational mother who carries the baby to term. Thus, these new technologies can increase the number of "parents" involved in the process of birth, gestation, and caregiving. Genetic parents, who have provided sperm and ova, may, for example, be different than the gestational parent who carries the neonate to term, or the caregiving parent who nurtures the baby from birth onward. These factors create the necessity of considering anew the meaning of parenthood and the genetic, social, and psychological meaning of family (Beauchamp & Walters, 1994).

The clinicians who respond to a family's request for emotional help, therefore, must become familiar with the clinical, physical, and emotional issues underlying ART. Clinicians working in this field have much to learn from the parents themselves as they reflect on the meaning of parenthood within the context of using socially and/or clinically new paths to family formation. They are the experts whose narratives can teach us much about the emotional and psychological aspects of the new technology.

This chapter attempts to weave together the medical and clinical processes of ART and the meaning of complex birth heritage and family identity for the developing child. We review some of the clinical aspects of ART, including the dynamic impact of these new forms of human reproduction on the social and psychological formation of a family. Two primary developmental tasks faced by all parents are the establishment of a sense of family identity and the achievement of a secure relationship with their child. For families, these tasks are made more difficult by the sometimes complex biological origins of the child and the subsequent impact of ART on family relationships.

THE COMPLEX MEANING OF "FAMILY"

The very definition of "family" is undergoing a transformation in response to a wide range of changes in society (Mintz & Kellogg, 1988). The social norms that define what is "normal" or "acceptable" in family life have always been in a dynamic state of change as family structures respond to the social and economic conditions of the times. For example, historian Lawrence Stone (1979) has provided some perspective on the shift in the meaning of "family" over time by focusing on the social changes in British family life and the evolving social role of the family from the 16th century onward. As Stone points out, in earlier times, the family was more likely to be thought of as a legal and economic unit, with sharply defined work and gender roles. Children were seen primarily as important members of the economic household. The parents were viewed as having ultimate authority over their offspring, and child care was often repressive and harsh. In addition, children's biological ties to their parents were a major legal criterion for family belonging and an important factor in children's rights to the family name and inheritance.

Over time, however, family cultural norms adapted to the changing economic, cultural, and social life of the community. In comparison with earlier conceptions of the family, the modern Western nuclear family has greater autonomy over itself, according its members a greater degree of privacy and freedom of choice over the formation of their own families. Furthermore, families came to have greater latitude as to how to raise children as long as the children were taken care of within reasonable, protective limits. In addition, there came to be a greater emphasis on the affective or emotional ties between parents and their children (Stone, 1979).

More recently, new forms of childbearing made possible by the evolving science and clinical potential of ART have presented a particular challenge to the narrow biological definitions of parenthood. An increased understanding of the concept of psychological parenthood challenged the narrow biological definition of the family (Macklin, 1994b). The psychological parents, who will be known to the child, are those intentional parents that claim the child as a part of their ongoing family and eagerly look forward to establishing a special, long-term psychological relationship with that child (Levine, 1990).

With the advent of new forms of ART, the biological birth narratives of children are often more complex, as their genealogical roots can be more elaborate. In adoption and certain types of ART, biological relationships are no longer an adequate basis of family identity. As a result, the legal definition of the family is being expanded to deal with the many new forms of parentage occurring through complex adoption and various forms of ART. For example, where there are different sets of biological and psychological parents, society must decide who will be considered to be the "legal parent" of the child. Some scholars have suggested that family adoption law be used as a model for solving the new legal problems arising from the use of ART, such as the rights of the gestational mother vis-à-vis the rights of the intentional parents (Capron & Radin, 1988; Levine, 1990).

Despite the growing cultural acceptance of nontraditional families, current laws continue to provide support primarily to heterosexual couples in marriage. Lesbian and gay families, for example, do not have the right to marry at this time, although in April 2000, Vermont established a "civil union" that provides some legal recognition to this new family form (Goldberg, 2000). These nontraditional couples have frequently faced difficulties in forming families through adoption and in many cases have been denied access to the clinical services of reproductive clinics. Nevertheless, lesbian and gay couples and individuals are slowly being accepted as adoptive parents and are now also gaining access to ART clinics (Andrews, 1999; Hodder, 1997; Sullivan, 1995a).

Many observers believe that the significant changes now occurring in family formation require a broader social and psychological view of the family and expansion of the biological, legal, and cultural frameworks currently being used. For families who wish to have a child, and use ART to do so, the act of forming a family requires much long-term effort, thought, and financial resources. Moreover, the process of becoming a parent can in these cases include physical risk for the birth mother and emotional pain for the intentional parents. Whether the intentional parents are a married couple dealing with infertility problems or a lesbian or gay couple or individual wishing to safely have a biologically related child, the act of creating a new infant is a very active one. As with traditional families, the family has a prebirth psychological commitment to claim the child as its own. The meaning of the family in this sense is thus a subjective commitment; it is certainly this commitment that forms the basis of the parents' definition of their family (Capron & Radin, 1988; Levine, 1990).

The Importance of Having a Child

Many scholars and clinicians who study the family have tried to understand the deep personal and emotional reasons that underlie the importance of having a child, and the special meaning that may be attached to bearing a child (Murray, 1996; Strong, 1997). Developmental perspectives across the lifecycle, for example, consider parenthood an important role in identity formation and a step in the process of growing into mature adulthood (Benedek, 1959; Erikson, 1950). It is also an empirical fact that both men and women who realize that they may not be able to have their own biological children may experience a sense of shock, deep loss, and a long period of mourning (Domar, 1997; Tobin, 1998). Those families who have not been able to conceive a child through the medical resources available sometimes readjust their yearning for a biological child and move on to consider the possibility of adoption. Others remain emotionally committed to go to any and all lengths to have a child that is at least partially biologically related (Bartholet, 1993).

The philosopher Carson Strong (1997), who has studied the variety of reasons that people actually give for having a birth child, has identified the following six interrelated reasons:

1. *Participation in the creation of a person.* The idea of creating a child has certain spiritual overtones that go beyond the drive for biological reproduction. There seems to be great satisfaction in the opportunity to create a new human being and thereby contribute a new life to the long stream of human history. Having a baby is symbolic of establishing one's own self as a separate part of the family heritage, as well as identifying with the parental role.

2. *Affirmation of mutual love within a relationship.* Having a baby with another can be an affirmation of a couple's mutual love and acceptance. There is anticipation that by choosing a partner with whom to conceive a child, the couple's bond will be strengthened. These issues are present in both heterosexual couples and lesbian and gay couples, although conception and or gestation relies on very different circumstances in the latter families.

3. *Contribution to sexual intimacy.* Sexual intimacy is deepened when

a couple makes love in a manner that is open to procreation. The loss of this intimacy when conception is separated from sexuality and achieved through artificial insemination, or in a laboratory through IVF, is a concern to some couples and to some religious doctrines. The Catholic Church, for example, believes that the use of such technologies undermines the unity and the procreative purposes of marriage and sexuality and, indeed, violates the sacramental covenant of marriage (McCormick, 1981).

4. *Link to future persons.* Many couples feel that through their children, they will have a link to future generations and immortality, although certainly this link is only one way individuals can contribute to future generations.

5. *Experience of pregnancy and childbirth.* Many women desire the experiences of pregnancy and childbirth for a wide array of reasons. While there are many physical strains related to pregnancy, increased social and emotional support are often present during this period. The responses by family, friends, and society at large communicate approval and validation of the traditional role of motherhood. Finally, pregnancy often provides a significant opportunity for maturation and identity formation. The arrival of a grandchild is often much sought by awaiting grandparents, and this need frequently influences the intentional parents.

6. *Experience of child rearing.* Child rearing, a creative act, is felt by some to be one of life's most rewarding experiences. The relationship with their dependent child provides parents with a new opportunity for self-fulfillment and a broader self-identity.

These social, psychological, and philosophical reasons partially explain why the experience of having children is so highly valued. It is clear that the experience of parenthood is so important that people who face barriers to childbearing often experience this news as a personal wound and suffer deep grief reactions (Leiblum & Greenfeld, 1997). Furthermore, the desire to have a family may also be deeply felt by persons in untraditional marriages, namely, single, unmarried women and lesbian and gay couples. The new forms of ART and the broader social acceptance of different forms of families have given rise to these persons' ability to pursue the possibility of parenthood (see Chapter 10).

Access to ART is not always a straightforward matter. There is an ongoing debate in this country as to whether infertility is an impairment or a disease. At the moment, many health insurance plans do not provide coverage for infertility treatment. There is no federal framework that assures the rights of families' access to ART clinics. This has diminished the ability of poorer families to deal with infertility problems. In addition, some ART clinics still do not accept single parents and lesbian or gay parents as candidates for treatment (Institute for Science, Law, and Technology Working Group, 1998).

In summary, some bioethicists believe that the "freedom to procreate" should be available to all who wish to try to bear a child, because having a child has deep existential meaning for many individuals and can contribute to life satisfaction and the full realization of self-identity and self-fulfillment (Strong, 1997).

AN OVERVIEW OF MEDICAL AND PSYCHOLOGICAL ISSUES IN INFERTILITY

Because infertility is relatively widespread, many couples must cope with the realization that becoming pregnant and having a family will not come easily. In 1995, the National Survey of Family Growth (NSFG) found that in the United States, an estimated 2.1 million married couples were infertile (Abma, 1997). This particular definition of infertility applied when a family had not conceived after at least 12 months' unprotected intercourse. Using this definition, 7.1% of the almost 30 million married couples with wives of childbearing age were deemed infertile. However, if a 2-year period is considered, the number of families reporting infertility decreases significantly (Abma, 1997).

The reasons for infertility are many, and prospective mothers and fathers must undergo extensive diagnostic procedures to pinpoint the specific nature of their problems. It is estimated that male infertility is the primary cause in one-third of couples with infertility problems and a contributory cause in another one-third (Swerdloff, Overstreet, Sokol, & Raifer, 1985). Although many social observers have the impression that infertility has been on the rise, the overall fertility rate in the United States has remained relatively stable during the last 30 years. There is some indication that primary infertility or difficulty in having a first child, has increased due to delays in the age at which women may begin to start a family and the possible effect of untreated sexually transmitted infections.

New York State Task Force on Life and the Law (1998) offers the following definitions commonly used in studies of infertility:

- *Fertility:* The ability to conceive a pregnancy.
- *Fecundity:* The ability to conceive a pregnancy and carry it to term.
- *Infertility:* The difficulty in achieving conception.

- *Impaired fecundity:* The difficulty in carrying a pregnancy to term, including situations in which pregnancy has been deemed medically risky for the woman and/or her offspring.
- *Primary infertility:* Infertility in persons who have never had children.
- *Secondary infertility:* Infertility in persons who have already had children. This condition increases with age and difficulties inherent in the production of healthy ova.
- *Female sterility:* Permanent infertility due to structural problems.
- *Surgical infertility:* The inability to conceive or carry a pregnancy to term as a result of surgery, such as a tubal ligation of the woman or a vasectomy of the male, or other medical conditions, such as endometriosis, fibroid tumors, or cancer.
- *Male infertility:* Sperm may be abnormal in density, shape, or motility and in some cases be unable to penetrate and fertilize the ova. In other cases, genetic conditions may cause the absence of sperm.

Female infertility problems can occur in all phases of conception and gestation, that is, during the 9 months of pregnancy. The diagnostic procedures to assess the reasons for female infertility are often lengthy and painful. Hierarchy of diagnostic and treatment approaches, from less intrusive to more intrusive methods, may be required to assess and treat the problem fully. There are many reasons for female infertility, such as hormonal deficits that affect the production of a healthy ovum in the monthly cycle; structural abnormalities; untreated infections; scarring; blocked fallopian tubes, and other genetic medical conditions. Furthermore, as a woman ages and approaches menopause, both the production of healthy ova and the ability to carry an infant to term may decrease, resulting in a higher frequency of miscarriages. It has also been found that lifestyle habits, such as smoking, anorexia or obesity, excessive alcohol, caffeine, or drugs, as well as environmental toxins, can cause both male and female infertility. Each condition requires a special approach to treatment, often including a lengthy process of successive clinical interventions (Keye, 1999).

Before the advent of ART, physicians offered a range of treatments to infertile women: prevention strategies; education regarding sexually transmitted diseases; safer contraceptive planning; reproductive education; medical treatments, such as the treatment of infections; hormonal treatment to increase ovulation; and the treatment of structural problems through surgical repair. If traditional approaches fail, couples may now consider ART procedures that seek to establish a pregnancy without necessarily correcting the basic structural problems that previously prevented pregnancy from occurring.

In the past, artificial insemination by donor was the only way families could deal with male infertility. In the late 1990s, new discoveries enabled pregnancies to occur, the most promising being intracytoplasmic sperm injection (ICSI), in which a viable sperm is identified and, using microsurgery, directly injected into an ova that has been retrieved from the birth mother. These methods are costly and researchers are still assessing the risks to the fetus and the child (New York State Task Force on Life and the Law, 1998).

ASSISTED REPRODUCTIVE TECHNOLOGY

In Vitro Fertilization: A Watershed in the Treatment of Infertility

In 1978 the birth in England of Louise Brown—the world's first "test tube baby"—marked a turning point in the treatment of infertility. Her birth history captured the world's attention. For the first time, a woman with blocked fallopian tubes, who could not be helped by conventional surgery, conceived a child through a process that became known as *in vitro* fertilization (IVF). Louise's father's sperm and her mother's ova were placed in a petri dish in a laboratory setting, fertilization occurred, and the resulting embryo was implanted in her mother's uterus. Since Louise's birth more than 20 years ago, 300,000 children have been created through various techniques of IVF (Institute for Science, Law, and Technology Working Group, 1998).

IVF generally refers to a group of procedures that involve the fertilization of an ovum outside the human body. In the standard form of IVF, a woman's ovaries are stimulated by drugs to produce 10–20 eggs rather than the usual one or two produced monthly. When mature, these ova are surgically "harvested," or removed, from the ovaries. These ova are exceedingly small, so that the process of retrieval requires considerable skill and experience. The use of drugs to hyperstimulate the ovaries can produce significant emotional and physical side effects in the woman, and the surgical removal of the eggs can be painful.

Each egg is then combined with 75,000 to 100,000 sperm in a glass petri dish—hence *in vitro*, or in "glass"—where fertilization may occur. If two nuclei are visible in the egg overnight, fertilization has occurred. Two or three days later, the embryos are ready for transfer back to the woman's uterus, or to the fallopian tubes, depending on the medical diagnosis. Considerable scientific and medical expertise is required to complete the procedure of embryo implantation successfully.

Clearly, the birth mother must be involved as an active participant in the preparations required for ovulation and the harvesting of her ova and in the process of implantation of the eggs into her body. The procedures are strenuous and often interfere with her life or work on a daily basis. She needs to be available for the medical technicians to monitor her status, so that the harvesting of her eggs occurs at the right moment. After fertilization of the egg, reimplantation, or embryo transfer, is attempted. This sensitive procedure also requires special monitoring of the prospective mother in order to ascertain the optimal time for implanting the embryo into the uterus. Timing is critical to the success of sustaining the pregnancy (Caplan, 1994; Leiblum, 1997).

For the intentional parents, waiting to see if implantation is successful is extremely anxiety provoking. Women who are involved in infertility programs using IVF usually participate in more than one monthly cycle, and the rate of success varies between 23% and 29%, depending on the nature of the problem, the procedures used, the age of the woman, the skills of the clinicians, and other technical determinants. It has been shown that emotional factors such as depression and anxiety can have an impact on the process, indicating that women undergoing these procedures often need significant emotional support (Hodder, 1997).

Other Procedures

Other procedures have been developed to increase the chance of successful implantation and pregnancy. In gamete intrafallopian transfer (GIFT), the gametes—unfertilized ova and sperm—are procured and transferred to the fallopian tube, the natural site for fertilization. In zygote intrafallopian transfer (ZIFT), the ova and sperm are mixed *in vitro*, and the resulting zygotes are then transferred to the fallopian tube. Statistics reveal that there is a slightly greater chance that implantation in the uterus will occur with these procedures (New York State Task Force on Life and the Law, 1998). In addition, new techniques for freezing embryos created *in vitro* enable clinicians to implant them in the intentional mother's uterus at a later date. Thus, if the first implantation attempt fails, the woman does not have to continue to undergo the difficult process of harvesting eggs, and transfer of the embryo can occur at an appropriate time. A key issue in infertility is the differential diagnosis in matching the procedures with the unique needs of each patient (U.S. Department of Health and Human Services, 1999).

THE PSYCHOLOGICAL AND PHYSICAL EXPERIENCE OF PREGNANCY THROUGH ASSISTED REPRODUCTIVE TECHNOLOGY

Many couples experience infertility as a deep psychological wound, and the realization that the problem lies with one partner or another is painful. It is not unusual for husband and wife to experience a time of anticipatory mourning for the loss of biological parenthood. The road to parenthood is now unclear, and many couples face a long and often uncertain journey as they try numerous cycles of treatment or consider other alternatives, such as adoption or putting aside their wishes to have children. Clinicians observe that men and women often deal with this difficult news in very different ways. Generally, established patterns of defenses that are used to cope with loss and disappointment come into play as each partner copes with the unexpected narcissistic injury he/she experiences (Domar, 1997).

The symbolic meaning of infertility is also often different for men and women. The hopeful father may feel that his virility has been diminished, while the hopeful mother may feel that she has lost the central core of her feminine identity. Clinicians observe that there is a tendency for men to keep their feelings more to themselves and for women to express their sadness and anxiety, and reach out for comfort (Meyers et al., 1995a, 1995b). The tension between husband and wife may increase as the process of treatment becomes more difficult, and family or individual treatment may be sought. About half of the couples who receive a diagnosis of a major infertility problem seek further medical help (Tobin, 1998).

The use of ART often subjects the intentional birth mother to prolonged exposure to difficult procedures, including hormonal treatment, continuous monitoring of blood levels, daily hospital visits, ultrasounds, and the precise regimen needed for the harvesting of eggs and conception. These treatments affect her both physically and psychologically. Intimate feelings of sexuality, generally part of the act of conception, may become secondary to the more mechanical *in vitro* methods used. The emotional tone of the family is likely to change during this time of complete devotion to the goal of conception, as husband and wife cope with their separate burdens. The separation of sexuality from conception can begin to interfere in the feelings between husband and wife; at times, the family is overwhelmed by the effort. Nevertheless, despite the hardships, IVF gives approximately one-fourth of infertile couples the opportunity to deliver a healthy infant and to enter a phase of their life that they have sought—genetic and psychological parenthood (Braverman, 1997; U.S. Department of Health and Human Services, 1999).

Case Vignette

The experiences of Tom and Katherine Canfield illustrate the enormous effort it takes for a family to have a child through IVF. One of the most advanced IVF techniques helped Mrs. Canfield and her husband to have a child. After enduring two miscarriages and 4 years of arduous and expensive hormone therapy, Mr. and Mrs. Canfield were in a state of loss and despair because of their inability to have a baby. They were encouraged to approach a fertility and endocrinology clinician. After diagnostic testing, the physician decided to try one of the newer IVF techniques, cryopreservation, or the freezing of embryos, and started Mrs. Canfield on drugs to stimulate ovulation. The eggs were harvested, and fertilized with her husband's sperm *in vitro*. The resulting embryos were frozen to await the right moment for implantation. The physician used this technique to allow the drug-induced imbalance in Mrs. Canfield's body to abate, so that the embryos would have a better chance of implantation in her uterus. Mrs. Canfield gave birth to a healthy little girl, Emma, and later on to a son, through the same process. Despite the long, multiple hardships, she felt that the births of her daughter and son were miraculous (*People* magazine, 1998).

The family needed to have strength to sustain both their psychological and physical health during the 4 difficult years of extensive hormonal treatment and the processes of IVF. They had experienced the painful loss of two miscarriages and spoke of their despair "in their quest to have a baby" ("Miracle Babies," *People* magazine, 1998, p. 69). Their adaptive resilience, excellent medical care, and financial resources helped sustain them. They joyfully became the biological and psychological parents of their daughter and son, but the resonance of both the wonder and the endurance needed in overcoming infertility remains a part of their family narrative and parental senses of self (Tobin, 1998).

IVF: ETHICAL, MEDICAL, AND LEGAL ISSUES

As soon as IVF procedures became accepted practice for treating infertility, researchers raised questions as to the potential ethical implications of this new form of parentage and expressed concern for the health of the parents and infants. Some observers worried that the "asexual" reproduction would forever change the relationship between parents and children. In addition, many ethical and legal issues have arisen regarding the moral and legal status of created embryos. Three particular areas of concern were described by the New York Task Force on Life and the Law (1998): (1)

multiple births, (2) disposition of unused embryos, and (3) the legal status of frozen embryos.

Multiple Births

A serious issue in IVF procedures is the high probability of multiple births because of physicians' practice of placing a group of embryos into the uterus of the mother, in order to raise the chances that at least one will implant and a pregnancy will occur. Multiple pregnancies present significant risks to the birth mother and the fetus, including a high risk of premature birth and medical complications. Data reveal that of all ART births, 38% are multiples compared to less than 3% in the general population (U.S. Department of Health and Human Services, 1999). Many ethicists now recommend that physicians limit the transfer of embryos per cycle to four (Andrews, 1999). The Association for Reproductive Medicine has suggested that quadruplet pregnancy, or higher, should be discouraged because of the health hazard to the fetus and the birth mother. Physicians may ask the parents to consider reducing the number of embryos by a technical process of selective reduction (i.e., some of the embryos will be aborted). This is a difficult choice, and some parents cannot agree on religious or moral grounds (New York Task Force on Life and the Law, 1998).

The new clinical field of human reproduction exists in an environment where there are no federal regulations regarding the oversight of clinical procedures, and no federally financed research that focuses on this arena. While many states are developing guidelines for clinics regarding certain dimensions of care, only Virginia and New Hampshire have enacted regulations to protect families from potentially harmful situations. For example, until recently, clinics were not asked to disclose success rates of various procedures so that families did not have adequate information upon which to make decisions (Institute for Science, Law, and Technology Working Group, 1998).

Disposition of Unneeded Embryos

Sometimes, more embryos are produced than are used, and no federal standards outline how fertility clinics may use left over embryos or the nature of the role of parental consent in this regard. Some states recommend that clinics should be required to disclose all options for dealing with the "excess" embryos to the intentional parents who should be empowered to choose between indefinite storage of the embryo, use by another couple, use in medical research, or destruction. Clearly, these choices raise many ethical and legal issues.

The Legal Status of Frozen Embryos

The questions here concern the legal status and ownership of the embryos either following a divorce or the death of one of or both donors of the gamete or ova and sperm. A number of unusual cases have been brought before the courts, in which a gamete donor sued for custody of the embryo following divorce or the death of a partner. These are very complicated issues, and state ethics committees and the courts are working through the many ethical, legal, and personal issues involved in developing policies that keep in mind the interests of the various parental figures.

COLLABORATIVE PARENTHOOD: IMPLICATIONS REGARDING FAMILY IDENTITY

In nonstandard IVF, the intentional parents are helped to create a child through a form of collaborative parenthood. As we have already noted, infertility problems can exist in either parent and affect the different phases of conception and gestation. The intentional parents may need to use the sperm and/or ova of a donor, or may require the use of a surrogate and/or gestational mother to carry the baby to term. In this sense, the "collaborative" experience may be either "partial" or "full," but in either case, it often requires *in vitro* methods for conception.

In the full collaborative effort, a child may have five parental figures: a genetic sperm donor; a female ova donor; and a surrogate/gestational birth mother as well as the intentional parents waiting to claim the baby as their own. These distinct roles are sometimes called the *genetic parent*, the *gestational parent*, and the *social parent*. Thus, the biological heritage and genealogical roots of the child are complicated (Macklin, 1994a). The particular ART procedures that are used will have an imprint on the child's birth narrative. There are actually 16 different sets of procedures by which the genetic, gestational, and psychological parents can engage in the cooperative effort to create a child using various forms of IVF (see Appendix 8.1).

Fatherhood and the Use of a Sperm Donor

In the past, when male infertility was diagnosed, the family's only solution to having a child was to consider artificial insemination by donor (AID). The technological advances in ART, however, have changed the process of sperm donor insemination. The current success rate of donor insemination is relatively high, with 45–75% of fertile women becoming pregnant within nine cycle attempts (Emond & Scheib, 1998). In previous practice, the donated sperm was "freshly produced" and quickly used. The new ability to freeze donated sperm has improved the safety of this approach by allowing certain screening procedures. The frozen sperm can be stored in a sperm bank, giving the clinic time to ascertain the health of the donor for medical illnesses such as AIDS and/or particular genetic risks. Reputable donor clinics now usually take a lengthy medical and social history of the donor, including racial, religious, physical, medical, and academic attributes. When a family selects a particular donor, the sperm can be injected into the woman's uterus by a physician or by the intentional parents themselves, in the privacy of their home. Some families select a sperm donor whom they know; others have only the biographical information provided by the donor clinic.

Usually, the psychological meaning of the use of AID within the family has different meanings to the husband and wife. The birth mother and her husband may face different concerns about the urgency of having a child. Because of the mother's sensitivity to her own "biological clock," she may wish to become pregnant before her husband has had time to resolve his grief about his own infertility. Many partners bear this experience privately and cannot easily talk to each other about their feelings. For the husband, it may be especially hard to find the words to explain his grief reaction to the loss of the experience of biological fatherhood. Clinical experience suggests that if the parents can express their feelings to each other and find a way to come to terms with the compromise they have had to make in forming their family, both father and mother may be more attuned to each other regarding the advent of parenthood and the joy of relating to their child (Meyers et al., 1995b).

The use of AID has a psychological impact on the family in that parents have to deal with the symbolic meaning of infertility. The psychological father has a special task in establishing a secure sense of his paternal role. This may be difficult given the absence of biological relatedness to his child and the meaning this has for him. In addition, two new questions emerge in this context: What is the legal status of fatherhood for the husband and the sperm donor? How open will the family be about the child's birth heritage?

Legal Issues

Within a marriage in which AID is used, the husband of the birth mother is declared to be the legal father of the child, and his name is on the birth certificate. Moreover, the donor is legally absolved of all parental responsibility. The sperm donor's identity is safeguarded and will be protected indefinitely. His medical history often can be accessed by the family if a particular concern arises in the future. Therefore, for all intents and purposes, the husband is the primary legal and psychological father of the child. This practice of sealing the identity of the father is similar to sealing the identity of birth parents in adoption. Just as open adoption practices have changed, however, so may practices regarding sperm donor identity change in the future (Andrews, 1999; Macklin, 1994a).

Disclosure to the Child

In all cases, parents need to consider whether they will disclose the shared genetic parentage to their child (Klock, 1997). The issue of keeping the genetic history of the child a secret is a difficult one. On the one hand, parents may wish to preserve their privacy about a very sensitive issue; on the other hand, they may worry about the future effect on the child and the family if such an important issue is concealed. It might become important to share this knowledge if an illness required a full genetic medical history.

A hypothetical case illustrates the ways in which many nonbiological fathers cope with their preparations for the psychological role of fatherhood. This vignette is a composite of accounts in the literature (Burns & Covington, 1999; Leiblum, 1997; Meyers et al., 1995b).

Case Vignette

Mr. Davids had a strong grief reaction when he learned of his infertility. His wife, dealing with her own fears that she was getting older and might have waited too long to become pregnant, decided to become impregnated with the help of a sperm donor clinic before Mr. Davids had time to resolve his grief and ambivalence. The couple sought therapeutic help when Mr. Davids expressed his ambivalence about creating a family through a sperm donor.

Mr. Davids articulated his unease and anxiety about the fact that he would not be the genetic father of his child. Although he said that he had always wanted a family, it was disturbing to him that his wife was carrying a baby that was an outcome of sperm donated by another man. He was unsure whether he could become attached to the child or the child would become attached to him. He felt that he needed the child to know, almost at birth, that he was not the biological father. He did not want to keep this a secret for fear that the child would eventually find out and feel betrayed.

The family sought therapy and painful issues emerged, but the therapy was also helpful in that both husband and wife could share the depths of their feelings and the very different ways they felt about their losses regarding the issues of infertility. They dealt with many questions about their relationship as a couple and the husband's worry that they might be accepted unequally by the baby. Mr. Davids, however, became involved in helping his wife through the pregnancy and attended the prenatal classes for parents. Gradually, this involvement helped him to feel a part of the process of becoming a father.

When the infant was born, Mr. Davids was entranced by his healthy and appealing son and, as he said, "fell in love" with him. Even in the hospital, Mr. Davids began to tell the baby about his birth history. He became involved in the caregiving, and father and son became attached to each other. When the boy could understand language, his father was surprised that he did not seem to really care about his "birth story" but preferred instead doing the things he loved to do with his father. Obviously, the boy would understand the meaning of his birth heritage in different ways as he matured, just as in adoption, children's understanding of its meaning changes over time.

This vignette illustrates the importance of therapeutic assistance to help fathers work through the many issues that occur when they confront the reality of their own infertility problems. Parents may need help in resolving their grief and ambivalence about the use of collaborative parentage in order to claim fully their roles as psychological parents. Education, guidance, and therapy may be helpful, for example, to the fathers in deciding whether or when or how to share the birth narrative with their children. In this respect, it is important to consider the maturational capacity of children to understand the narrative of their birth heritage (Pruett, 1992). The past history of the parents and their patterns of dealing with painful subjects may shape the route they take in trying to resolve the symbolic meaning of collaborative parenthood. Many clinicians believe that families can benefit by exploring issues of whether to tell or not to tell their children. They must come to a decision that is informed by their own values, beliefs, and capacities (Klock, 1997; Leiblum, 1997).

The Formation of Single, Gay, and Lesbian Families through Collaborative Parenthood and Assisted Reproductive Technology

Cultural changes and ART have enabled a single woman or a gay or lesbian couple to consider having a family that is at least partially biologically related to them. The decision for a single person or lesbian or gay couple to proceed in the creation of a family is a difficult one. This is especially true when the intentional parents know that they and their child may face social prejudice and a potential lack of social support (Lamb, 1999). However, women and men can now create a family through asexual reproduction, with the result that collaborative parenthood is now possible through various forms of ART. In Chapter 10, we more fully explore the evolution of family identity in single, gay, and lesbian families.

Usually, great attention is given by single and/or lesbian mothers to the selection of a sperm donor. In general, these birth mothers pursue donors they believe to have positive inheritable characteristics such as health, desirable physical attributes, and intellectual abilities, even though one cannot be sure such characteristics will be genetically transmitted (Scheib, Kristiansen, & Wara, 1997). While character also is deemed important, birth mothers tend to believe that character is more a product of environment than genetics. In some families, the characteristics of race and religion are very important factors in creating a family identity similar to the birth mother's own identity. For a single-parent or lesbian family, if there is no surrogate psychological father involved, the choice of a sperm donor father may take on more meaning as the mother hopes to select the best potential inheritable characteristics to pass on to her child.

Men now are able to reach out to a gestational birth mother who is willing to become pregnant using their sperm. Intentional parents, whether men or women, can decide whether they wish to create a child with a known donor or an anonymous one through a donor clinic. Some men seek out women who wish to provide the ova and also carry the fetus to term. Often, surrogate/gestational mothers may desire to have a continuing relationship with the family. As we shall see in Chapter 10, single mothers by choice and gay and lesbian couples constructing new forms of social parentage are trying to resolve new questions that arise when children are born to single- or sex-parents (Pruett, 2000).

Children in single-mother or lesbian families will inevitably raise the question: "Who is my father?" Many birth mothers, anticipating this question, have developed birth narratives that offer an explanation to their children regarding birth heritage. These narratives reveal the importance of the cherished children. When the children are young, these narratives generally suffice, but when they go to school, classmates and teachers may ask more about their family history, raising sensitive questions that are not easy for children or parents. Talking with parents about being "different" is an important part of children's exploration of questions about their biological and psychological heritage (Wind, 1999). However, the "not said" may linger silently in the minds of all members of the family and emerge suddenly at different times of stress or developmental crisis (Wind, 1999) (see Chapter 10). The new forms of family formation also require that teachers promote acceptance of differences in families, in order to protect the self-esteem of all children. This is true for the many different forms of families discussed in this book (Casper, Schultz, & Wickens, 1992).

As children mature they may wish to find out more about their unknown genetic parent. The meaning of the "missing parent" may have a much deeper impact as children enter adolescence; for some youngsters, the realization that they may never know anything about their birth parent is experienced as a shock at this time. Some young adults are finding ways to identify their genetic parent and begin a search similar to that of adopted children who need to know of their biological roots and birth parent (Andrews, 1999). In the future, perhaps fertility clinics will encourage the genetic ova and sperm donors (the birth mother and father) to be open to contact when their children reach the age of majority. Such potential changes in practices are much like those in the new practice of open adoption policies and the decisions by some states to allow adoption records to be unsealed. The rights of children to know their genealogical history and to learn about their roots is a concern of clinicians and ethicists who study family law (Andrews, 1999).

Motherhood through the Use of Ova Donors

The reality that one cannot produce a healthy ovum and may need to use another's egg to create a child is often a stunning blow to a woman and her family. One intentional mother said, "When you take away being able to have a child biologically, it is like having to face death; almost like having half of you die" (Hodder, 1997, p. 57). This loss of a part of one's identity can be so severe that it is not unusual for many women to experience reactive depression as they integrate the meaning of this new reality. Many clinicians encourage the intentional mother to become involved in therapeutic treatment to help her cope with her grief and explore decisions about how to proceed. Women are often ambivalent about the possibility of using an egg donor, and education and support are helpful in clarifying decisions.

The number of women using ova donations, however, has been increasing; in the last 10 years, approximately 6,000 women in the United States gave birth to babies using ova donations (Stolberg, 1998). The chance of a successful pregnancy through the use of an egg donor compares favorably with the success of standard IVF methods. Ova donations are suggested for three types of reproductive problems: (1) women who lack functioning ovaries and cannot produce ova; (2) women who cannot achieve a pregnancy despite the use of advanced reproductive techniques such as IVF; and (3) women who face a genetic risk that may result in chromosomal defects in offspring. In addition, older women in their 40s or 50s may be able to overcome infertility through ova donations, although the chances for successful pregnancy decrease with age (New York State Task Force on Life and the Law, 1998).

The ability to use donor ova requires that both the birth mother and the ova donor undergo IVF treatment, often through a series of monthly cycles. The physical and emotional process of becoming pregnant through an egg donation is a difficult experience. Before a donor cycle is initiated, the recipient's health is evaluated for her capacity to carry a pregnancy to term. Physicians usually first simulate a pregnancy through drug treatment to determine whether the woman's uterine lining can be prepared for embryo transfer. This evaluation of the woman's womb includes repeated blood tests, ultrasound examinations, and, if needed, biopsy to assess the potential of supporting embryo implantation. During the transfer of the embryo, the recipient is treated with hormone therapy to enhance embryo transfer. These treatments may cause significant physiological reactions, such as high blood pressure, that may endanger the birth mother. The maternal recipient may also experience fatigue, headaches, and depression. If the uterus is not ready for implantation, the embryo can be frozen and transferred in a later cycle. After the embryo transfer, the recipient continues the same protocols as other women in the IVF programs. Once the difficult conception is completed, the mother has the chance to experience fully pregnancy and childbirth.

Being an ova donor also is physically difficult, involving many of the hormonal and monitoring procedures of an IVF cycle in order to produce ova, which are harvested by a surgical procedure. Once harvested, the ova are fertilized *in vitro* with the sperm of the genetic father, who may or may not be the intentional caregiving father. The resulting embryos are subsequently transferred to the gestational mother's womb.

A number of medical, legal, and ethical issues have arisen regarding the use of ova donors. These include the protection of the health of the ova donor and the legal status of payment for ova and the relationship between the birth mother and her child. These new questions are being explored through many special state task forces such as the New York State Task Force on Life and the Law (1998). This particular task force has recommended the following guidelines:

- Despite the physical risks to the egg donor, the practice of egg donation should be allowed. All egg donors should undergo medical and genetic health screening, and this information should be made available to the intentional parents.

• Egg donors should be informed of the health risks and provided with sufficient information to help them make informed decisions. Donors should not make a commitment to more than one cycle at a time.

• Women who donate eggs should provide written consent at the time of donation to relinquish their parental rights and responsibilities.

• The law should provide that a woman who gives birth to a child is the legal mother, even if the child is not conceived using the woman's egg.

• Clinics should consider an age limit on egg donor recipients because of not only the risk to the mother's health but also of the ethical implications of childbearing at an age at which the probability of being able to raise the child to adulthood is not realistic.

• Although it is illegal in this country to sell a baby, most states should allow egg donors to receive payment for their medical care and time committed to the process. Payment is usually determined between the ova donor and the parents, and the amount of payment varies broadly; however, it is often very expensive and prohibitive to anyone with a modest income.

• At the same time that recommendations are being made about the ethics of excessive payment to egg donors, some commercial donor clinics advertise that they have highly desirable donors, whose eggs are valued at very high prices. These clinics try to urge intentional parents to "buy" certain valuable characteristics for their children. This process overestimates the promise of certain genetic transmissions to children and underestimates the importance of psychological parenthood and nurturance.

The following advertisement appeared in the February 18, 1999 issue of *The Stanford Daily,* hoping to capitalize on the attractiveness of Stanford University students:

> Egg Donor Needed; Large Financial Incentive; Intelligent, Athletic Egg Donor Needed for Loving Family; You must be at least 5′10″, have a 1,400+ SAT score, possess no major family medical issues. 50,000 Dollars, Free Medical Screening, All Expenses Paid.

This advertisement, similar to many at campuses across the United States, plays to the fantasies of prospective parents about their expectations regarding the as-yet-unborn child. Most responsible organizations, such as the Association of Reproductive Medicine, are opposed to excessive payment for ova and recommend compensation only for time, expenses, risk, and inconvenience.

The ability to become pregnant through the assistance of an egg donor still allows the birth mother to play a major role in the birth of her child. As the gestational and intentional psychological mother, she makes a significant contribution to the neonate's health and to the safe birth of her child. The hormonal changes of pregnancy prepare her to breast-feed and nurture her infant, and the child will know her smell and voice, aiding the development of attachment. For some mothers, the subjective identity of being both the gestational and psychological mother will attenuate the loss of having had to share biological parenthood.

Just as with the families who have used a sperm donor to create a child, parents who have used an egg donor will also have to decide when and what to tell their child. While there are many experts who think that openness about a donor is likely to be helpful, many parents do not tell for fear that it might create confusion and stress for the child. Clinically, it is important to help parents explore the symbolic meaning of the shared parenthood, in order to establish comfortably a secure relationship with their child (Klock, 1997; Stolberg, 1998). We will discuss the issues "to tell" or "not to tell" in Chapters 9 and 11.

Surrogate/Gestational Parenthood

Some women have medical problems producing ova and/or difficulty carrying a baby to term. Although many authors do not distinguish between a surrogate and gestational birth mother, we use the term "surrogate/gestational mother" to refer to a birth mother who both provides the ova and carries the baby to term, with the understanding that the baby will be raised by the intentional parents. A "gestational mother" refers to the birth mother who will carry the fetus to term for the intentional parents. The intentional parents are the ones who have made a commitment to raise the child(ren) and who may or may not be the genetic donors (Beauchamp & Walters, 1994). Each family arrangement brings unique ethical, legal, and family dilemmas. The procedures involve a variation of the complex *in vitro* techniques that have already been described. Once again, this method of constructing a family requires a very active effort on the part of the intentional parents, as they must seek out a person or persons they can trust to provide the gametes, if needed, and/or a healthy gestational birth mother to carry the fetus (Macklin, 1994a).

Gestational parenthood involves extremely complex legal and psychological questions. The case of Baby M heard in the New Jersey Supreme Court in 1988, starkly brought the legal problems of surrogate parenthood to public attention. Dr. Stern and his wife, who also was a physician, approached Mrs. Mary Beth Whitehead to be the ova donor and surrogate/

gestational mother. Dr. Stern was the sperm donor, and although his wife was unable to contribute ova or carry the baby, she intended to be the baby's psychological mother. Although the family had a "monetary contract" with Mrs. Whitehead, when the baby was born, she could not part with the newborn infant, who became known as Baby M. A lawsuit was filed by Dr. Stern, and the baby became the subject of an intense and protracted custody dispute. In the end, the Supreme Court of New Jersey decided that Dr. Stern should be registered as the father of the baby, and that the baby be raised in the Stern family. Mrs. Whitehead would have visitation rights. This case galvanized the country into considering the relationship of the gestational mother to the baby (Andrews, 1999).

A special New York State Task Force made the following recommendations for public policy regarding the rights of both the surrogate/gestational parent and the intentional psychological mother (New York State Task Force on Life and the Law, 1998):

- Surrogate contracts should not be legally binding in that the surrogate or gestational birth mother should be able to change her mind about keeping the baby. Payment of fees to women who serve as surrogates and their brokers should not be allowed beyond medical expenses and reasonable fees.
- Voluntary, and noncommercial surrogate parenting should be permitted to continue. For example, a woman can carry a baby for her sister or a close friend.
- When the surrogate gestational mother has been impregnated with the intentional father's sperm, the gestational mother should be considered to be the child's mother in all respects. If she decides not to relinquish the child, she retains the legal rights and responsibilities of any mother.
- When the gestational mother is carrying an embryo created by the egg of the intentional mother, the child has two biological mothers. The recommendations in the special New York Task Force study suggest that if there is a dispute between the two mothers as to who has the right to be the legal caregiving mother, each woman should have the right to seek custody through the court. As in other family disputes, the determination of who is the legal mother should be based on the best interests of the child.

Where disputes occur, lengthy court cases may cast the family in limbo and endanger the early psychological life of the child. States differ in their decisions about custody; some rule in favor of the genetic mother, whereas others favor the gestational mother; still others favor the intentional parents. Only two states, Virginia and New Hampshire, have actual legislation governing these disputes (Macklin, 1994a).

In disputed custody cases, children may have begun to have a relationship with their birth mother and/or intentional parents. If the intentional parents are given legal custody and conflict persists, the task of establishing family identity is now more difficult and may affect the child's sense of security. If visitation with the birth mother is permitted, the two families become involved in a process similar to that of an open adoption. In this situation, children may need help to differentiate the various levels of relationship to their extended "kinship family," their birth parent and their psychological parents. Ideally, a child therapist should be assigned to help the child cope with the confusing situation. Capron and Radin (1988) suggest that family law, rather than contract law, is most appropriate in these judicial determinations. The "best interests of the child standard" can help the court to decide the custody issues. Uncertainty and protracted conflict inevitably have a detrimental effect on the child, who does not know where "home base is" and must cope with extended periods of anxiety and loss (Goldstein et al., 1996; Paret & Shapiro, 1998).

DISCUSSION

The new advances in human reproduction have introduced a broader concept of the family. This concept reaches beyond our traditional legal, biological, and cultural perspectives, and places a greater emphasis on the family as an essentially *subjective entity*. In all families, the intentional parents make a strong commitment to become the psychological parents to the unborn infant. In families created through collaborative parenthood, this commitment becomes the core basis of the future family identity (Macklin, 1995b). A broader definition of the idea of a family has been proposed by Carol Levine (1990, p. 35):

> Families should be broadly defined to include besides the traditional biological relationships, those committed relationships between individuals which fulfill the functions of the family. Family members are individuals who by birth, adoption, marriage, or a declared commitment share deep personal connections and are mutually entitled to receive and obligated to provide support of various kinds to the extent possible, especially in times of need.

The importance of having children is the driving force that underlies the willingness of many couples and individuals to undertake the difficult and rigorous course of infertility treatments (Zelizer, 1985). Many infertility clinics recognize the extraordinary emotional crisis that infertility presents and have developed a range of individual, family, and group therapeutic programs to assist families enduring its painful realities (Leiblum, 1997; Stanton & Burns, 1999). The therapeutic programs offer a broad range of approaches, including education and guidance, support, and a range of therapeutic services. These services are attuned to the interwoven medical, psychological, and social issues involved in infertility treatment. Group and family intervention programs are often found to be very helpful. Many families find that sharing their deep feelings of pain with others allows them both to grieve and to gain hope as their invisible pain becomes visible.

Some intentional parents will finally have a child through various processes of ART. Others may decide to abandon treatment and adopt a child, and still others may decide to forgo having children. In all of these situations, the participants must go on with their lives. The opportunity to have received empathetic therapeutic treatment will benefit many couples and individuals by enabling them to move forward with a greater sense of self-understanding and self-acceptance. The complex human issues that the families have confronted and their attempts to overcome the problems of infertility, will have a significant and enduring impact on their lives.

If a couple has a child, the parental focus shifts from a preoccupation with the pregnancy to attention to the real baby. As with all parents, the arrival of a healthy baby is an adjustment in the life of the family. However, recovery from the strenuous efforts to have a child takes time. Parents who cannot have a biologically related child may need to resolve their feelings of the loss regarding the genetic child they wished to have in order to fully claim the child who is now theirs (Brodzinsky, 1997).

The baby, however, like all healthy infants, has an active need for his/her psychological parents and draws them into a real and important caregiving relationship (Stern, 1985). The psychological parents can begin to experience a sense of attachment through the satisfaction they experience in holding, feeding, and soothing the baby. They soon can come to feel that *they* know the baby best, and the baby's first smile reinforces the feeling that they are very special in their baby's life. The signs of attachment between infant and parents begin to strengthen the parental self-concept and establish the boundaries of family identity (Benedek, 1959). This budding relationship begins to build a sense of closeness between them and can help mediate the difficult questions that may arise later regarding identity issues inherent in the new forms of parentage.

Over time and at different phases of development, children begin to ask questions about their birth heritage and family roots. Families who have used complex forms of ART, such as collaborative parenthood, often struggle with the question of whether to tell their children about their genetic heritage (Klock, 1997). Parents must find a way to tell the birth narrative in a manner that matches their child's level of understanding and their own readiness to talk about these sensitive issues (see Chapter 11). Therapists can help families explore these issues and offer guidance in the context of a therapeutic relationship that offers empathy and is informed by the complex, interrelated knowledge of the medical and psychological issues in the treatment of infertility.

APPENDIX 8.1. Genetic Roots and ART Procedures

TABLE 8.1. Options for Married Couples

	Gamete source			
	Sperm	Ova	Site of fertilization	Birth mother
1	Husband	Wife	Wife	Wife
2	Sperm donor	Wife	Wife	Wife
3	Husband	Wife	Laboratory[a]	Wife
4	Sperm donor	Wife	Laboratory[a]	Wife
5	Husband	Ova donor	Laboratory	Wife
6	Husband	Ova donor	Surrogate mother	Wife
7	Sperm donor	Ova donor	Laboratory	Wife
8	Sperm donor	Ova donor	Surrogate mother	Wife

[a]Embryo transfer.

TABLE 8.2. Options for Married Couples Who Require the Use of a Surrogate/Gestational Mother

	Gamete source			
	Sperm	Ova	Site of fertilization	Birth mother
1	Husband	Wife[a]	Wife	Gestational mother
2	Husband	Wife	Laboratory	Gestational mother
3	Sperm donor	Wife	Wife	Gestational mother
4	Sperm donor	Wife	Laboratory	Gestational mother
5	Husband	Ova donor	Laboratory	Gestational mother
6	Sperm donor	Ova donor	Laboratory	Gestational mother
7	Husband	Ova donor	Surrogate/gestational mother	Surrogate/gestational mother
8	Sperm donor	Ova donor	Surrogate/gestational mother	Surrogate/gestational mother

[a]Embryo transfer.

Tables 8.1 and 8.2 are adapted from Weil and Walters (1994, p. 203) in Beauchamp and Walters, *Contemporary Issues in Bioethics.* Copyright 1994 by Wadsworth Publishing Company. (The original tables were first published in the *Journal of Medicine and Philosophy,* August 1985, p. 210, and then in the *Journal of Fertility and Sterility,* September 1986, p. 175.)

9

Family Identity and Emerging Psychological Issues

> Infertility teaches you about yourself, about what's important, about marriage, about what is fair and just—being infertile makes you question the purpose of marriage and life. . . . Nothing is left unaffected by this experience. . . . It changes you, subtly but profoundly. . . .
>
> —LEIBLUM (1997, p. 103)

Throughout the ages and across many cultures, infertility has been recognized as a serious life crisis. The inability to have a biologically related child touches on deep emotional, social, cultural, and familial factors; therefore, the distress resulting from infertility can be profound. For those men and women who dreamed of having a family, infertility often results in anticipatory mourning for the loss of parenthood and continuity across the generations (Burns & Covington, 1999; Leiblum, 1997; Tobin, 1998). Hence, infertility blocks a major development in the lifecycle, namely, parenthood. For many adults, parenthood offers an opportunity to consolidate identity formation and brings an increased sense of personal fulfillment and satisfaction (Erikson, 1950). Infertility affects not only the individual but also the relationship between the couple, the extended family, and the social perception of the couple in society (Menning, 1980).

Anthropologists report that even before modern science created a more effective understanding of the etiology and treatment of infertility, many cultures developed their own interpretation of its causes. Over time, various cultures adopted social, spiritual, and/or medicinal approaches to help families cope with the personal, biological, and social crises of infertility (Burns & Covington, 1999).

During the last decades of the 20th century, scientific advances in human biology have led to successful new procedures for the treatment of infertility. These treatments, known collectively as assisted reproductive technology (ART), have made new forms of parentage possible (American Fertility Society Ethics Committee, 1994). For the first time, fertilization can be achieved outside the human body (i.e., in the laboratory) through a group of techniques called *in vitro* fertilization (IVF). IVF has helped couples and individuals overcome barriers to conception, pregnancy, and the birth of a full-term infant (see Chapter 8).

In the pantheon of ART treatments, 16 different sets of procedures are available to deal with specific infertility problems (American Fertility Society Ethics Committee, 1994) (see Chapter 8, Appendix 8.1). Depending on the differential diagnosis, some families can try to use IVF approaches to give birth to their own biologically related child. Other couples, however, may need to try to have a child through more complex procedures involving collaborative parenthood, in which other donors may be required to provide the gametes, the sperm, and/or ova needed to form the embryo. In still other situations, the intentional parents may require a surrogate and/or gestational mother to carry the fetus to term.

In collaborative parenthood, therefore, a child may be conceived, carried to term, and nurtured by three different sets of parents: the genetic parent who provided the gametes (sperm or ova), the gestational parent who carried the infant *in utero,* and the intentional parents who nurture the child after birth (Macklin, 1994b; Snowden, 1990). In these cases, the intentional parents face unique developmental tasks in claiming their new infants as their own, in building a strong sense of family identity, and in helping their child deal with any issues that arise from the particular and unique birth history (Brodzinsky & Schechter, 1990).

These new forms of parentage have raised legal, ethical, and social issues regarding the definition of the family and attitudes about family identity (Capron & Radin, 1994). Most importantly, the definition of the family has been broadened from an emphasis on the biological basis of family to include the concept of the family as a subjective entity. In the nonbiologically related family constructed through ART, psychological nurturing alone, rather than a combination of psychological nurturing and biological relatedness, is central to the formation of family identity. As in all families, however, it is the parents' emotional cathexis of their child that provides the impetus to create a secure holding environment within which the child can thrive (Freud, 1965; Winnicott, 1965b).

The phases in achieving parenthood through ART are an unfolding process. First the family must deal with its own deep reactions to the facts of infertility. Second, the couple must decide whether to make a commitment to undertake fertility treatment, including, perhaps, various forms of ART. Because families may find it difficult to take these steps, therapeutic intervention is often suggested. Counseling, guidance, and education can help families deal with the emotional impact of infertility and the burdens that treatment exacts on families' psychological and social world. The complexity and diversity of these problems have led to the development of new holistic models of supportive treatment that focus on the dynamic relationship between personal, social, medical, and family forces. Treatment is often provided by social workers, nurses, psychologists, and other professionals attached to infertility clinics (Applegarth, 1999; Leiblum & Greenfeld, 1997).

This chapter reviews the phases of family development in the special pathways to parenthood that occur through ART. According to clinical studies, families that have had a chance to explore their feelings about their unique experiences are likely to be better prepared to consider the choices they confront and to respond to the special questions that emerge as they undertake their parental role. This chapter discusses infertility as a medical and psychological crisis, the new social and biological issues in family formation, the role of supportive therapy, and issues of family identity in the child's psychological world.

THE PSYCHOLOGICAL CRISIS OF INFERTILITY AS A PRELUDE TO PARENTHOOD

The Psychological Impact on Women

Historically, some viewed the etiology of female infertility as related to a woman's unconscious psychological resistance to childbearing (Benedek, 1952; Bos & Cleghorn, 1958). In the 1940s and 1950s, the *psychogenic infertility model* suggested that infertile women subconsciously reject pregnancy, childbirth, and motherhood. This model implied that, for many women, pregnancy was "psychologically blocked" because of unresolved identity conflicts, conflict between motherhood and career, negative identification with their own mother, and the negative symbolic meaning of "motherhood." Many infertile women were referred for psychotherapy as a way to help them overcome their emotional barriers to "psychological infertility."

New medical insights reveal, however, that infertility primarily results from complex *physiological* barriers to pregnancy (New York State Task Force on Life and the Law, 1998). The *psychological sequelae model* now suggests that the symptoms of anxiety and depression follow the news of infertility and are a grief reaction to the potential loss of parenthood (Menning, 1980). This has led to the realization that focused counseling or psychotherapy is useful, if not critical, for families undertaking fertility treatment.

Women may respond to the news of being infertile with deep emotion. In some studies, infertile women are found to be more depressed than their fertile counterparts. Indeed, the level of their depression and anxiety is similar to the degree of depression found in women with heart disease, cancer, or HIV-positive status. In one study, 11% of infertile women met the criteria for a current major depressive episode (Domar, Broome, Zuttermeister, Seibel, & Miedman, 1992). Other studies report that women experience infertility as the worst crisis of their lives, worse than divorce or the loss of a parent (Daniluk, 1997).

Moreover, during infertility treatment, anxiety can increase dramatically and the resulting stress can trigger the reemergence of preexisting symptoms, such as major depression or an eating disorder (Applegarth, 1999). When women come to infertility clinics with anxiety and depression, a differential diagnosis is required to assess whether or not the symptoms are reactive to the news of infertility or whether they represent a more chronic state of a previous disorder (Domar et al., 1992; Mai, Munday, & Rump, 1972; Noyes & Chapnick, 1964).

Female infertility is often experienced as a major biographical discontinuity, as it disrupts a core sense of gender identity. Symbolic and real losses are intrinsic to the experience of female infertility. These include loss of health, self-esteem, self-confidence, social status, friendships (particularly with peers and family who have children), as well as the potential for intergenerational continuity (Daniluk, 1997; Mahlstedt, 1985). Furthermore, the intentional parent may experience both the loss of an important fantasy and life dream, and the loss of a relationship with a future child who holds great symbolic value (Brinich, 1990).

The potential loss of motherhood may also interfere with the consolidation of female identity and the opportunity to establish a more mature relationship with one's own mother (Notman & Lester, 1988). Pregnancy and motherhood can provide a woman with an opportunity to fulfill an unconscious, powerful wish to form a new kind of identification with her own mother. Symbolically, the wish to have a child is partly related to a daughter's hope to repair maternal failures of the past. The developmental crisis of infertility may block the opportunity for a woman to work through past psychological losses by preventing her from carrying out positive wishes and hopes for a child of her own (Benedek, 1959; Bibring, 1959; Klempner, 1992). These deep psychological reasons and feelings may drive many intentional mothers to go to great lengths to have a child.

A personal loss of self-esteem may also be experienced because the intentional mother cannot meet the social expectation of motherhood, which is "the" defining role of women in our culture (Chodorow, 1978; Rich, 1976). In fact, many women report that being with young mothers who have children is too painful and causes them to withdraw, exacerbating their sense of isolation and diminished sense of self (Daniluk, 1997). Of course, not every woman is strongly influenced by the prevailing cultural view, and many feminists have decried the emphasis on childbearing as the defining measure of femininity (Tobin, 1998).

In addition to the problems of becoming pregnant, a woman may face failures in completing pregnancy. Loss can occur at any phase of the process including problems in fertilization of the ova through IVF treatment; implantation of the embryo in the mother's uterus; miscarriage during gestation; and premature birth. Each loss can be experienced symbolically as the death of the anticipated child. In addition, many couples do not share their infertility problems with others and often suffer in isolation without adequate support from their families, physicians, or friends (Cooper & Glazer, 1994).

For intentional mothers, pregnancy failures also raise doubts about bodily integrity. The experience of a bodily defect is intimately tied up with feminine identity, and this particular loss may be very difficult. Women often undertake reflective life searches based on past sexual relationship histories to explore the reasons for their infertility. Often, this results in feelings of guilt, self-blame, and inadequacy (Applegarth, 1999).

In addition, the infertility treatment itself interferes with every aspect of marriage, including the sexual and emotional relationship between the couple, social relationships with other families and friends, and disruption of job and career plans. The anxiety that many women experience during treatment is exacerbated further by the knowledge that more than half of all women in IVF programs never conceive or bring a child to term (Leiblum, 1997 pp. 1–12). Tobin (1998, p. 110) describes the "addiction" of some women who "shut out all external life and narrow their focus, living from menstrual cycle to menstrual cycle, from fix to fix, in a desperate commitment to having a child."

The Psychological Impact of Infertility on Men

The study of the psychological impact of infertility on men has not been as extensive as that on women (Wright, Allard, Lecours, & Sabourin, 1989; Wright et. al., 1991). Male infertility accounts directly for approximately 35% of infertility cases. Artificial insemination by donor (AID) is still the primary method of dealing with male infertility. Until the new IVF technique known as intracytoplasmic sperm injection (ICSI) was developed, in which a single sperm is retrieved and directly inserted into the ovum *in vitro,* no medical treatment for male infertility existed. Even with this new procedure, however, the success rate of a pregnancy is less than 50% (New York State Task Force on Life and the Law, 1998).

The studies that do exist note that men and women often express their feelings and thoughts about infertility in very different ways (Daniluk, 1997; Snowden, 1990). Women lament that their husbands appear to be less sensitive to, and less distressed by, the couple's childlessness. But studies suggest that in dealing with infertility problems, men may utilize different defense mechanisms than women and cope with their feelings in a less openly expressive way (Greil, 1991). Women are more likely to want to share their feelings with others, while men are generally more private about their sadness. Men more readily use defenses such as denial, distancing, and/or avoidance in dealing with the narcissistic blow of infertility. Their tendency is to deal with sensitive feelings internally rather than expressively, and these behaviors often obscure their deeper feelings of loss and injury (Abbey, Andrews, & Halman, 1991; Snowden, 1990).

If husbands and wives have different styles of coping with loss, the husband's adaptive response of withdrawal can be misinterpreted as "not caring," creating a sense of separation and isolation within the marriage. One husband expressed his inability to comfort his wife in the following way:

> "If my wife was sobbing at night on one side of the bed, I would just turn over and not be any comfort. . . . I couldn't really listen to her . . . to what she was communicating and the feelings and emptiness, the feelings of being alone, of feeling hurt. . . . My reaction was to be very silent, withdrawing, and not wanting to talk about it because I couldn't fix it." (in Daniluk, 1997, p. 107)

Clinical interviews with infertile men reveal that infertility is as deep a narcissistic injury to their self-esteem and identity as is the woman's experience of her own infertility (Meyers et al., 1995a, 1995b). The subjective experience of infertility is often experienced as a major disruption of the sense of male identity and virility. In men's narrative accounts, loss is also a pervasive theme: not having a biologically related child, not continuing the family lineage, the sense of personal failure, and feelings of guilt, shame, anger, and isolation (Abbey et al., 1991; Mahlstedt, 1985; Webb & Daniluk, 1999).

One infertile father said, "My major hang-up really was based on this rather metaphysical notion of genetic immortality. What depressed me most of all, and overwhelmed me mentally, was the idea that at this point my genetic channel stops. That's the end. And that was the most chilling thing I had to take on board" (Snowden, 1990, p. 75). It may be because of these deep feelings, and because of the fear that their masculinity will be diminished in the eyes of others, that most men, unlike women, choose to keep their infertility problems private (Klock, 1997).

Gender differences affect the ways in which men and women experience and respond to sperm and ova donation. A woman who deeply wishes to have a child and uses ova or sperm donation has the opportunity to experience a "normal" pregnancy and childbirth, with all its internal meaning. In addition, she is valued by the outside world and treated just like every other pregnant woman. On the other hand, many men express ambivalent feelings about the use of AID in creating a child. A man may feel uncomfortable about his wife becoming pregnant with the sperm of another man. He may worry that if the child knew he was not the biological father, the child would not admire him or feel he was the real father. Some men may feel that the role of the biological father is valued above the role of provider and can express neither their "shame" nor their loss in the presence of others (Snowden, 1990). Their imagined derision of infertility by other men increases their own feelings of inadequacy.

Family Conflict in Infertility Decision Making

Often, couples have different views on important decisions that they must make with respect to their infertility. The different degree of commitment to continuing treatment, for example, is related to many factors. The biological "clock" looms larger in the woman's childbearing years, and she may feel more social pressure exerted upon her by the perceived social importance of the cultural role of motherhood. For men, the social emphasis is often on the career roles of men rather than the role of fatherhood (Kaufman, 1993).

Furthermore, the significant emotional, financial, and physical strain on the family caused by fertility treatment can have a negative effect on marital, sexual, and family relationships (Daniluk, 1997; Leiblum 1994). Couples will, therefore, experience these strains differently, and this will affect how far they may wish to go in the pursuit of complex infertility treatments (Epstein & Rosenberg, 1997; Leiblum & Greenfeld, 1997). In addition, if theirs is not a first marriage, the husband and wife may have had different life trajectories affect their feelings about parenthood—differences in age, children from previous marriages, and other personal factors that may cause asymmetrical feelings about having children and about the value of "putting life on hold" while pursuing treatment. In addition, for families without health insurance coverage, the financial burden is often so onerous as to endanger future goals, such as providing for a reasonable retirement (Epstein & Rosenberg, 1997).

Thus, one of the central therapeutic issues in fertility counseling is the disagreement between partners in deciding whether to use ova or sperm donors, and whether or not to tell their child about his/her birth roots (Klock, 1997). Women and men generally have very different thoughts and feelings about the meaning of collaborative parenthood. Often, women are less threatened by the use of donor ova and/or donor sperm, and/or the possibility of using a gestational birth mother (Epstein & Rosenberg, 1997). Men often prefer to protect their privacy regarding their infertility more than women, who are more likely to reach out to others for understanding and comfort. If husbands feel strongly, many women respect their wishes for privacy, but keeping the secret may add an undercurrent of anxiety and discomfort within the relationship and cause isolation from friends and the extended family.

The road to parenthood is thus a long and winding one for many infertile couples, and the intentional parents can often benefit from psychological and supportive help. If serious disagreements persist, the ambivalence toward becoming a parent through ART may continue and unresolved feelings may interfere in the relationships between the parents and that between the parents and their future child (Epstein & Rosenberg, 1997; Snowden, 1990).

THE ROLE OF SUPPORTIVE THERAPY, GUIDANCE, AND EDUCATION

Therapeutic intervention is often suggested to help the family deal with the emotional impact of infertility and the burdens that infertility treatment exacts on its psychological and social world. The complexity of the problems families encounter has led to new holistic models of treatment that include supportive therapy, guidance, and education. Treatment usually focuses on the dynamic relationship between personal, social, medical, and family factors. Given the dynamic interaction between medical and psychological factors, the models of treatment are eclectic and draw on various psychodynamic, biomedical, and behavioral perspectives (Burns & Covington, 1999; Leiblum, 1997; Tobin, 1998).

Hospital-based infertility clinics are developing programs staffed by interdisciplinary treatment teams composed of social workers, psychologists, nurses, and physicians to meet the ongoing needs of families. For example, crisis intervention and short-term treatment methods help families adjust to the initial diagnosis of infertility; longer-term therapy methods deal with the interactive psychological and physiological stress of ongoing medical treatment (Applegarth, 1999; Braverman, 1997; Domar, 1997). Many families need long-term support to mourn the loss inherent in infertility and to achieve a more beneficial psychological balance, which includes a broader perspective on their predicament. This support can enable the couple or individual to develop a wider view beyond the single, life-fulfilling dream of a biologically related child (Applegarth, 1999; Klock, 1997; Tobin, 1998).

Women especially value therapeutic group support and find that sharing their despair, grief, and "shame" with others in similar circumstances often results in a decline in their sense of helplessness and depression, and an increase in their ability to feel empowered. They report becoming more proactive in influencing their medical treatment. In some instances, reduced depression and anxiety are thought to improve the chances for a successful pregnancy, although this relationship is uncertain and the subject of ongoing research (Domar, 1997; Hodder, 1997). Family treatment is also thought to be important and can improve the ability of prospective parents to communicate with each other and arrive at meaningful consensus regarding critical decisions (Epstein & Rosenberg, 1997).

Accumulating therapeutic experience has stressed the importance for the couple to arrive at a mutual consensus, if possible, regarding important treatment decisions. As we have discussed previously, two difficult issues for couples are the decisions regarding the use of donors and other aspects of collaborative parenthood, and the question of secrecy or openness regarding their child's genetic birth heritage. The following five therapeutic objectives have been identified as especially important in expanding the couple's mutual understanding (Stanton & Burns, 1999).

1. To discuss the personal significance of infertility, including grief and loss, to each partner, and to explore any personal differences in feelings, values, and meaning with regard to the importance of having a child.

2. To discuss their perception of the effects infertility has had on their broader life and their individual feelings about the amount of family resources, personal effort, time, and energy that should be devoted to continued treatment.
3. To help the partners reflect on their own relationship and the difficulties they may have in sustaining relationships with each other, family members, friends, and others. To provide guidance related to the importance of sustaining social relationships for their own emotional health, as isolation is a risk for couples coping with infertility.
4. To help the partners understand the need to maintain a reasonable emotional balance in the relationship by engaging in pleasurable and meaningful activities, and not simply focusing on the monthly cycle of treatments.
5. To help the partners mourn their experiences of reproductive failure and to put this experience in some perspective in relation to success in broader aspects of their life. This relative perspective on other accomplishments may help each partner preserve the more satisfactory self-image and sense of competence achieved before the crisis of infertility.

The success rate of live births through the ART treatment cycle is below 30% and is dependent on the particular type of infertility problem, the age of the mother, the treatment needed, and the skill and experience of the fertility clinics (Assisted Reproductive Technology Success Rates 1997, 1999). If the couple does not achieve a pregnancy, the partners need to grieve the immediate loss and think through whether or not they wish to continue treatment.

Some clinical paradigms have been developed to help couples work through the difficult decisions about whether or not to continue, and if needed, whether or not to use a donor or the assistance of a surrogate or gestational birth mother, and if a donor is chosen as the biological parent whether or not partners plan to tell their child about his/her genetic heritage (Burns, 1999; Epstein & Rosenberg, 1997; Klock, 1997). Many clinicians have found that being able to talk about these issues and come to a consensus before decisions are made is essential, in order that each parent be able to claim the child as their own, if a pregnancy occurs.

It is often recommended that if one of the parents is not ready to have a child through collaborative parenthood, the family should take more time to discuss the decision. This is especially important for infertile fathers who object to the use of a sperm donor. In this situation, it is suggested that the family wait at least 3 months before choosing to use AID. If a consensus cannot be reached, the therapist may suggest exploring other possibilities, such as adoption or the decision not to have children (Epstein & Rosenberg, 1997). Zoldbrod and Covington (1999) have developed a list of issues for discussion with the intentional parents that can be helpful in assessing the pros and cons of either having a child through donor insemination or considering adoption. This list is available in Table 9.1 of Appendix 9.1.

Another important issue concerns whether to tell or not to tell the child and others of the use of ova or sperm donors. Many experts think that while they as professionals may feel that openness is better in the long run, the partners must come to their own consensus on this issue, based on their emotional feelings, their thoughts of how this knowledge might interfere in the relationship between them and their child, and their religious, cultural, and personal beliefs (Daniluk, 1997; Klock, 1997; Snowden, 1990). Some of the pros and cons for the basis of these discussions are available in Table 9.2 of Appendix 9.1.

No matter which decision is made before the child is born, discussions of these issues will have helped intentional parents to explore feelings and ideas that can be painful. Often, parents may change their minds about an initial decision not to disclose as different questions emerge, and they do not want to embellish the "not true" narrative. If the parents decide to tell their child, it is important to recognize that the child's ability to grasp the meaning of his/her birth story will change over time. The main consideration for the parent is the need to match the content of the narrative with the emotional and cognitive ability of their child (Pruett, 1992). As we shall see in the following vignettes, the decision to tell or not to tell is not simple; it affects each family differently and can have a powerful effect on the evolving relationship between parents and their child (see Chapter 11).

PARENTAGE THROUGH THE HELP OF AN OVA DONOR

The first baby conceived with donated eggs was born in 1984. The demand for the procedure reached a peak in 1990, when some clinics made the procedure available for women approaching menopause (Greenfeld, 1999). Intentional single mothers or couples face difficult choices in selecting or finding a suitable ova donor. Both the donor and the intentional mother go through rigorous hormonal and other medical treatments. Embryos are created in the laboratory through IVF with the donated ova and either the husband's or a donor's sperm. A number of embryos are then transferred to the uterus of the intentional mother, and if implantation occurs, she will then undergo a traditional pregnancy. The reason for multiple transfer of embryos is to increase the chance that at least one will implant and a pregnancy occur. However, multiple embryo transfers carry risks for a full-term pregnancy and, depending on the number of fetuses, risks to delivery of full-term, healthy infants. From the mother's point of view, however, such multiple transfers increase her opportunity to experience pregnancy and become a birth mother (see Chapter 8). The psychological meaning in acceptance of an ova from another woman is different for each intentional mother and depends on her own psychological history, her sense of self-confidence, the support she feels from her family and husband, and the importance to her of having a child.

As we have previously stated, one of the most important decisions a family faces in gamete donation is whether or not to tell the child about his/her genetic birth heritage, and if so, at what age, and in what words. Some parents feel that by not telling the story they can help their child avoid potential confusion and unnecessary doubts about family belonging, thus creating a clear sense of family boundaries. On the other hand, some parents feel that not telling may interfere with the establishment of spontaneous and open communication within the family. They may also feel that the child has a right to know of his/her biological roots for medical and social reasons (Klock, 1997). Table 9.2 of Appendix 9.1 lists the advantages and disadvantages of telling children about their birth history (Zoldbrod & Covington, 1999).

Case Vignette: Mr. and Mrs. Kelly's Decision to Tell Tilly about Her Birth Heritage

Mr. and Mrs. Kelly were in their 40s when they conceived their first child, Tilly, through ova donation from a nonrelated donor named Sally, who was selected from a clinic's roster of screened donors. Mr. and Mrs. Kelly, both social workers, decided before Tilly's birth to tell their family, and eventually their child, about her birth heritage. Knowing that even toddlers love to hear stories about their birth, they developed the narrative they would tell their daughter. It had the components of most stories about birth histories: a loving Mommy and Daddy, a family who wanted a baby to love, and the joy they felt when Tilly was born. Putting their narrative in a normative frame, they said this was all true for "Tilly" except that a nice lady named Sally helped Mommy by giving her the egg that was needed. Mommy carried Tilly in her tummy for 9 months and gave birth to her in the hospital. She and Daddy would love Tilly forever.

Mr. Kelly said that although they knew the story would take on different meaning as Tilly matured, they did not want to dwell on the personhood of Sally or magnify her role as the biological mother. They wanted their daughter to know about her birth history but did not want to overemphasize its meaning or raise confusion about having "two" mothers. Mrs. Kelly has been clear about the fact that she is Tilly's psychological mother and strongly claims her sense of entitlement and attachment to Tilly. She said to the interviewer, " I am Tilly's mother, the one she knows. Sally is not my daughter's mother. I carried her, I nurtured her, I'm the mother. It's so complicated, I try to balance the reality of her birth narrative with the strong emotional feelings I have towards Tilly and my wish to make her feel secure in knowing we are her parents" (Stolberg, 1998, p. A-1).

Mrs. Kelly clearly feels entitled to being her daughter's mother and consciously addresses the sensitive issues for herself and her child. It is clear, however, that she feels that the issues of genetic heritage and family identity will need to be dealt with in different ways over time. For example, during the elementary school years, teachers often ask children to tell about their family tree, and Mrs. Kelly anticipates needing to respond to new questions that reflect Tilly's growing understanding of the role of the ova donor. The Kellys clearly believe that the strength of the relationship between themselves and their child will help to mediate sensitive questions that may arise (Stolberg, 1998).

Case Vignette: Mr. and Mrs. Cross and Their Toddlers, Barbara and Gail

Mr. and Mrs. Cross, both in their 40s, decided to ask their friend and neighbor, Mrs. Lane, if she would provide the ova so that they could have a child. The Lanes had their own young children but because of friendship decided to respond to the Crosses' difficult situation. After a successful IVF with Mr. Cross's sperm and Mrs. Lane's donated ova, the embryos were transferred, and Mrs. Cross became pregnant with twin daughters. Before the twins, Barbara and Gail, were born, the Crosses and the Lanes decided that they would not reveal to family, neighbors, friends, or the children that Mrs. Lane had been the ova donor.

The two couples had made the decision not to tell because they thought the relationship between the families would become confusing and problematic if the children knew about their shared genetic heritage. For the sake of clarity, and to protect the children from confusion around parenthood and the curiosity of others in the community, the decision not to tell about their maternal ova donor seemed right to both couples.

Mrs. Cross notes that at the age of 5, the children were strongly attached to her and her husband, and resemble them both in many ways, so much so that others often commented that the twins looked like her. The perceived similarity pleased Mrs. Cross but she could not tell anyone why she was amused at their comments. She felt that her daughters identified with her in many ways. In the long run, Mr. and Mrs. Cross knew that it was the strength of their relationship with their children that gave them the greatest pleasure (Stolberg, 1998).

On the other hand, Mrs. Cross reports that at certain times, the children's genetic heritage became an issue. For example, when the pediatrician asked her about her own medical history, she described the history of the genetic mother and not her own. She recognized that this might not always be an adequate strategy. She did not address the fact that the children's closest "friends" were in reality their half-siblings. Questions remain for the future, for example, the unlikely but possible romantic relationships that could develop between these half-siblings. If disclosure became necessary, the knowledge might disrupt the children's perception of their relationships, both to their own parents and to their friends. This biographical disjuncture could cause a break in the continuity of their internal representation of their family and themselves. As we shall see in Chapter 11, keeping important secrets about birth identity can be problematic if disclosure is abrupt and related to family crises.

Therapists acknowledge the potentially complicating factors that openness or secrecy can present to the establishment of a secure sense of family identity and generally agree that their role is to help the family work through the issues and come to a decision that they believe is in the best interest of their child.

THE PSYCHOLOGICAL MEANING OF FATHERHOOD AND ARTIFICIAL INSEMINATION BY DONOR

The roles of fathers in the lives of their children have recently become a focus of interest to those who study the well-being of children. In the past, primary attention was given to the importance of both the father's genetic role and his provider role in supporting the family household. More recently, however, social scientists and clinicians have begun to focus on the psychological meaning of fatherhood in the developmental lives of their children (Cath, Gurwitt, & Gunsburg, 1989; Pruett, 1992).

The "psychological" father is an important figure in the internal life of the child, as he is emotionally supportive of the infant's mother and offers the child a separate social relationship (Lamb, 1999; Snowden, 1990). Fathers, for example, often support their child's developing autonomy and assist him/her in moving beyond the intense early dyadic relationship with the mother to develop a broader set of social relationships. The child benefits from the alternative relationship and the often different styles in thinking, play, and emotional reactions of the two social parents. Thus, the child can develop a qualitatively different relationship with each parent.

For all fathers, the development of paternal identity takes time and occurs as they establish a relationship with their young children through sustained and mutually satisfying interaction. It is important for wives and extended families to support the psychological relationship between fathers who are not biologically related and their children.

Snowden (1990) interviewed 70 families in which the children had been conceived through AID. The study was designed to focus on the issues these fathers faced in the development of their paternal identity. Since the children in Snowden's study were not told about their genetic heritage until they were young adults, he was also able to evaluate how disclosure affected their views of their fathers (Snowden, 1990).

From Snowden's study, the following six themes emerged, providing insights into factors affecting the development of paternal identity in fathers whose children were conceived through AID (Snowden, 1990). We refer to the fathers in the study as psychological fathers.

1. *The supportive role of the psychological father in pregnancy was important to paternal identity formations.* In fact, the psychological father has an important creative role in the birth of the child. While AID does not cure infertility, the future psychological father participates in the creation of the baby in a social sense and can experience the emotional phases of pregnancy through the support of his wife during gestation and birth.

2. *Despite their supportive role, some psychological fathers experience confusion regarding their paternal role and identity.* One father spoke about this confusion as follows: "The fact that they were not mine—they are, I know that they are mine—but it was in the back of my mind that it was never mine, never my child—I wasn't the one, the father—but I know they are mine now, they will always be mine" (Snowden, 1990, p. 77).

3. *All of the psychological fathers benefited from their wives' affirmation of their paternal role.* It was important to the fathers that their spouses were strongly supportive of their paternal role. As the children grew older, the fathers themselves began to minimize the importance of insemination by the donor and stressed the importance of their roles in supporting their

wives during pregnancy and labor, and the long-term care and responsibilities they had taken on for their children.

4. *The acceptance of the child by grandparents and or other family members was important.* At times, the maternal grandparents welcomed the baby with greater acceptance than the paternal grandparents, and this was hurtful to the fathers' paternal identity. This narcissistic injury to the fathers often created a complex and painful set of issues. The dilemma often led to a reconfiguration of the emotional relationships with the extended family and the establishment of stronger boundaries of family identity for the couple and child.

5. *Many of these psychological fathers had to cope with social attitudes that were critical of fatherhood achieved through AID.* Cultural and broader family attitudes toward AID affected the fathers' self-esteem and parental sense of worthiness. The protective sensitivity of their wives and family helped to reinforce the importance of their contributions and the meaning they held for their children. In the study, many wives agreed with their husbands' wishes not to tell about their infant's genetic origins, to protect both their husbands' sense of virility and their families from negative public attitudes.

6. *The attachment relationship between these psychological fathers and their children was more important than genetic heritage.* The fathers and mothers believed that their most important efforts were informed by their decisions to keep the *best interests of the child in mind.* The families in this study had decided to disclose to their children their biological roots when they became young adults. Although more research is needed before any generalizations can be made, the results in Snowden's study indicated that when family relationships were strong, the disclosure in young adulthood did not seem to present a crisis for the adult children. Many of the children expressed concern for their "dad" after disclosure and empathized with his having carried the secret for so long. They did not regret being born through AID, they felt special and glad to be alive to have been able to fulfill their parent's wish for a child. They considered the father they knew to be their "father" and felt a full sense of family belonging.

The adult children claimed that family identity was based on their continuing relationships with important attachment figures such as mother, father, siblings, if any, and the extended family. The researchers noted that the families in the study were intact, with positive levels of family functioning and children who had achieved young adulthood without significant problems. The impact of delayed disclosures in *these* families did not evoke a critical crisis in the lives of the children. For families with troubled histories, however, the outcome of late disclosures of AID may be different. Further research is needed in this area.

The following examples illustrate some of the problems that can arise when a father is unable to establish a nonconflicted relationship with a child born through AID. The fathers in these two vignettes had not resolved their grief about their own infertility and the ambivalence about the choice of collaborative parentage that continued to interfere in the relationship with their children.

Case Vignette

Mr. and Mrs. Morley, who had two sons and a daughter conceived through the help of different sperm donors, had kept the birth heritage of their children a secret. From the start, Mr. Morley had difficulty connecting with his children, who developed a close relationship with their mother but were less involved with him and sensed his estrangement from them. Continuously disappointed that they could not fulfill his expectations, he was often critical of them—how they looked, what they enjoyed, and their abilities. The children's mother died when they were in late adolescence. At that time, Mr. Morley told them of their real birth heritage and said that he did not really feel like a "father" to them. A break in their relationship occurred. The children were grief stricken and angry that they had suffered their father's rejection for so long, at great costs to their own self-esteem and personal autonomy. They realized that they could never have pleased him because, sadly, he was still grieving the loss of his own biological children. He could not accept them for who they were. This insight brought some relief in that they felt there was a reason beyond themselves that he could not accept them.

Case Vignette

Mr. and Mrs. Calhoun gave birth to a son, Bill, who was conceived through AID. The baby was born prematurely and experienced many medical problems and prolonged hospital stays. Homecoming was difficult, as the baby needed intensive caregiving and the father felt "shut out" because he was uncomfortable in handling his fragile son. Bill exhibited significant developmental difficulties. Mr. Calhoun was unable to establish an empathetic relationship with his child. Perhaps this related to earlier narcissistic wounds in Mr. Calhoun's own past (Fraiberg et al., 1975). Perhaps, on the other hand, his inability to accept his child related to the grief over not having his own biologically related child and his inability to talk about his feelings. Mr. Calhoun believed that his son's atypical development was due to inherited characteristics and had fantasies about the "bad seed" of the genetic father. He was embarrassed about his son's development and confused about his own role as father.

At the urging of Mrs. Calhoun, the family sought out treatment for their son. A broad biopsychosocial assessment pointed to the dynamic interaction of a number of contributing factors: the possible genetic contribution to developmental delays; the impact of prematurity, illness, and early hospital stays; the unresolved ambivalence of the father; and the mother and father's feelings of isolation because of their secret.

SURROGATE/GESTATIONAL PARENTHOOD

With the advent of IVF techniques, complex forms of surrogate and gestational parenthood have become possible. If a woman is not fecund and is unable either to become pregnant or carry a baby to term, families may now become parents through the help of surrogate and/or gestational birth mother. The intentional parents can seek a volunteer, a relative, or a friend to be the gestational or surrogate mother. The surrogate parent is both the ova donor and the birth mother. The gestational mother, on the other hand, receives the embryos created through IVF and carries the fetus to term. Through IVF procedures, the embryos may be created *in vitro* via the gametes of the intentional parents, the ova of the surrogate mother, or other gamete donors.

The practice of surrogate and gestational parenthood has become more widespread since its origin in the 1970s but the process still has potential complications. Many intentional parents and surrogate or gestational parents seek, legal, medical, and psychological advice (Hanafin, 1999). Intentional parents who use this pathway to parenthood face important tasks in the formation of their family. A first major task is to choose the surrogate/gestational birth mother. Infertility clinics suggest that a thorough mental, physical, and genetic evaluation precede this choice. Some clinics require the chosen birth mother already to have had children, in order that she be able to give truly informed consent regarding her intention to give the infant to the intentional parents (Macklin, 1994b).

Research on the mental health of surrogate and/or gestational carriers reveals that these women show no significant psychopathology. Some do it for altruistic or familial reasons and/or financial help; others participate because helping to create infants has for them special, personal symbolic meaning. Gestational mothers often report satisfaction with their role.

Their level of satisfaction, however, correlates positively with the establishment of a respectful and comfortable relationship with the intentional parents (Hanafin, 1999).

The intentional parents' second major task is to provide for the financial and psychological support of the gestational mother to enable her to receive the medical care and guidance to provide a positive prenatal holding environment for the growing fetus. In this sense, the intentional parents share in the process of pregnancy. Clinicians note that the capacity of the intentional parents to trust, to contain their anxieties, and to be sympathetic with the experiences of the gestational carrier can help in avoiding future conflicts with the birth mother (Hanafin, 1999).

The third task of the intentional parents is to have a clear understanding with the gestational birth mother regarding the following relevant issues:

- Agreement over the conditions of prenatal care such as diet, lifestyle, travel, medical care, and prenatal testing
- A legal contract regarding issues such as appropriate behavior of the surrogate mother during pregnancy to protect the baby; financial responsibilities of the intentional parents as to medical care and other needs of the birth mother before and after birth or miscarriage; clear lines of authority in decision making if complications arise, such as the willingness of the surrogate to follow the doctor's orders if the baby is in distress. While payment to the surrogate or gestational mother is not legal per se, because baby selling is not allowed in this country, many families make their own private financial relationships (Andrews, 1999).
- Agreement on the decision-making roles of the intentional parents if emergencies or a crises occur. For example, who decides about fetal reductions, if the mother is carrying multiple fetuses, or abortion, if the neonate is found to have severe abnormalities (Macklin, 1994a)?
- Agreement as to the future relationship between the surrogate/gestational parent and the child after birth. Will the child be told about the surrogate/gestational mother? Will the surrogate continue to have contact with the child? Will there be a formal exchange of medical information? Will there be a long-term relationship between the two families (Macklin, 1994a)?

As we discussed in Chapter 8, surrogate and gestational motherhood raise legal, ethical, and moral questions regarding the use of payments in contracts with gestational birth mothers, and their rights to keep the children they have carried to term if they so wish. Family law, used in disputes in custody and adoption cases, is being used in many states to resolve disputes that may arise regarding surrogate or gestational parenthood (Capron & Radin, 1994). Moreover, many of these issues are being deliberated in state ethics commissions and state courts across the country.

The following vignette illustrates the potential psychological confusion that can develop when the gestational mother is a close relative and highlights the identity confusion that can arise. This composite case illustrates a variety of issues noted by clinicians.

Case Vignette

Mr. and Mrs. Owens were unable to have any children. The infertility diagnosis revealed that, although they each could produce viable ova and sperm, Mrs. Owens was not able to carry an infant to term. Coming from a large and close family, Mrs. Owens asked her sister if she would be willing to become pregnant with embryos created by the couple through IVF procedures. Mrs. Owens's sister Marion and her husband Eddy had two of their own children but agreed to the undertaking for a variety of reasons. Marion wanted to help her sister, because children were an important part of the family's values and the Owens's had promised to pay for all the medial expenses and help Eddy to start a small business.

The pregnancy went well and the resulting twins, Mary and Tommy, were full term and healthy. However, many unexpected difficulties emerged. Marion's own toddlers found their mother's pregnancy difficult and became aggressive about the pregnancy, sometimes hitting her stomach in anger because she was not as responsive as usual to them. They did not understand why she was going to give the babies to her sister. The pregnancy interfered in her role as wife and mother, and created stress in the marriage. When the twins were born, Marion found that she had a greater attachment to the children than she had expected, and it was difficult for her to visit her sister without reaching for them. Her attachment went beyond the role of just being their aunt. Marion's children continued to have negative feelings toward the twins. The roles of grandmother, grandfather, mother, father, aunt, uncle, and cousin were confused within these two families, who lived closely together.

While the babies' psychological parents were also their biological parents, the complex social family relationships and confusion in family boundaries were difficult to manage. The typical expectations of roles within families (mother, aunt, sister-in-law, and wife) became confused and led to interpersonal conflicts. As preschoolers, the children began to feel divided loyalties, and their parents felt threatened by the unclear status of their roles with their children.

The complex social dynamics that emerged for this family were not anticipated, and the children showed signs of insecurity and confusion in identifications with dual sets of parental figures. They were unclear as to which family they actually belonged to and which parental figures were their primary parents. Furthermore, how, for example, were the children to understand the intense sibling rivalry that existed between themselves and their cousins? As the children reached school age, the family sought help to cope with the unusual and enmeshed set of family relationships that had evolved.

THE SHIFT TO PARENTHOOD: IDENTITY AND ATTACHMENT RELATIONSHIPS

When pregnancy occurs for the infertile couple, it is often a surprise. Many parents anxiously await the passing of the first trimester, which may signify that the baby will be carried to term. At times, the "unexpected" pregnancy can create an abrupt shift in psychological focus, before family members have been able to resolve their remaining conflicts and ambivalence about the specific form of family formation they have chosen (Burns, 1999; Epstein & Rosenberg, 1997). They may, for example, carry their feelings of uncertainty and anxiety with them as they adjust both to the fact of pregnancy and the transfer of their care to a new medical team (Brodzinsky, 1997).

Clinical reports reveal that many families and their children adjust in a healthy, positive way (Kovacs, Mushin, Kane, & Baker, 1993). The advent of parenthood achieved through IVF has also been found to affect parental perceptions of their child for the better. Greenfeld (1999) and her colleagues found that over half of the mothers reported having special, positive feelings of attachment toward their children but also noted unease about separations.

However, for infertile couples, some risk factors exist for both children and parents in the formation of family identity and attachment relationships (Abbey et al., 1991; Greenfeld, Ort, Greenfeld, et al., 1996). For example, there is a higher rate of cesarean deliveries in women who receive ova donations, making recovery from pregnancy more difficult. Multiple embryo transfers in IVF procedures often result in the birth of twins, triplets, and larger sets of children. These infants are more likely to be premature, with low birthweight, and caregiving is difficult following cesarean section (Applegarth, 1999).

In addition, the psychological recovery of parents involved in long years of infertility treatment is often slow. They often face a number of special problems in the development of parental identity and the establishment of a secure attachment relationship with their children (Glazer, 1993). For these parents, establishment of an attachment relationship with their child is often colored by residual anxiety and grief that may be evident in the ongoing mourning of the difficult losses previously endured. While happy about the arrival of their infant(s), they may unexpectedly feel depressed, exhausted, and ambivalent. These feelings may interfere with their ability to become emotionally attuned to the early needs of their infant.

One mother, Mrs. Andrews, expressed in an interview her unexpected reaction of depression following the delivery of her daughter, who was born through IVF, and for whom she and her husband were the genetic parents.

> I was supposed to be so happy, but I felt so depressed and so washed out. I don't know what I was expecting. The baby cried all the time; he was beautiful, but motherhood was not what I expected. After all we went through, I realized how much care the baby needed, how hard it would be for me to go back to work. The sadness I had been feeling during the many years of trying did not easily go away, even though I thought the baby was beautiful.

The literature on the effects of maternal depression following birth indicates that depression can interfere with the richness of maternal interaction with an infant. If the mother is too depressed to provide attuned nursing and holding, for example, the baby's affect can become muted and both mother and father will miss the satisfactions of gaze seeking and special smiles that often represent the first signs of attachment to the parents (Fraiberg et al., 1975). Usually, when interactions go well, the parents develop a sense of parental competency that supports the process of attachment and parental identity (Benedek, 1959). On the other hand, the dynamic of withdrawal on both sides may create distance rather than reciprocity and hinder the development of the attachment relationship (Beebe & Sloate, 1982; Glazer, 1993).

Many parents who have had a child through ART experience anxiety about the loss of the anticipated child during the years of treatment. If it persists, this anxiety can have an impact on the mother's behavior in that she may feel a need to watch over her baby at all times and worry that he/she will be at risk if any separations occur. Sleep disorders among infants are often associated with intense anxiety of new mothers (Paret, 1982). One recent study of ART infants reported higher than normal sleep disturbances at 9 months, and corresponding evidence of maternal depression (Greenfeld, Ort, Greenfeld, Jones, & Olive, 1996). The new mother and father need extensive support from their extended family at this time and may seek therapeutic help to understand their reactions to the birth of their child(ren).

The use of ova and/or sperm donors, multiple embryo transfers, and gestational/surrogate birth mothers can affect the psychological issues with which caregiving parents must deal. For those parents who conceive a child through collaborative methods, the attachment relationship is often complicated by the parents' feelings about the loss of their own ability to have a genetically related child. Letting go of this loss is essential in order to accept the real baby who is now theirs. Part of the process of relinquishing the sorrow of infertility is the ability to grieve. Parents who have had a child through gamete donation and/or a gestational mother may still unconsciously mourn the hoped-for child who carries their "genes and their dreams" (Brinich, 1990, p. 46). This unresolved mourning may interfere with parents' acceptance of their child, to the detriment of the child's evolving sense about him/herself.

Many new parents have a fantasy about being "perfect parents," especially those who have had a child following great loss. Often, this subconscious feeling is a mystical belief that they must show their gratitude for fulfillment of their wishes to have a child. In most families, this idealized sense of parental identity is modified as parents experience the complex realities of parenthood: the ambivalence, disappointment, frustration, worry, discouragement, confusion, and joy that occur in the process of raising a child. If the parents are afraid to recognize or express their own feelings they may not be able to assume fully their roles as authority figures who use their adult judgment to support their child's developing autonomy and to help him/her accomplish age-appropriate developmental tasks. Parents who have had a child following years of despair may especially fear the loss of their child and go to extreme lengths to avoid conflict with him/her.

When parents cannot express their own ambivalence toward their child, they may not be able to help their child manage his/her own negative feelings and conflicts. If parents cannot convey to their child that he/she remains the same person across different states of feeling, the child may not experience a relational model that helps achieve the needed synthesis of anger and love toward the parents. This ability to know that one can have both loving and angry feelings toward an important attachment figure, and that continuity of the relationship is possible, is an important key to the maintenance of future intimate relationships and mental health (Brinich, 1990; Freud, 1965).

For psychological parents who have experienced the loss of genetic motherhood or fatherhood, the risk of loss is perhaps more frightening, and they may be inhibited in expressing their feelings when normal developmental conflicts arise. Such parents may consciously or unconsciously fear the strength of their raw feelings and therefore inhibit any actions that they fear might cause a break in the relationship with their child. Or they may find themselves in the grip of unconscious dynamics, such as unresolved ambivalence, that interfere with their rational intentions of caring for their child.

When children express anger and disappointment toward their parents, for example, many parents may feel hurt. Parents who have children through shared genetic parentage, however, may be less likely to have confidence that their child will reconnect with them at a later time. In such situations, parents may need to seek guidance and support to deal with the unresolved narcissistic wounds of their infertility problems and the interference with confidence in their own importance to their children.

Parents who have formed their families through collaborative procedures, including surrogate/gestational motherhood, must find ways to develop a family identity and narrative that is satisfactory to themselves and their child (Brodzinsky, 1997). The family has to choose either to tell the child about the reality of his/her birth heritage or to create an alternative narrative that subsumes within it the use of donor or gestational parents. In either situation, the parents will have to cope with this extraordinary narrative throughout life. Finally, all parents have to come to terms with the reality that their child may not be, and probably will not be, "just like them." For parents who are not biologically related to their child, however, the need to accept the child's differences may be difficult, as it can be a reminder of their own infertility and vulnerability. Often, therapeutic help can assist parents in dealing with the narcissistic blow that is experienced when they fully realize that the child will not be congruent with their own image.

Self-esteem in children is related to the internalization of parental attitudes over the years. If the parents reject aspects of the child that do not match their idealized hopes, the child must either disown his/her own behavior (part of him/herself) or distance him/herself from their parents (also part of him/herself). In either case, the identity formation of the child is adversely affected and may be compromised (Brinich, 1990; Hoopes, 1990).

This process of acceptance of the real child is important for all children, but in adoption and shared parentage, the lack of biological relatedness between parent and child sometimes stretches the differences in temperament, physical attributes, and other characteristics. In this situation, parents may have difficulty empathizing with the child whose characteristics are significantly different from their own and carry important symbolic meaning.

DISCUSSION

Every child develops an internal representation of his/her place within the family (Beebe & Sloate, 1982). In other words, regardless of the structural context of the family and whether or not children are biologically related to their caregiving parents, they need to know that they are valued for themselves and wanted by their parents. Moreover, children are sensitive to signals by their psychological parents of positive feelings toward themselves. They are also especially sensitive to conscious or unconscious, spoken or unspoken, *negative* feelings toward themselves, especially in relation to parental rejection and disappointment in their abilities and accomplishments. These overt and latent feelings can be internalized by children and impact their sense of self-esteem and self-worth. Regardless of whether children know about their complex birth history, emotional and empathetic acceptance by the psychological parents is critical for their developmental progress and the formulation of positive self-identity.

When a child's parents have gone through the traumatic experiences of coping with infertility, the pathway to parenthood is complex and often filled with despair and a loss of expected fantasies and dreams. Many parents struggle for years to have a biologically related child, and, often, this dream is not fully realized. Intentional parents frequently have to take advantage of new forms of ART which that may include the use of collaborative parenthood, that is, sharing genetic parenthood with other sperm and ova donors. For these families, emotional and therapeutic support is essential to resolve their grief and ambivalence regarding the loss of their ability to continue their genealogical heritage.

Most parents do succeed in finding great satisfaction in their role as psychological parents to their children. If they can accept their loss and the different pathway to parenthood they have taken, and establish a sense of joy and achievement in the family they have created, they can receive great satisfaction from nurturing their child. If they can establish a trusting and empathetic relationship with their child, he/she is likely to feel love and strong attachment to them. From the child's point of view, acceptance as a wanted child helps supersede any matters of particular birth heritage.

Many questions related to the consequences of new forms of parentage for children and the consequences of secrecy or openness in sharing birth heritage with children have yet to be explored. These questions await further clinical and basic research. As parents undertake new ways to form their families through ART, they often require the assistance of informed and empathetic clinicians who will listen to their narratives with compassion and wisdom.

APPENDIX 9.1. Alternative Considerations in Family Decision Making

TABLE 9.1. Deciding between Donor Insemination and Adoption

Advantages of donor insemination	Disadvantages of donor insemination
Wife and/or husband genetically connected to child.	Inequity of husband's and wife's genetic relationship to the child.
Able to have more genetic information about the child than adoption.	Inability of parent to accept child who is not biologically related to father or mother.
Husband and wife able to share pregnancy experience.	Legal concerns in some states.
Able to control the prenatal environment.	Religious, ethical, or moral obligations to this means of family building.
Typically more expeditious than adoption.	Pressures of unique method of parenthood: secrecy, lack of genetic information.
Typically less expensive than adoption.	
More "normal" or typical means of family building, therefore, less stigma for whole family.	

TABLE 9.2. Considerations Regarding Openness versus Secrecy

Advantages of openness	Advantages of secrecy
Avoids burden of deceiving child (and others) over a lifetime.	Infertility to remain secret, protected.
Avoids burden of others deceiving child over a lifetime.	Avoids stigma of unique conception for child.
Avoids chance disclosure by others or discovery of secret by child.	Avoids potential stigma for other family members or family as a whole.
Acknowledges ethical right of child to know circumstances of his/her conception.	Avoids potential legal problems.
Allows child to integrate truth of conception into his/her identity in normative fashion.	Extended family or friends unable to respect boundaries have potential for destructive or retaliative behavior; or believe choice is sinful and will, as a result, treat child badly.
Information about child's genetic parentage available for later circumstances.	Current practice of donor anonymity means child unlikely to have information or access to donor.

Tables 9.1 and 9.2 are adapted from Burns and Covington (1999). Copyright 1999 by Parthenon. Adapted by permission of the authors and the Publisher.

10

Single, Gay, and Lesbian Parents

New Family Perspectives

The growing diversity of family structure in the United States is reflected in part by the increasing numbers of single-parent, gay, and lesbian families (Lamb, 1999; U.S. Bureau of the Census, 1990). The increased acceptance of the rights of individuals to have children regardless of marriage or sexual preference reflects many important social and political changes (Fadermen, 1991; Miller, 1992; Parks, 1999). Within these new family structures, however, parents must often cope with distinctive biological, legal, and psychological issues (Kammerman & Kahn, 1988; Miller, 1992; Patterson & Chan, 1999).

While nontraditional family life is slowly meeting with more social acceptance, bias and prejudice still exist with respect to single-parent, gay, and lesbian families. Prejudice and bias can intrude on family life, often causing greater burdens to the parents as they try to care for themselves and their children. Moreover, their "nontraditional" family status often requires them to face parenting and family challenges with less access to social support (Jacob, 1997). As in all family structures, single parents by choice and gay and lesbian parents vary greatly with regard to the social, emotional, and financial resources they can bring to bear on parenting and family life. And, when single, gay, and lesbian parents choose complex adoptions or assisted reproductive technology (ART) as pathways to parenthood, they may encounter additional challenges in parenting and the formation of family identity.

Outcome studies of children in single-parent, gay, and lesbian families address two primary questions: First, to what extent does growing up in these nontraditional families influence the child's development? Second, how does the nature of relationships between parents and children in these families compare to that of parents and children in traditional marriages (Miller, 1992; Patterson, 1992; Tasker & Golombok, 1991)? While many outcome studies have focused on psychosocial factors within the family system, it is also important that practitioners consider the broader social surround of these children and families. Not all of the institutions that provide important services to children, such as school systems, have developed a receptive and open environment for children from these diverse backgrounds. When children encounter bias toward themselves or their parent(s), they may go through painful processes that include the experience of ambivalent feelings toward their parent(s) and/or distress about being seen as different.

In this chapter, we explore the special issues that arise in complex adoption and ART as pathways to family formation in single-parent, gay, and lesbian families. To this end, we integrate research findings and clinical insights in order to understand more fully the implications for children and parents alike. As experience accumulates, practitioners, researchers, and parents themselves are *learning not only about the issues common to these pathways to parenthood, but also about the great individual differences* that exist both within and across these diverse family structures and life experiences. It is our hope that clinicians will utilize the accumulating research and clinical experience with respect to individual differences to avoid the overgeneralizations sometimes associated with efforts to describe these families. We begin our discussion with a focus on gay and lesbian families. Within these families are both single- and dual-parent households. For the purposes of our discussion, we examine the experience of both complex adoption and ART from this perspective.

A SUMMARY OF RECENT RESEARCH ON LESBIAN AND GAY PARENTS AND THEIR CHILDREN

Although firm statistics are not available, it is believed that well over 6 million children live with gay or lesbian parents (Green & Bozett, 1991; Lamb, 1999; Turner, Scadden, & Harris, 1990). Early research on gay and lesbian families focused primarily on children born within heterosexual traditional families whose parents divorced following the mother or father's self-identification as a homosexual. Early outcome studies, initially undertaken in response to custody cases, focused on the adjustment of children in these circumstances. Often, in these cases, the decisions rested on the rather personal perceptions of the court as to the effect of parental homosexuality on a child's development (Achtenberg, 1990; Falk, 1989; Flaks, 1995; Patterson & Chan, 1999; Rivera, 1991). Gay and lesbian parents were confronted by entrenched biases regarding whether they could provide a healthy environment for their children (Sullivan, 1995a).

However, accumulated findings of research studies and our growing clinical experience seem to indicate that, by itself, homosexuality of a parent is not sufficient grounds for limiting visitation or blocking custody rights. Of course, within any particular family, mental and physical health can vary, and relationship problems within a family can occur. A number of studies, however, using a wide variety of assessment modalities, have found few differences between homosexual and heterosexual individuals in terms of their psychological adjustment and levels of psychopathology (Bell & Weinberg, 1978; Flaks, 1995; Gonsiorek & Weinrich, 1991). In addition, Patterson and Chan (1999, p. 212) find that "the results of empirical research provide no reason under the prevailing best interest of the child standard to deny or curtail parental rights of lesbian or gay parents on the basis of their sexual orientation, nor do systematic studies provide any reason to believe that lesbians or gay men are less suitable than heterosexuals to serve as adoptive or foster parents."

A primary focus of many of these outcome studies has been the question of whether a child's gender identity is influenced by a parent's sexual orientation. Gender identity encompasses three psychological components: a person's self-identification as male or female; a person's identifications with prescribed female and male role behavior; and a person's sexual preference (Wind, 1999). Many recent studies find no significant differences in gender-identity or gender-role behavior of children raised by a homosexual parents as compared to children growing up in heterosexual families (Bailey & Dawood, 1998; Bozett, 1989; Golombok & Rutter, 1983; Golombok & Tasker, 1996; Gottman, 1990; Green, 1978; Green & Bozett, 1991; Miller, 1979).

On the other hand, recent studies suggest that there may be some modest positive correlation between the gay or lesbian status of parents and the homosexuality of their children (Bailey, Bobrow, Wolfe, & Mikach, 1995; Pattatuci & Hamer, 1995). As with all aspects or indices of human behavior, it is hard to disentangle the many genetic and environmental factors that combine to form important contexts for child development. Still, researchers believe that, on the whole, the accumulated evidence shows that the great majority of children who have a homosexual parent grow up to have a heterosexual identity.

More recently, additional research has expanded the scope of these studies to consider a broader range of adjustment outcomes for children. Mirroring the bias that limits research on fathers in developmental research, these studies have explored mainly the impact of being raised in lesbian families on children's psychological and personality development. Overall, the results show that these children do as well as children in heterosexual families in relation to personality development, self-concept, locus of control, the capacity for moral judgments, age-level adjustments, and the presence of behavior problems (Patterson & Chan, 1999). Furthermore, in a longitudinal study, Tasker and Golombok (1997) found that the mental health and work status of adults raised by lesbian parents compared well with adults from heterosexual families.

In light of the accumulating research, early hypotheses suggesting that children of gay and lesbian parents suffer deficits in personality development appear to be without empirical foundation (Flaks, 1995; Lamb, 1999, p. 207; Patterson & Chan, 1999). Researchers acknowledge, however, that the generalizability of the research findings is limited by relatively small samples and homogeneous ethnic, class, and geographic distribution in the samples, and the lack of longitudinal studies (Flaks, 1995; Lamb, 1999; Patterson & Chan, 1999).

Below, we discuss different patterns of family formation in gay and lesbian families, drawing a distinction between families in which children are born into a heterosexual marriage that ends in divorce when one parent openly comes out as a homosexual and those gay and lesbian families formed openly by choice. In the former case, the child's adjustment is complicated by a disruption in the family surround and the need to cope with the associated losses. In the latter case, we are more likely to find families formed via either complex adoption or some form of ART. In the case of complex adoption, the child's early history may have been traumatic and may present special caregiving challenges to the adoptive parents. In the case of ART, the family may face a different set of medical, social, legal, and psychological issues.

THE TRANSITION FROM A TRADITIONAL TO A NONTRADITIONAL FAMILY: PSYCHOLOGICAL IMPACT ON THE CHILD AND PARENTS

In the past, many children were born within heterosexual marriages to a mother or father who later "came out" as lesbian or gay. With the growth of the Gay Liberation and Gay Rights movements, many of these parents came to affirm more openly their sexual preference and separated from their spouses in order to live a more internally consistent life (Parks, 1999).

All children of divorce have to adjust to significant changes in their lives: loss of their familiar surround, the break in the continuity of a parental relationship, and, often, loss of financial and psychological security provided by their family (Wallerstein & Kelly, 1979). For children who experience divorce related to the "coming out" of their mother or father, additional issues arise, including a shift in their view of their parents' former relationship to each other and the overt change in sexual preference (Wind, 1999). The psychological impact of this new knowledge about their parent depends on the age of the child, his/her comprehension of its meaning, and the potential disruption that occurs in the child's family life. In addition, the manner in which the parents handle the transition will also shape the child's adjustment (Wallerstein & Kelly, 1979).

Some clinicians recommend that it is best for the child if parents "come out" sooner rather than later. Adolescence is a particularly sensitive period for children, and often the "coming out" of a parent at this time is more threatening given the child's own emerging sexuality (Clunis & Green, 1995). Secrets in a family can interfere with open communication and spontaneity, creating secondary anxieties and interference with trust and intimacy (see Chapter 11). In any case, the child's first and most significant awareness of his/her parents' sexual identity should come from conversations with their parents (Clunis & Green, 1995). If children can have open and sensitive discussions with their parents, they are more likely to be able to deal with their own worries, the strain of the family separation, and the critical attitudes they may encounter in school or with peers (Casper et al., 1992).

On the whole, children most fear the loss of a relationship with their parents. One fear is that the "new identity" will mean that the parent is not the same person as before. They may feel displaced by the new partner and his/her relationship with their parent. Parents' ability to talk about these issues often depends on their level of comfort regarding their own homosexuality and their ability to understand the potentially painful implications for their child. Conversely, some parents worry about losing the love of their child, and perhaps losing the child in a custody suit. Many parents wisely seek therapeutic help at this time to deal simultaneously with their own conflicts and their children's needs (Clunis & Green, 1995).

Thus, the emotional impact of divorce has special overtones in the family when it occurs in the context of a revealed lesbian or gay identification. Two vignettes illustrate the ways in which this acknowledged shift in a parent's identity can precipitate an identity crisis for the child entering adolescence.

Carol and Her Mother, Ms. Todd

Carol was in elementary school when her mother, Ms. Todd, identified herself as a lesbian and the parents separated and divorced. Carol grieved the loss of her father at home even though she continued to see him. She experienced the loss of her mother's love when her mother's partner moved in with them. Carol was further threatened when her father established a relationship with another woman. Carol first entered treatment because of a reactive depression following the multiple losses in her internal view of herself and her family, despite the continuing real relationships with them. She needed reassurance that both of her birth parents would still care for her. As a latency-age child, she was angry at the disruption and overturning of her life, but was more concerned about the continuity of her relationships with her parents than about the issues of her mother's homosexuality.

In adolescence, however, gender-identity issues became more central. Carol was sensitive about her peers' reaction to the "difference" in her family. She could not easily share her feelings with others or comfortably bring friends home. Her own emerging sexuality created additional anxiety. Dating and social experiences made her wonder about her own gender identity. She returned to treatment to work through both her identification with her mother and her differentiation of herself from her mother, while still being able to retain the emotional tie with her.

Chad: A Developmental Crisis in Adolescence Following a Transition in Family Context (Wind, 1999)

Chad's parents were divorced when he was 9, because of his mother's revelation of a lesbian relationship. Although he had coped with the initial divorce without undue reaction, at the age of 13, he began to have both emotional and achievement problems in middle school. Chad was referred for treatment, and a broad-based assessment revealed that he was experiencing concerns similar to those of many adolescent children of divorce. The clinical social worker found that Chad's school performance was hindered by his inability to concentrate due to of his depression.

The issue of his mother's sexual preference became a theme in treatment. He expressed anxiety and confusion regarding his own sexuality, compounded by feelings about the sexuality of his mother. Chad could not communicate with his parents because of the sensitive issues involved and his fear of alienating them. He was upset because of the difference between his family and other families, and his concerns about other children's views of his mother and her partner. He felt powerless to improve his situation.

During the therapeutic work, Chad became more comfortable with himself, his family, and his peer group. The therapeutic strategies included education on sexual matters, support, and an informed empathetic therapeutic relationship with Chad, his mother and her lover, and Chad's father. Chad expressed his fears about his own sexual maturity and sexual identity, his sense of isolation from his peers, and his discomfort in expressing his feelings and worries to his family. During the therapeutic work, both parents became more aware of Chad's needs for reassurance and changes in their behavior that would display sensitivity to his adolescent world. The communication in the family became more open and enabled all members of the family to feel more comfortable and more accepting of the situation.

As these vignettes illustrate, therapeutic work with children needs to be embedded within the context of developmental theory and family dynamics. Normally, for example, latency-age children, like Carol, are not necessarily consciously aware of the sexual relations between their parents. When confronted with the issues of a parent's sexuality, a disruption of the child's view of the family world often occurs, causing confusion, anxiety, and a sense of loss of family identity. Adolescents, on the other hand, are just beginning to become aware of their own sexual feelings and to reconsider the meaning of their own sexual identity. As in Chad's experience, when a parent overtly presents a different sexual preference, the impact may have significant ramifications on normal phases of adolescent development. The psychological and emotional issues for the child can be compounded by the bias encountered in the external world, and the child can become more isolated.

The therapist often has to establish a working alliance with the child, the parental caregivers, and, if needed, relevant others, such as teachers and support staff in the child's school. Children must cope with a range of feelings that may include anger at their parents for the disruption in their lives, fear of loss of love, the burdens of dealing with the meaning of homosexuality in a biased world, questions about their own sexuality, and a longing for the earlier sense of the intact, traditional family they lost. However, a dominant need of children is to be able to retain relationships with the parental figures to whom they are attached, and these connections need to be supported in therapy.

LESBIAN AND GAY PARENTS: NEW ROUTES TO FAMILY FORMATION

Increasingly, gay and lesbian couples are choosing to have children within more open homosexual relationships (Patterson & Chan, 1999; Savage,

1999; Wind, 1999). When lesbian and gay couples begin to plan a family, they must decide between adoption and new forms of collaborative parenthood (Jacob, 1997). If they adopt, they are likely to have to form their family through complex adoption given the few children available for adoption at birth and the prejudice and bias that still exist in many adoption agencies toward gay and lesbian couples (Sullivan, 1995a). If they decide to have a biologically related child, couples faces many questions as to who will be the genetic mother or father, how they will achieve a pregnancy, and how they will divide parenting roles.

The social acceptance of homosexual families is ambivalent at best. Legal marriage is still prohibited for gay and lesbian couples, although the state of Vermont now provides for legally recognized "civil unions" for these couples. In most states, however, whether the family is formed through adoption or biological parenthood, only one parent is initially identified as the legal parent. The other parent, referred to as the co-mother, or co-father, or co-parent, has no legal standing until adoption can be arranged at a later time. For these and other reasons, many co-parents feel invisible. Their role is undefined; often, teachers, pediatricians, and others do not recognize them as parents who can make decisions. Furthermore, without legal parental status, the co-parent cannot include the child as a dependent in relation to health benefits, social security, inheritance, or other income maintenance programs (Sullivan, 1995a). Should the couple separate, the co-parent is also at a disadvantage in terms of custody, visitation rights, and the continuation of a relationship with the child (Horowitz & Maruyama, 1995).

Many aspects of adoption law are relevant to our discussion of gay and lesbian parenthood, and the most salient of these are summarized below:

- Bias and prejudice regarding the lifestyle of gays and lesbians have caused some states to rule against adoption and custody and visitation rights for gays and lesbians. The prohibition of gay and lesbian adoption, however, has recently been deemed unconstitutional in several states on the grounds that it is an infringement of the individual's rights to privacy, equal protection, and due process of law. At present, only Florida and New Hampshire explicitly prohibit by statute gay and lesbian adoption of children, presumably on the grounds that a heterosexual marriage is a better context for child care (Horowitz & Maruyama, 1995).
- In states where adoption is not prohibited by law, adoptive gay and lesbian parents may be required to show evidence that their sexual orientation will not be harmful to a child, and that their sexual preference has nothing to do with their ability to be good parents. In this respect, judicial

interpretations of "the best interest of the child" vary a good deal across different localities and states.

• Adopting jointly is a benefit to the security of the child, but most state statutes still do not allow joint adoption outside of marriage. The courts in some states, however, have gone to great lengths to interpret the laws so that gay men and lesbians who are "coupled" can have the same rights to joint adoption as married couples (Horowitz & Maruyama, 1995). In 1993, in the legal case *Adoption of Tammy*, the Massachusetts Supreme Court allowed a lesbian couple jointly to adopt their daughter, saying, "Adoption would enable Tammy to preserve the unique filial ties to her mother's life partner, would make her eligible for the health insurance and Social Security benefits of her mother's partner, and would allow her to inherit from the partner" (Horowitz & Maruyama, 1995, p. 15).

MATERNAL IDENTITY AND PARENTAL ROLES IN LESBIAN FAMILIES

Literature on the experience of lesbian parents is beginning to emerge. The sea change in the understanding of the complexity of gender issues has altered the previously accepted view that a lesbian woman would not wish to be a mother, and that motherhood should begin within a heterosexual marriage (Laird, 1993).

For lesbian women, pregnancy and motherhood set in motion profound processes that affect their sense of their own identity (Laird, 1993). Planning to have a family causes lesbian partners to expand their understanding of the complex dimensions of gender identity and to differentiate among the related issues of feminine identity, parental role identifications, and sexual preference (Wind, 1999). Important questions for lesbian couples include "Who will bear the child?" and "Who will be the sperm donor?" Assisted conception for lesbian couples generally involves the use of therapeutic donor insemination (TDI). The donor might be anonymous, obtained through a sperm bank or a friend or third party (Jacob, 1997). Couples have to decide whether they wish the donor to be involved with their child, and this may complicate the relationship between the two women.

Deciding who will be the birth mother may not be simple for the couple. Physical problems such as infertility or other medical considerations will affect this choice. Psychological issues may also determine the choice (Muzio, 1993). For example, the decision to have a child can precipitate strong reactions on the part of the prospective grandparents. Disapproval of the pregnancy by the potential grandparents can deter a daughter from becoming the birth mother. On the other hand, some prospective grandparents grasp onto the prospect of a grandchild with anticipation that the pregnancy will provide an additional bond between themselves and their daughters (Miller, 1992). In some cases, both partners will have a child, so that they can each experience pregnancy, birth, biological motherhood, and the opportunity to provide continuity across the generations (Jacob, 1997; Wind, 1999).

For lesbian women, pregnancy and motherhood may be associated with unexpected psychological changes, as well as change in the relationships with their partners and their wider social network. For example, feelings of attachment to the future infant usually begin during pregnancy and are reinforced by hormonal and physical changes in the birth mother's body. These changes may be disturbing to the mother and partner. A shift may also occur in the reaction of others toward the expectant mother as a pregnant woman. This increased focus on her maternal identity raises new questions about gender identity (Muzio, 1993).

The relationships between the pregnant mother and her partner are bound to undergo significant changes, as is true for all expectant parents. In addition, relationships between each woman and her family of origin and wider social network may also undergo significant change (Laird, 1993; Rohrbaugh, 1989). For example, some grandmothers may be threatened by the overt identification of their lesbian daughters with them as women and choose to disengage. Other grandmothers may wish to reconnect with their daughters around the birth of a child. As in all families, the grandparents acceptance of their new role is often of great importance in sustaining the confidence of the new mother and provides an opportunity to build a new and more satisfying relationship between mother and daughter (Anthony & Benedek, 1970).

The birth mother and her partner face different issues in the development of an attachment relationship to their new infant. The birth mother is physiologically primed to breast-feed and nurture her infant. The baby seeks the body, face, and smell of the birth mother, and frequently can be best comforted by her (Stern, 1985). During this phase, the co-parent may be disappointed when she realizes the difference in the birth mother's attachment relationship with the infant and longs to be recognized as an equally wanted parent. Each partner may yearn to be the primary attachment figure to whom the child turns when seeking comfort or companionship. Both have to negotiate sharing the maternal role, a complex task often so painful that it may precipitate a break in the relationship. The two mothers are often not prepared for the powerful emotional meaning that the child creates in them.

The difference in the relationships between the two mothers and their infant is visible in the names each mother uses to define her role. The birth mother's traditional name, "Mama" or "Mommy," signifies her legal, biological, and psychological relationship to her child, but it is not easy to decide the maternal name for the co-parent. Many partners come to refer to themselves by their first names, such as Mommy Emily, and Mommy Beth. Until the co-parent can adopt the baby, her legal status with regard to the child is unrecognized and can also contribute to her feeling like a shadowy figure (Sullivan, 1995a). If a known sperm donor is the genetic father and remains involved with the family, the co-parent can feel further distanced from recognition as a parental figure (Jacob, 1997).

The parenting and work roles of mothers and fathers in the modern family are less strictly defined and structured than in past generations. Often, parenting and economic support of the family are shared and the contributions of each parent must be negotiated. With the birth of the baby, the lesbian couple, too, must adjust the family work and nurturing roles. Mothering, however, may be unexpectedly important to both co-parents as they seek closeness with their child. Issues of maternal identity, self-esteem, and self-definition often arise.

Often lesbian couples are committed to the idea of equality in the partnership. After a child is born, they must construct new models for themselves (Allen & Demo, 1995; Rohrbaugh, 1989). In some lesbian families, the co-parents may each feel the need to nurture the baby. In other families, some co-parents may wish to undertake the role of primary breadwinner. Generally, role definition is a process of negotiation. Often, conflicts may develop over primary roles within the family, and these conflicts may continue as the child gets older, raising new questions at different developmental phases (Laird, 1993; Muzio, 1993). As the child begins to understand the special nature of the family, the parents may need guidance and support in constructing a realistic picture of the family that is attuned to the developmental age of the child.

Therapeutic issues with lesbian families are sensitive, and the therapist must be aware of his/her own bias and comfort with lesbians and their efforts to form a family. Laird (1993) has suggested that the therapeutic holding environment must include an empathetic understanding of the special issues that arise between the co-parents. The therapeutic alliance must be based on trust and acceptance which enables the parents to voice safely their often subjugated feelings about themselves and each other, and to feel that the therapist can bring an informed and objective readiness to listen to their ambivalence, concerns, conflicts, and pleasures as a couple and as parents (Sussal, 1993). This context can best enable couples to work through the unexpected crises they may experience, while providing the attuned and protective care their child needs.

PATERNAL IDENTITY AND GAY FATHERHOOD

There are an estimated 1 to 2 million gay fathers in the United States, most of whom became parents within the context of heterosexual marriage. Major issues for these fathers and their children revolve around divorce and the breakup of the family. The threat that father and child may be separated forever because of bias and prejudice in court custody decisions is frightening, and this potential loss is a central issue (Pruett, 2000).

An increasing number of gay couples choose to form their families through complex adoption or through ART with the use of surrogate/gestational birth mothers (Bruni, 1998). Research on the social dynamics in families headed by gay fathers is limited but provides an optimistic view that gay couples can appropriately nurture their children. Studies of children born within marriage and then cared for by their gay fathers conclude that, on the whole, the children achieve both developmental and psychological competence (Bailey et al., 1995).

Bozett (1989) found that gay fathers' parenting compares well with that of single, heterosexual fathers, and that they are especially sensitive to their children's needs (Bozett, 1989). One of the major problems these families face is prejudice in the broader community. Children benefit when their fathers can communicate with them openly and empathetically about these issues and help them develop skills in coping with external bias. Gay couples who seek to form a family through complex adoption must often make strenuous efforts to do so.

Case Vignette 1: Adam

Jon Holden and Michael Gallucio, after living together for 15 years, became the foster parents of 3-month-old Adam (Smothers, 1997). Adam was born to a cocaine-addicted, HIV-positive mother. The child required extraordinary care and, together, Jon and Michael nursed him back to health. In 1996, when Adam was 2 years old, they applied to adopt him but found that under New Jersey law, nonmarried parents could not jointly adopt. They went to court, and in December 1997, a New Jersey judge ruled that the joint adoption was "in the best interest of the child" (Smothers, 1997). This case set a new precedent in adoption law in New Jersey and reinforced the idea that the capacity for psychological caregiving was to be a major criterion in adoption decisions.

Fathers who form their families through ART can have a biologically related child through collaborative parenthood by seeking a surrogate/gestational birth mother to provide the ova and carry the baby through pregnancy (Bruni, 1998; Savage, 1999). In many situations, the surrogate/gestational birth mother becomes involved in the future life of the child; thus, the family takes on the characteristics of an extended family, including some elements of an open adoption. This process is too financially costly for many men, as the medical and support costs for the surrogate mother may be many thousands of dollars. Fathers who choose this approach need to negotiate contracts with birth mothers regarding medical treatment, prenatal testing, questions of unanticipated birth defects, the possibility of abortion, and other medical issues. Although the law varies by state, the birth mother retains the parental rights to the child in most states and can make the decision either to keep or to give the baby to the genetic father as planned. The father usually has to ensure his custodial status as parent through the courts.

As with the experiences of lesbian motherhood, it can be expected that the fathers' experiences of parenthood set in motion a new phase of identity formation, including the realization that they have profound and satisfying nurturing feelings. The relationship between the partners may be transformed as each father seeks to cope with his work and the task of parenting. Early reports suggest that grandparents, other family members, and friendship groups are important to the fathers in providing concrete support and nourishing a sense of acceptance of the child within the extended family (Savage, 1999).

THE EFFECTS OF PREJUDICE AND BIAS

Homophobia and heterosexism remain present in many aspects of social life, and children are hurt when they experience negative attitudes toward themselves or their parents (Casper et al., 1992; Wind, 1999). Prejudice and criticism are significant factors in increasing the emotional distress of parents and children in nontraditional families and place an additional burden on parents in their efforts to provide a positive context for their families. Some gay and lesbian parents themselves have internalized homophobic attitudes and may find it difficult to feel competent as parents (Crawford, 1987; Patterson, 1992).

Moreover, children in nontraditional families may encounter bias and prejudice in the schoolyard, the classroom, society at large, and through the social construction of single, gay, and lesbian families in the media. It is important, therefore, that professionals working with families be aware of their own biases and the way in which such biases can become manifest in work with single, gay, and lesbian parents and their children. Clinicians must bring an ethical, nonprejudicial, and open approach to their efforts to understand the family's experience and to support the family's strengths (Laird, 1993). This can be difficult considering the powerful, not always conscious reactions some practitioners may have toward diversity with regard to family structure and pathways to family formation.

Helping the Child Cope with Bias

All gay and lesbian parents have to attend to the impact on their children of bias in the external world. On the one hand, most lesbian and gay parents wish to live openly and be truthful to their children about their identity. On the other hand, secrecy and privacy may be a protective response for their children, as they may fear external reprisal at work or at the children's school (Wind, 1999). Bank Street School, in New York City, aware of a "dialogue of silence," between the school and nontraditional families, reached out to lesbian and gay parents. They established new programs and policies in the hope that all children at the school could feel more accepted and communicate more openly about their family life. However, many parents remained reluctant to identify themselves because of fear of social repercussions to themselves and their children (Casper et al., 1992).

As one might expect, family members' hesitancy to "come out" depends on the degree of acceptance they feel. One parent said, "I mean, with all our practice and skills, I'd say that every time we have to do it (i.e., identify themselves) you feel your blood pressure go up, you feel your heart pound, your palms sweat. It isn't easy. . . . We get the lowered eyes, and the muffled clearing of throat, and the back-turn" (Casper et al., 1992, p. 120). Today, in cities with a large number of gay and lesbian families, the gay and lesbian community itself creates a strong supportive network, helping to mediate bias in schools and other institutions.

MATURE SINGLE PARENTS BY CHOICE

As we enter the 21st century, we are witnessing a new form of single parenthood; namely, the mature, older, professional, unmarried woman. Three factors have accelerated the acceptance of mature single parenthood. First, the Civil Rights, Feminist, and Gay Rights movements have underscored individual rights to privacy in broad spheres of personal life. Second, ART has provided effective ways for a single parent to have biologically related children. Finally, the increasing need for adoptive homes for foster children and children living abroad has pushed many states and private adoption agencies to reconsider earlier barriers that restricted both single parents and gay and lesbian couples from consideration as adoptive parents for these children (Sullivan, 1995a).

Women decide between the options of adoption and ART for different personal reasons, including the symbolic meaning to her and her parents of having a genetically related child; the positive or negative feelings about accepting insemination by a known or unknown sperm donor; the confidence to be pregnant without a partner for support; assessment of the ability to undertake infertility treatment, if needed, and to cope with miscarriages and the disappointment of pregnancy failures; the potential conflict of religious and cultural bias; and the reality of one's financial resources and emotional stability. The wish to adopt may also be influenced by the personal meaning of giving a home to a needy child (Jacob, 1997; Miller, 1992).

For a single parent, forming a family through complex adoption or ART involves a matrix of different contextual factors. The mother must be able to provide for the financial and emotional needs of her child as well as deal with the special repercussions of complex adoption or ART. Three case vignettes describe specific clinical problems that emerged in single parent families who sought treatment: enmeshment of mother and child; a child's depression and anger about the unknowable father; the impact of preadoption trauma and loss combined with the absence of a father.

Case Vignette 2: Margaret

In some instances, demands on single parents to provide total emotional and financial support for their children can be overwhelming and create serious conflict between them. Margaret, a child conceived by sperm donation, and her mother, Ms. Post, became enmeshed in a great struggle in the preschool years of Margaret's life. Mrs. Post worked unusually long hours each day, and felt such guilt over her absence that she gave in to all of Margaret's demands in the evening. They had regular fights over what to eat, what television program to watch together, what time to go to bed, even where to sleep.

Although these issues can develop with many mothers who work full-time, the absence of a partner intensified Margaret and her mother's neediness for each other. Inevitably, they could not totally fulfill each other's wishes, and disappointment and frustration mounted. Ms. Post resented her inability to satisfy Margaret and blew up in anger when, for instance, Margaret could not accept any of the many choices she was offered for supper.

In the Post family, the underlying conflicting longings for closeness and separateness grew stronger each day, and the struggles on both sides spilled over into Margaret's life at school, where she became aggressive and uncooperative. Although Margaret had a room of her own, she slept in her mother's bed every night—an arrangement about which her mother was ambivalent but that she permitted. Margaret both wished to be intensely involved with her mother and have more autonomy for herself. She tried to control her mother and feared that if she separated even a little bit, her mother would leave her. Both she and her mother were angry at the situation and needed help to find ways to cope more effectively. An additional available family figure, whether a relative or friend, might have lessened the intensity of the struggle. The therapist helped by differentiating between the developmental needs of a child Margaret's age and the psychological needs of the mother. Family therapy allowed Margaret and her mother to express and understand their different feelings within a relationship that was supportive of both their independent and mutual needs.

Case Vignette 3: Martin

Martin, a 16-year-old boy conceived by a single mother through the use of anonymous sperm donation, had known of his birth history since the age of 4 and intermittently expressed longings for a father. He had a good relationship with his mother, on whom he was consistently able to rely for emotional support. Suddenly, because of something he saw on television, he became acutely aware of having a genetic father "out there somewhere." He was deeply upset for a few days and began to think about the possibility of having half-siblings and other relatives. He felt that he did not even know important aspects of his own heritage, such as religion and ethnicity. With his mother's encouragement, he entered therapy to explore these issues. He was enraged at the thought that his biological father existed but did not seek him out. Martin's feelings and distress led to a crisis, in which for the first time he attempted to integrate the missing father into his picture of himself. The long-standing good relationship with his mother sustained him as he experienced this new anxiety.

Case Vignette 4: Matthew and Tanya

Matthew and Tanya were both adopted by Ms. Smith. Matthew was adopted at the age of 7 following years of foster care and uncertainty about his permanent placement. Tanya was adopted from an orphanage in Eastern Europe at the age of 2½. She had been born prematurely and because of illness remained in various hospitals or in institutional care until adoption. Being a single parent of vulnerable children is difficult, since the children have emotional scars from the past; often, the mother has to bear the intense feelings of the child without sufficient support.

At ages 10 and 8, respectively, Matthew's and Tanya's development remains delayed even though they had made significant progress (see Chapters 4 and 5). The impact of their preadoptive history emerges in the vulnerability that quickly surfaces when challenging situations arise. They easily felt that they were outsiders at school and spoke of their family as being "different" given the history of adoption and the absence of a father. Despite the stability of their adoptive home and the loving care of their mother, anticipation of rejection and fear of failure were recurrent themes (Beebe et al., 1997; Fonagy & Target, 1998b; Hurry, 1998). One of the more painful issues for both children was the absence of a father.

Matthew worried about his masculinity and often felt less worthy and different than other boys. His play, reading, and drawings often elaborated on military themes. This preoccupation represented both his need to identify with powerful male figures who could master danger and his efforts to master worries about being able to cope with danger. Matthew's level of knowledge about history and his competence as an artist reflected important internal strengths and avenues through which he could express his internal feelings. He missed the availability of a "father figure" with whom he could identify to support his efforts to cope with his often frightening internal world (Cath et al., 1989). Although treatment for Matthew was helpful, he had always lacked a father figure who might help modulate his intense anxiety and aggression. His mother attempted to support his involvement in Boy Scouts and summer camp, but he has missed any ongoing, enduring relationship with a man (McLanahan & Teitler, 1999).

At 8, Tanya expressed great interest in and wishes for a father. When asked what a father meant to her, Tanya said, "A father is someone who can carry me on his shoulders, who I can send a father's day card to, and who can teach me things." In therapy, she imagined what kinds of relationships could exist between a husband and a wife, and a father and children. Often the father is seen as protecting the children from danger and setting limits on their behavior. She worried about growing up, and her fear of being alone was represented in her nightmares about death and separation. She sometimes felt that no one would want her and feared she would never marry. Despite Tanya's difficulty experiencing such frightening affect, she was able to use therapeutic support to modulate her emotional life and experience.

Single parenthood through complex adoption or ART is difficult, and therapeutic work with these families addresses many painful topics. The therapist cannot undo the past, and must acknowledge to the children that he/she cannot fulfill wishes or supply the missing parent. The therapeutic holding environment makes it possible for children to mourn their losses, to express fantasies of what could have been, and to discuss their present reality. Individual and family sessions are helpful in supporting the further development of family identity and children's adaptive capacities.

As the previous vignettes illustrate, it is always important that clinicians understand that each family is unique and the particular family dynamics in each single parent family shape the psychological context for the children (Lamb, 1999; Sullivan, 1995). A special concern in some families is separation anxiety. As with gay and lesbian parents, it is essential for single parents to realize that the establishment of a trusting relationship with their children will help them cope with the special nature of their family and the new questions that emerge as they grow. This relationship is the foundation that supports developing autonomy and resilience (Anthony, 1981; Beebe et al., 1997; Fonagy & Target, 1998b; Stern, 1985).

Single Mothers by Choice (SMC), a national organization founded in 1981 to provide information and support for single mothers and single women considering motherhood, offers formal and informal support networks that are especially helpful to single mothers (Jacobs, 1997; Kammerman & Kahn, 1988; Miller, 1992; Pakizegi, 1990). This support helps mediate the bias and prejudice that single mothers may experience, as they often must bear the long-standing stigma that was directed toward unwed parents in the past. The available social support and acceptance by the extended family, and external resources such as schools, community centers, and pediatricians, are important in sustaining the single mother's efforts to manage work, family, home, and personal life, while being the sole psychological parent to her child. When joining groups such as SMC, parents and children feel accepted by each other, and find both companionship and respite from the day-to-day intensity of single parenthood. For the children, relationships formed within these groups can improve identity formation and self-esteem.

DISCUSSION

For single, gay, and lesbian couples who are becoming parents, the family beginning is unlike beginnings in most traditional families. The parents must choose between adoption and ART, both of which present significantly different challenges to caregiving and the establishment of family identity. The complex beginnings set in motion special dynamics in the family's life. Each family has its own specific circumstances, but single- or same-sex parents may have increased difficulty adapting to family life as they face the combined impact of new forms of parentage, external prejudice or lack of support, and new psychological shifts related to parental roles.

The single-parent, gay, and lesbian families using complex adoption and ART as pathways to family formation teach us about the ways in which a range of family structures can support developmental health. However, we await further research that focuses on the dynamics of family life and the process by which single-parent, gay and lesbian families try to help their children negotiate the various phases in development. As more and more children grow up in these new forms of families, they, too, may help us to understand the special nature of their family life and its particular impact on their personalities as adults. These family structures have already brought new insights into the ability of fathers to nurture, the sustaining role of a second parental figure, and the importance of the support of extended families (Cath et al., 1989; Miller, 1992).

If and when these families seek therapeutic help on behalf of their children, the therapist must consider the presenting problems within the context of the child's phase of developmental growth. A developmental framework that includes attention to the attachment history of the child as well as to the relational dynamics within the family can be helpful to the therapist. The issues of difference, of growing up without a second parent or growing up with same-sex parents will echo throughout childhood and present different challenges at each phase of development. The process of identification with and differentiation from parental figures may be impacted by the distinctive nature of the family with structure.

Effective therapeutic approaches must include a working relationship with parents and their children. Often, both the parents and children have difficulty communicating about the sensitive issues that arise related to "being a different kind of family." When parents reach out for help on behalf of their children, it is important for clinicians to respect the parents' "informed subjective knowledge" and listen to the voices and narratives of their children as well. Those in nontraditional families have knowledge about their lives in a world that often expresses bias and prejudice unknown to outsiders. This subjugated knowledge is part of the narrative that parents and children often suppress. Clinicians who bring an informed, empathetic, and objective perspective to therapeutic work can help parents and children express their specific, personal, subjective knowledge of the experiences and history of their family life and undertake new adaptive pathways (Shapiro, 1995). These pioneering families are learning about their lives from the "inside out," and clinicians will need to understand parents' experience as they work with them on behalf of the developmental well-being of their children (Brinich, 1990).

IV

Implications for Practice, Training, and Research

11

A Clinical Look at Knowing and Telling

Secrets, Lies, and Disillusionments

MARSHA H. LEVY-WARREN

I met David when he was 15. Both he and his parents felt that relations in the family had become untenable. David and his father were constantly at odds with each other. Everyone in the family contended that the two of them were completely different personality types and had always clashed; it was just worse now, because David was older, bigger, stronger, and more able to hold his own in a fight with his very bright, articulate dad.

David was born from a pregnancy that resulted from his mother being artificially inseminated with a combination of her husband's sperm and an anonymous donor's sperm, following a determination that her husband had poor sperm motility. David's parents never told him that his father might not be his biological father.

Imelda was adopted at 8 months. Her adoptive parents had found her in an orphanage in South America. Her biological mother, a 13-year-old girl who had been raped, had brought her to the orphanage when Imelda was a few weeks old.

Marsha H. Levy-Warren, PhD, is Associate Director of Training at the Institute for Child, Adolescent and Family Studies in New York City. She has published extensively in the field of adolescence, cultural perspectives, and gender studies.

She and her parents came to see me after they had found 14-year-old Imelda and a young man having intercourse in her bedroom. Imelda was tied to the bedposts at the time.

The Desais tried to have a baby for 6 years. They experimented with a variety of drug treatments, they tried sperm donation. Musaf had a poor sperm count. Pilar had endometriosis. Nothing worked.

When Pilar turned 40, the Desais decided to proceed with ovum donation and a mixture of Musaf's sperm and that of a donor. Pilar became pregnant and carried the baby to term. Both of their extended families were told that Pilar was pregnant and were thrilled for this couple they knew had so wanted to have a baby.

The Desais, who were dark-skinned and dark-haired, had been able to find donors described as being of similar complexion and hair color. They planned to keep their baby's parentage a secret.

In their consultation, they said their world shattered when Leila was born with blond hair and blue eyes. They were concerned about whether they could keep themselves from conveying the degree of disappointment, alienation, and betrayal they felt toward her.

With the new and varied forms of parentage, family situations such as those that I just described seem to be almost commonplace. Time and time again in clinical practice, the changing developmental needs of children bring identity issues to the fore that require clinicians to think through the complex communications about family origins that inevitably take place: the secrets, the lies, the disillusionments that parents may harbor on the one hand, and the ways that children may come to know and understand these on the other.

It is critical to clarify issues such as how open to be with children about their origins, when to be open, and how information might be understood at different developmental stages. This chapter is an effort in the service of such a clarification. It begins with the three clinical situations I briefly described and the problems each presents, and continues with an elaboration of the issues such cases challenge us to consider.

Others have made significant contributions to this subject (Burns & Covington, 1999; Klock, 1997; Weider, 1977, 1978), especially among those researchers who have studied issues related to the counseling of families who have struggled with infertility and its aftermath. This chapter is designed to address not the general issues related to counseling of families who have experienced infertility but the specific issues related to children's readiness to know about their origins in families formed in nontraditional ways.

SECRETS

David, a tall, lanky, laid-back kind of guy, has long eyelashes, a quick and broad smile, and a twinkle in his eye. He is soft-spoken, thoughtful and open, bright, and artistically talented.

David began our initial meeting.

DAVID: I really feel like Dad and I are from different planets. Warring planets, I suppose . . . since we completely rub each other the wrong way. These fights that we are having are out there right now, but—truthfully—I feel like we've always fought. It's just that he was so much bigger than me until recently and he talks so much more logically. I felt like I could never speak up with him. He kind of scared me. Not so sure it wasn't better before, though. This has been hell.

LEVY-WARREN: What *has* it been like recently?

DAVID: Lots of screaming. Feels like we're going to slug each other sometimes, it gets so loud. We get on each other's nerves all the time. I look at him and get aggravated—and, frankly, I think he looks at me and just hates my guts. I feel like I'm just a big disappointment to him. Just by being who I am. It's not like it's something in particular.

LEVY-WARREN: Have you ever been able to tell him that you feel he hates you or is disappointed by you?

DAVID: No way. He and I don't talk to each other that openly . . . never have. I *have* said something about it to my mother, and I assume that she talked to him about it, but I can't be sure. I think she's intimidated by him, too.

LEVY-WARREN: So there's a lot that's left unsaid at home?

DAVID: Yeah, definitely.

I did not know about David's family origins when he and I met, but—from the first moment—what was happening but undiscussed was a major theme in his description of family life. Some weeks later, when I broached the subject of having a session with his parents, either with David or without him, so that they could meet me and give me their sense of what was happening at home, David was apprehensive.

DAVID: You're not going to tell them what I have been talking about, are you?

LEVY-WARREN: Absolutely not. I will only tell them what you and I agree on ahead of time. I just think that it is important for them to get a chance to meet me and to say something about what they think is going on.

DAVID: Well, I guess it makes sense . . . because I don't think what's going on is only about me.

LEVY-WARREN: Do you think it might make sense for you to be there when they come in?

DAVID: It might make sense, but I don't want to do it. The whole thing seems too weird to me.

It was in the meeting with David's parents that I found out that he was conceived by an artificial insemination that mixed David's father's sperm with the sperm of a donor. It was his mother who brought it up. His father became immediately uncomfortable when she did.

FATHER: What difference does that make? I have always treated him as my son, whether he is or not. For all practical purposes, he is and always has been.

LEVY-WARREN: And what about the nonpractical purposes? Are you aware of ways in which you may be affected by the possibility of his having been conceived with another man's sperm?

FATHER: (*appearing very uneasy*) Look. I don't like thinking about this. I don't like talking about it. In fact, I don't think it should even have been brought up. It makes no difference.

LEVY-WARREN: I wonder if that's possible. It is hard to imagine that it doesn't have any impact on you and your wife whatsoever. At the very least, not knowing may well create questions that lead you to look at David very carefully for signs of genetic linkage or its absence.

MOTHER: I know that's true. We have talked about it, in fact . . . but my husband is very uncomfortable with this subject.

LEVY-WARREN: Yes. I can see that. But perhaps we can ease some of the tension by talking about it. Keeping such thoughts and questions inside doesn't make for very fluid conversation or relations, either in the family or in talking about it.

FATHER: But I don't see how talking about it is going to do any good, either. There are questions that we can never answer in this. We simply can't know whether he is my genetic makeup or not, without telling him that he might not be . . . and that's never going to happen. I wouldn't want to hurt him that way.

LEVY-WARREN: Are you also concerned about how it would affect you? Either his knowing that you might not be his biological father or his knowing that you had poor sperm motility?

FATHER: This isn't easy, you know. You're being very direct, which I appreciate, but this is a really tough thing for me—and has been since we first started trying to have a kid many years ago.

LEVY-WARREN: I can certainly appreciate how difficult this is. But I think that some of the trouble between you and David may well be related to it, so I feel compelled to encourage you to think out loud with me about it all—in the hope that we can find a way to think and be about it that will make life at home more harmonious. As you know, at the very least, David feels that the two of you are very, very different and have always had trouble getting along. Perhaps there's some underlying communication that he has picked up on, or some distance that you feel because all of this has not been brought to the surface.

FATHER: Look. We made a decision a long time ago that we would not tell him or our daughter about this. I have no intention of changing that decision.

LEVY-WARREN: Please, if you can, bear with me for awhile. What do you think led you to the original decision not to tell the kids about their parentage?

MOTHER: We thought it might lead them to feel estranged from us in a way that was totally unnecessary.

FATHER: Look. That's not totally true, and she's trying to get us to be really honest. What's honest is that I felt so bad about my abnormality that my wife decided that there was no need to tell the kids about it.

LEVY-WARREN: (*looking at David's father*) I admire your courage in saying that just now . . . and I am struck by your referring to the poor sperm motility as your "abnormality." It seems a rather harsh way of describing what is actually a very common fertility problem that can stem from any number of sources.

FATHER: Yeah, yeah, yeah. I know. But, let me tell you, when you're a young guy looking to have kids, it just feels like you're a freak of some kind.

LEVY-WARREN: What kind?

FATHER: (*sounding bitter*) Look, I felt like there was something with my manhood, you know?

LEVY-WARREN: Sounds painful.

MOTHER: It was . . .

FATHER: You don't have to speak for me. It was probably the worst time in my life. I felt like we should get divorced, so she could be with a real man.

The meeting with David's parents was difficult and moving. We went on to talk about the situation at home between David and his father, including the father's assumption that he was not really David's father and how that might be leading to his heightened scrutiny and low-level antagonism toward his son. By the end of the meeting, the father said that David was a constant reminder to him of what he regarded as his compromised masculinity.

In our last exchange, I asked David's father to consider telling his son exactly what he had just said to his wife and me, that I felt that it would make what had been incomprehensible to David about their relationship understandable, and that he might be underestimating David's capacity to feel compassion for his situation. David's father was subdued in response to what I said to him but indicated that he would give some real thought to all that we had discussed.

Two weeks later, David's father called and said that he had concluded that it would be better for both David and his sister to know. He felt that having a family meeting about it with me present would feel comfortable to him and his wife. He then asked for my help in thinking through how to present it to David and his sister.

I suggested that he might want to say that he would like to have a family meeting in my office, that he had something he wanted to talk to the kids about that he had never talked about before and thought it might be helpful to have someone like me present for the discussion, since it involved a number of psychological issues. He agreed, and we set up a time to meet the following week. I suggested that he feel free to call in the interim, if he had questions or concerns. Two days later, he left a message on my machine. He was feeling really nervous about the meeting and would appreciate a chance to speak with me.

When I called him back, he expressed his concern that his children would lose all respect for him. When I responded that I thought they were likely to have a whole range of reactions but would ultimately feel greater respect for him, he calmed down immeasurably.

The day of the meeting arrived. I was struck by how David and his father looked as they came into the office next to each other. They were walking in step, animatedly talking with each other. It turned out that they were discussing David's father latest business deal, and David was suggesting a possible marketing strategy for a company in which his father considered investing. It was immediately clear that a different feeling now existed between them. Neither of them had described anything like it in our prior discussions.

The family meeting was very emotional. David's father began the session by saying that the meeting was his idea, and that he wanted to have it because there was something that he had never told them and thought it important for them to know. He said that he had never told them because he was afraid that they would be hurt by knowing, but had come to realize recently that he had never told them because he was afraid of how they would feel about him were they to know. He then related how he and their mother had experienced difficulty conceiving children and had been told that it might well be because his sperm was not sufficiently active to reach their mother's eggs, and that there were many men for whom this was true and no known, surefire medical intervention. He said that they had tried many medical procedures but—in the end—his sperm was mixed with donor sperm, and that their mother was impregnated by the mixture of the two.

David's 12-year-old sister spoke up.

SISTER: Wait a minute. Are you saying that you may not be my real father?

FATHER: Biologically, I may not be.

SISTER: (*with tears in her eyes*) But how could that be? You and I have the same-shaped eyes and eyebrows, the same-color hair, the same-shaped mouth.

MOTHER: That's true . . . and you may well be Dad's biological daughter, but it is also possible that you aren't. But, no matter what the biological situation may be, your father is your father and he loves you. He always has and always will.

DAVID: (*quiet, seemingly lost in thought*)

LEVY-WARREN: David, it's hard not to notice your silence. Can you say what's on your mind?

DAVID: Well, I was thinking that this explains some things to me . . . but I was wondering whether I sort of knew this without knowing it, or what. And I was thinking about why Dad didn't say anything about it a long time ago. Maybe it would have saved us a lot of years of being at each other . . . but, then again, I can see how he might have felt pretty shitty about this whole thing.

FATHER: (*loudly*) Watch your language!

No one said anything for a couple of minutes. The elapsed time seemed much longer, however, as David's father's words echoed in the room.

LEVY-WARREN: (*looking at David's father*) I don't want what is going on here to get lost in the shuffle of David's use of the word "shitty." I suspect that he was picking up on how messy and bad you might have felt about all this.

DAVID: Yeah. Sorry, Dad. I was really thinking about how bad you might have felt when you and Mom couldn't have a kid and it turned out to be because you had this problem. Seems kind of scary to me . . . but I still wish you had told me sooner, since you and I don't look anything alike . . . and we never have . . . and we are so different, as personality types.

FATHER: I think I was afraid . . . and, Dr. Levy-Warren would probably say, defensive about it all.

LEVY-WARREN: Actually, I would call it a state of being understandably unsure about what was best for all of you . . . but it certainly seems that some tension can be relieved by talking about it now.

SISTER: I don't know. I feel pretty weird, at the moment.

MOTHER: I can certainly understand that. I do, too. Dad and I have kept this secret for so long. I hardly know what to think about it all at this point.

DAVID: Well, I can't say I loved hearing this . . . but I do feel better somehow. Like I did kind of know it without knowing it, strange as that may seem.

LEVY-WARREN: There are stranger things . . . and communication is so complicated. You may well have picked up on something.

FATHER: I think I always wondered with you, more than with your sister, because you *are* so different. Maybe you just sensed that, in some way.

The family session was surprisingly calm, though at different moments all members of David's family members were moved to tears. We decided to meet again in a month to see how the family was assimilating this new exchange of information. David said that he wanted to come in on his own the following week.

When I saw David, he said that he had been upset all week by what he called "the revelation." On the one hand, he was relieved, since it helped him to understand why his father may have always overscrutinized him. On the other hand, he felt that he had been deceived his whole life. He also wondered what it would have been like to hear it when he was younger, and he was worried about what his sister was feeling. He and his sister had talked a lot about it all week, and he felt that she was okay, but part of why she was okay was because they had concluded that she *was* their father's biological offspring. However, they were sure he was not. David said that he knew that it was going to take a long time for him to *really* assimilate this information.

When David's family came in a month later, it was clear that they had been working hard to process the telling of the secret. As a result, there had been heated moments as well as some sad and tearful ones. Both David and his sister were able to express feelings of betrayal, anger, and distance. Most importantly, after years of discomfort and months of out-and-out hostility, telling the family secret had opened up the relationship between David and his father, as though each of them had been building up enormous resentment without having an opportunity to find common ground to discuss their differences.

I felt relieved about the outcome of "the revelation," since I had been uneasy about the position I took with the family. I was mindful of a number of factors in making the decision to encourage David's father to think about telling David and his sister about their origins. First, I sensed that the tension was partly motivated by David's father harboring the secret and David's awareness of his father's apparent distance toward him. Second, I knew that David was in the throes of thinking about what it meant to be a man, and that he felt that his father did not respect him as a man. I thought that both might well benefit from being able to discuss manhood in the context of how David's father felt when he was confronted with his fertility difficulties. My reservations were about what effect this might have on David's sister, with whom I was much less familiar, and how David's father might feel once the secret was revealed.

The work of assimilating the secret would have to continue for many years, but the immediate outcome left me feeling that the secret needed to be told.

The next case involves a complex mixture of secrets, lies, and enacted fantasies.

LIES: THE CHANGING OF THE LIFE STORY

Imelda and her parents arrived 10 minutes late for their first appointment. When they came into the office, the tension was palpable.

FATHER: Sorry we're late. We had trouble getting Imelda out of the apartment.

IMELDA: I don't see why I have to come here. I don't think there's anything wrong with me. You just can't deal with the fact that I'm growing up. That's your problem.

LEVY-WARREN: Can't be easy living in a situation in which you and your parents see things so differently.

IMELDA: It's not. They should move out.

MOTHER: Imelda!? How can you say something like that?

IMELDA: Okay. Then maybe I should move out.

LEVY-WARREN: I feel like I joined this discussion in the middle. What is all this about someone moving out? Why should anyone be leaving?

FATHER: As far as I'm concerned, no one should . . . but we *do* have to come to some agreement about what is appropriate behavior.

IMELDA: Translation—I have to do and be exactly what they want.

MOTHER: Imelda, that's just not true. But what we walked in on was absolutely shocking to us. Can't you understand that?

LEVY-WARREN: Seems that I *have* come in the middle of something. Could someone tell me what happened?

IMELDA: My boyfriend and I were having sex. My parents can't deal with it. They think I'm perverse or something.

MOTHER: It was a bit more complicated than that. She was having sex. . . . (*Her voice broke, and she became tearful.*)

IMELDA: Hey. It was no big deal. It was just a fantasy thing. I wanted Joey to make believe with me that I was kidnapped.

FATHER: Imelda . . . can't you understand that finding you having sex and tied to the bed was upsetting to us?! Do you have any sense at all of what it might have been like for us to see that?

IMELDA: I don't understand why you think it's such a big deal. It was make-believe, you know? I *wanted* to be having sex. I love Joey and he loves me. We were just having fun.

FATHER: First of all, you're only 14 years old.

IMELDA: So what? My real mother was 13 when I was *born.*

What quickly emerged was that Imelda had been adopted. Her adoptive parents had tried without success for a number of years to conceive a baby, then heard through friends that there were babies who needed homes in a particular orphanage in a South American country. They went to the orphanage and met Imelda when she was 3 months old but were not allowed to take Imelda home until she was 8 months old. In the interim, her adoptive mother went back and forth for several weeklong visits. They were told that Imelda had been brought there by her 13-year-old mother, who did not have the resources to care for her adequately.

Imelda was clearly of a different cultural origin than her adoptive parents. She was a slight, dark-complexioned, attractive girl with brown eyes and dark, straight hair. Her parents were both tall and of medium build; her mother had curly brown hair and green eyes, and her father had blond hair and hazel eyes. Imelda had been told from the time she was 2 years old that she had been "chosen" by her adoptive parents from a group of children who needed homes.

From the time she first spoke, Imelda asked many questions about her origins. She asked where she was from and wanted her adoptive parents to show her that country on a map. She asked many questions about her biological mother: for example, whether she was from the same place, whether she had a family, and whether her adoptive parents had met her and could therefore describe her. She desperately wanted to know whether she looked like her biological mother.

After I met with Imelda and her family this first time, I met with each member of the family alone, and then with her parents together. I said that in order to make sense of their situation, it was important to have each of their perspectives and that of the parents as a unit.

In the meeting with Imelda's father, he expressed long-standing concerns about his daughter:

FATHER: I have always worried about how Imelda would be as a teenager. She was stubborn from the time she was a baby, a big risk-taker, and very verbal. I used to say to my wife that she would be a hellion when she hit adolescence.

LEVY-WARREN: Is that how you would describe her now?

FATHER: Absolutely . . . if not worse.

LEVY-WARREN: Translation?

FATHER: This is tough . . . how fresh she is, how much she does things that we find outrageous . . . and how worried we are. Maybe that's the most important thing. . . . We worry all the time. Especially my wife.

LEVY-WARREN: What do you worry about?

FATHER: That she'll end up like her actual mother.

LEVY-WARREN: You mean, that she'll end up pregnant?

FATHER: It's not just that. Her mother was raped . . . and Imelda is just uncontrollable. She goes anywhere she wants, with all kinds of people. I just really don't know what kind of judgment she has.

LEVY-WARREN: Does she know about how her mother got pregnant?

FATHER: We've never told her. We always thought that she might be too upset by it . . . but she did ask about it, once.

LEVY-WARREN: What happened?

FATHER: Well, a few years ago, she got all concerned about how it was that a girl so young had a baby. She asked whether her mother had meant to get pregnant, or whether it was an accident. She said that one of her friends had told her that her brother was an accident. We explained we didn't think she was an accident . . . but that her mother was from a very different culture, and that girls there often had babies at a younger age there than they did here.

LEVY-WARREN: What made you decide to respond in that fashion?

FATHER: We just couldn't imagine telling her that she was the product of a rape. . . . Do you think we should have told her the truth?

LEVY-WARREN: You know, I simply am not yet sure. I need to learn more. But I am trying to make sense of what Imelda is doing, and I am struck by how her actual origins have resonance with her fantasies and actions.

In the meeting with Imelda's mother, it became clear that Imelda's father's concerns were echoed by his wife:

MOTHER: She has always been a challenge. I think her father and I have always been somewhat frightened of her.

LEVY-WARREN: Frightened of what, exactly?

MOTHER: That she would run away. That she would reject us. That she would become sexually active at an early age. We even worried that she would become pregnant.

LEVY-WARREN: Past tense?

MOTHER: No. Not really. We still worry about it. And we certainly found that scene with Joey profoundly upsetting.

LEVY-WARREN: What did you think when you saw her?

MOTHER: (*looking away, looking down, then looking back up with tears in her eyes*)The worst . . . what we imagined at our worst all along.

LEVY-WARREN: Can you put it into words?

MOTHER: I don't know why it feels like it could be bad luck to say it, but I do.

LEVY-WARREN: As in, saying it will make it actually occur?

MOTHER: I can hear how silly that sounds . . . but it does sort of feel that way.

LEVY-WARREN: I wonder whether Imelda has any idea that you have the thoughts that you do.

MOTHER: I wonder about that, too . . . especially because last year, she asked me straight out whether I thought that her mother was raped.

LEVY-WARREN: How did you respond?

MOTHER: I told her I didn't think so . . . in other words, I told her a white lie. Do you think that was the wrong thing to do?

LEVY-WARREN: I don't know, although it is something I think we need to try to sort out. Seems to me that Imelda is operating with partial knowledge and filling in the blanks with her fantasies and her behavior. I think we need to decide whether she is at a point at which it would be better for her simply to know the truth, inasmuch as you and her father know what the truth is.

MOTHER: I can't tell you how much it scares me to tell her.

LEVY-WARREN: Perhaps that is where we should start to sort it out, then.

Imelda's mother went on to talk about how she had felt intimidated by Imelda for some time and lived in constant fear that Imelda would run away and get raped and/or pregnant. I tried to explore with her why she had these particular fantasies and how Imelda's having been adopted fit into the overall picture. It was clear to me that Imelda's mother had considerable residual guilt and pain over not having been able to conceive. It also emerged that she was deeply concerned about whether she had bonded firmly enough with Imelda, and that she believed that she had not established sufficient limits with Imelda as she was growing up because of these other concerns.

It was apparent to me after the meeting with Imelda that she was aware that her parents were not telling her all that they knew about her origins.

IMELDA: Can't you tell that they're hiding something? That they are unbelievably uncomfortable around me?

LEVY-WARREN: I certainly could see that there was a great deal of tension in the room when we all met, but I wasn't sure whether it was a product of being with me or the usual family atmosphere. Is that what it's like at home, too?

IMELDA: Yeah. Sometimes better, sometimes worse.

LEVY-WARREN: What do you make of it?

IMELDA: I think I am *so* different from them that they don't know how to deal with me. I completely freak them out.

LEVY-WARREN: What's *that* like?

For a moment, Imelda looked like a sad young girl. Then, she seemed to gather herself together and said: It's totally cool. I do whatever I want.

LEVY-WARREN: I don't know. I think if I were in your shoes, I might find it a bit more of a mixed experience . . . but that's just how I would feel.

IMELDA: Yeah . . . well, sometimes it makes me feel like I don't have real parents.

LEVY-WARREN: Speaking of real parents, your mother and father did tell me that you were adopted . . . though, admittedly, you look so different from your parents that I had already assumed this was the case.

IMELDA: (*clearly annoyed*) So what?!

LEVY-WARREN: You tell me. Certainly it must have *some* meaning for you if you react this way to my asking about it.

IMELDA: Well, actually, I think I was surprised that you asked me straight out about it. Most people make believe they don't notice.

LEVY-WARREN: Definitely not my style.

IMELDA: To be honest, I think about it a lot . . . especially lately. I feel like my parents just don't get who I am.

LEVY-WARREN: What kinds of things don't they get?

IMELDA: My social life. My relationship with Joey. The fact that I'm growing up. The fact that school just isn't that important to me.

LEVY-WARREN: Pretty big issues . . . so how do you feel about *them* at this point?

Imelda's demeanor suddenly changed again. She became quiet, looked out the window, and seemed lost in thought. I decided to wait a moment, to see where she was when she emerged from this state.

IMELDA: You know, I love my parents. And I know that they love me. But I feel like they are both afraid of me, too. It makes me feel pretty strange. I don't exactly know what it is that they are afraid of, but it kind of makes me afraid of myself. Like I just don't know myself very well or something. I can't explain it.

LEVY-WARREN: It makes me think of what you said when you came in today . . . about feeling that they are hiding something. Are they related?

IMELDA: Maybe. I guess so. Maybe whatever they're hiding is what makes them afraid of me. I don't know. . . .

This felt to me like a pressure cooker family—and Imelda was the one who let out the steam. Her parents were relatively controlled people, though each of them felt like a bomb ready to explode; Imelda, in contrast, was constantly being outrageous in her behavior and attitude—letting off steam left and right, shocking her parents and friends. It seemed to me that the family had to strike some better balance.

After meeting with each member alone, then the couple together, I felt that it was important that the truth about Imelda's origins be told—and why it was that her parents had felt so uncomfortable talking about it earlier in her life. I met with her parents, and they immediately raised the question of whether it now made sense to tell Imelda about the fact that her mother was raped. I told them that I thought it did, that she would understand it—and even be able to understand why they might not have felt comfortable telling her about it when she was younger. They said that they wanted to tell her but were unsure about *how* to tell her. They also thought it would be a help if I were there during the telling.

When we all met together the following week, the atmosphere was tense. Imelda's parents were anxious, and she was uncharacteristically quiet. After her father told Imelda that there were facts about her origins that he and her mother had not felt she was old enough to hear before now,

Imelda became very alert and focused. After her father had said what he had always known but never told her about her mother's life, she murmured, "I thought so." Then, the room was quiet.

It took several minutes for anyone to speak. But then the conversation took off, each family member animatedly participating. I was astonished at the quality of the change and—to some degree—the quality of the exchange. There was obvious intelligence, curiosity, love, and humor. It was extremely moving.

I continued to meet with Imelda for several months to try to help her to sort out her feelings and reactions to what her mother and father had told her, and to help her to come to terms with her own values and aspirations at this time in her life. I also met with her parents to help them with two issues in particular: how to set limits with kids Imelda's age, and how to assimilate telling the secret about Imelda's origins.

The next situation also poses questions about knowing and telling, both in families and in the consulting room. However, Leila Desai was a young child rather than an adolescent like David and Imelda. This raises a distinct set of questions and issues.

DISILLUSIONMENTS

The first time I met the Desais was shortly after Leila was born. They were exhausted, as new parents often are but also seemed subdued in ways that were unrelated to the sleeplessness that usually accompanies the first weeks of life. I began with "So, what brings you here?" They looked at each other, then Musaf nodded at Pilar.

PILAR: We are very worried. We look at our baby and feel that she isn't really ours. We cannot imagine how to talk to our families about what has happened. . . . (*Her voice broke; she became tearful, then looked over at Musaf.*)

MUSAF: This birth is the result of one of those medical miracles. Leila came from a mix of my sperm with a donor's and an egg donor, even though Pilar carried her. She doesn't look anything like us. . . . (*This time, Musaf looked over at Pilar. It seemed that each looked to the other to continue to speak when he/she was overwhelmed.*)

PILAR: We come from conservative families and a very traditional culture. We cannot imagine how to speak to them about having a baby that is clearly not of our background, even though I gave birth to her. We didn't tell anyone what we were doing, and now we have no choice but to tell them.

LEVY-WARREN: So, there are issues that involve how to talk to your families about Leila's origins and issues related to how you feel about her—and both of these are troubling?

MUSAF: Exactly. You see us—and Leila has light hair and light eyes. We feel. . . . (*His eyes filled with tears, then he bowed his head. He looked up, cleared his throat, and continued.*) We feel humiliated. We don't know how to talk about what has happened . . . in our families, to Leila as time goes on. . . . We hardly know how to talk to each other. . . .

PILAR: It is hard to admit even between us that we fear that we cannot love this baby because she is so very different from us.

LEVY-WARREN: It is as if the way she looks feels like a betrayal to you.

MUSAF: Yes. That is exactly what it feels like.

PILAR: And we do not know how to go on from here.

I immediately felt drawn to the Desais and to their plight. Their turmoil was palpable and I was moved by the integrity and courage with which they faced their struggles. In this first consultation, I talked about the necessity for them to allow the relationship with Leila to unfold—that they had to get to know her, and she had to get to know them—and that they should try to be patient. I told them that in my experience with families that had been formed in alternative ways (such as through adoption or medical intervention for infertility), it had seemed clear that there was a particular need for such a period of mutual adjustment, that alternative families were at a somewhat greater risk for feelings of alienation between parents and children, and the getting-to-know-each-other period was an important first step in coming to terms with the family's origins.

The Desais were interested in what I had to say. They said that it gave them some comfort to think that an immediate, "natural" bond was not always critical between parents and children; and that there could be a period of adjustment. They also said that they wanted to come back and have a lengthy consultation about how they might approach their families in talking about how Leila came into the world. We set up a double-session for two weeks later.

When they returned, the Desais seemed less subdued. Musaf began speaking upon entering the room: "We are getting to know Leila. She is so beautiful and alert. She follows us with her eyes wherever we go in the room. She quiets down as soon as we hold her. She is really a sweet baby."

PILAR: I enjoy nursing her. She molds to me in such a lovely way. And the pediatrician says that she is thriving. We feel so lucky.

LEVY-WARREN: This is not just about luck. She is reacting to the way you are acting with her.

PILAR: We found it very helpful to feel we had some time to get to know her. I think both of us have felt more relaxed.

MUSAF: We are still very concerned about how to talk to our families about Leila. So far, we have not even had them over, which is very unusual for us. We feel we need to have a way of talking to them.

LEVY-WARREN: Can you articulate some of your concerns? What are you anticipating will be the reactions of your families?

MUSAF: We have no way of really knowing. In our culture, having children is extremely important—and not having them may imply something about how good or pious we have or have not been. Pilar and I are not especially traditional, but many in our extended families are. We do not know how to approach this with them. We worry that we will be rejected, or Leila will be.

LEVY-WARREN: Perhaps we can talk about what might be the best way to introduce Leila to your families, but let's start with whose acceptance in your families is most important to you.

PILAR: I would find it terribly upsetting if my mother, father, and sisters couldn't accept us and Leila. I believe that my sisters will understand and accept what has happened—they were educated in the West. But I am concerned about my parents, who are really very traditional.

LEVY-WARREN: Traditional . . . but they supported you and your sisters' getting educated in a different society.

PILAR: True.

MUSAF: And they did that despite the fact that their sisters and brothers did not send their children away to be educated.

LEVY-WARREN: (*turning to Musaf*) And your family?

MUSAF: My parents would never have sent my sisters away to be educated. . . . Only the men were educated in England and the States. They are, overall, more traditional than Pilar's . . . much less open to new ideas of any kind. They are upset that I live here. It is hard for me to imagine their accepting Leila.

LEVY-WARREN: Has their degree of upset stayed the same over the years you have lived here?

MUSAF: No. It has lessened.

PILAR: In fact, they said they would come to visit us next year. This will be their first visit.

LEVY-WARREN: Perhaps news of Leila will have a similar trajectory. How do you imagine it would be best to tell them? In person, by a letter?

MUSAF: Since they so rarely come here—and we cannot afford to go there more than once a year—I think it would be a mistake to wait to tell them until we see them. I think a letter would be best in my family.

LEVY-WARREN: A letter might also give them a chance to process what you say and formulate a response rather than just reacting in the moment.

PILAR: One of my sisters is here. I think I want to tell her in person . . . but, for me, too, a letter would probably be a better way to inform my parents and my other two sisters.

We spent the rest of the time formulating a letter to Musaf's and Pilar's families, in which they spoke of their deep wish to have children, their disappointments in trying to conceive, and their eventual decision to use whatever means were available to them to produce a child. In the letter, they wrote of their desire to have a child together, to carry on the traditions of their families, and to create a family of their own. They said that Leila was a joy to them—though she clearly was at least partly of another background—and that through their relationship with her they felt they had been able to transcend their disappointments in conceiving. They also said that they looked forward to being able to introduce Leila to them.

The letter, an affirmative one, assumed that their families *could* come to terms with the fact of Leila's difference from them. The Desais were satisfied with the content of the letter and left, saying that they would each tailor the letter so that it fit their particular families but planned to send it out in the near future.

The Desais periodically consulted with me over the first few years of Leila's life, usually with questions about whether their frustrations with her and difficulties in setting limits were "normal" or a consequence of their reactions to the way that Leila had been conceived. Their concern was always that they had buried resentment toward her or feelings of betrayal that made these aspects of child rearing more difficult. They did not express further concern about bonding with her; each was clear that the bond was strong. They showed me pictures of Leila, who was absolutely adorable, but they never felt it was necessary to bring her into the consultation.

When Leila was 4 years old, however, the Desais came in with concerns about her and raised the question of whether it might make sense to bring her in to see me. They were troubled by the fact that Leila had developed a repetitive theme in her play.

PILAR: Leila insisted that we buy Playmobil figures in every skin color. Then, when she played with them, over and over again she played out the same story. In the story, there were two families. One family, which I feel represents our family, had two dark parents and a light child. Everyone in the other family was light. In the story, the mother from the light household goes next door to visit the father in the dark household. They go to a room, they dance together, and then she leaves. Leila loves this story. She plays it out almost every time she plays with the Playmobils. She sings along when the couple dances, then hums the tune most of the day afterwards.

LEVY-WARREN: What is the tune?

PILAR: It's an old Peter, Paul, and Mary song called "Leaving on a Jet Plane."

LEVY-WARREN: How does Leila know the song?

MUSAF: Pilar and I have always liked folk music. The song is from an album from the 70s that we have always enjoyed. So Leila has heard it many times.

LEVY-WARREN: Can you tell me what you make of this story of Leila's? Seems to me you have some thoughts about what the play means.

PILAR: (*Looked over at Musaf.*)

MUSAF: Leila has asked each of us why she is a different color from us. We think that she suspects that she comes from a union between me and a light-complexioned woman.

LEVY-WARREN: I can see why you might think that, but I need to know more about what has been going on with her before I can really come to that conclusion myself. Has she been having any difficulties of any kind—for example, sleeping, eating, or playing with other children?

PILAR: No . . . not that I can think of.

LEVY-WARREN: Have there been any changes in your everyday life? Have either of you changed your work situation or her school routine?

MUSAF: I changed jobs recently and have to leave for work earlier . . . so Pilar takes her to school on days that I used to take her. I also have to travel a bit more for this job.

LEVY-WARREN: Has Leila shown any reactions to these changes?

PILAR: Yes. She asks over and over again why Musaf goes to work before taking her to school, who the woman is that takes Musaf away in the morning, and about where he is when he is away overnight—and why he isn't at home.

LEVY-WARREN: Seems to me that Leila is concerned about his absence. In fact, I wouldn't be surprised if it had something to do with the repetitive story.

PILAR: The neighbor that picks Musaf up in the morning *does* have a lighter complexion than we do.

MUSAF: We hadn't thought about that. But is there another reason you are thinking that her story may be related to my new position and the attendant changes in my relationship with her?

LEVY-WARREN: Her choice of the song "Leaving on a Jet Plane" made me wonder about whether she had concerns about someone's comings and goings.

PILAR: That's one of the songs we sing in the car when we go away for trips over the summer.

As the conversation continued, it seemed clear to each of us that Leila's repetitive play was probably more about Musaf's new position and the consequent changes in his daily involvement with her than about Leila's origins. Simultaneously, it *did* seem that there might also be an unconscious fantasy about her origins getting expressed in the play, but it did not seem to me that this was the time to talk about it with Leila. She had yet to ask any questions about her origins, she was not symptomatic in any way that concerned me, and she had a recent change in her life with her father to which she undoubtedly was reacting.

I also did not think it was necessary to bring Leila in to see me, curious as I was to meet her. Instead, I suggested that the Desais talk with her more about Musaf's new job, his traveling, and his being able to travel to work with their neighbor—emphasizing that he leaves and returns more now than he used to and misses being able to take Leila to school. I also suggested that he make a point of spending time alone with Leila, perhaps on short trips.

The consistent message I brought to the Desais was that they should try to respond to Leila's specific questions or the issues she brought to them. I felt that, in time, the deeply buried questions about her origins would likely rise to the surface; but for Leila, these questions were not now in the forefront. I also cautioned them about superimposing an adult's way of looking at the world on Leila: I said, for example, that her asking about why her parents' complexions were different from hers was asking about exactly that—why people had differences—and not about her origins, and that more specific questions about her origins would come as Leila came to understand more about conception, birth, and the transmission of family traits.

KNOWING AND TELLING

These cases (and so many others) pose difficult questions about how to deal with all that is left unsaid in families. What *is* it that these children knew? And *when* did they know it? And how do we (as clinicians) take positions about revealing what is unsaid?

I felt that David, for instance, was just on the edge of knowing, and that the long-standing, escalating tensions in his family and his psyche were likely to be dissipated by revealing the secret of his origins. David's sense of being scrutinized by his father, the constant friction between them, and his feeling that they were so very different seemed one small but very frustrating step away from actual knowledge of his family secret. His parents were burdened by knowing but not telling the story of David's origins; it was on their minds a great deal and came up almost immediately when I first met with them.

After meeting with David for a couple of months, I also felt that he was both mature and caring enough toward his father to be compassionate about the fertility difficulties. The fact that he and his father were fighting so much, that he felt his father did not like who he was, and that virtually the first statement he made to me was that he and his father were from different planets led me to believe that he had preconscious knowledge of the family secret that was pressing into consciousness.

Imelda's actions also led me to believe that she had preconscious knowledge of her origins. The questions about her origins and about her mother, and her enacted fantasy of being forced to have sexual intercourse, demonstrated that her beginnings were right on the edge of conscious awareness. I am distinguishing between preconscious and unconscious knowledge in both David's and Imelda's cases because I believe that each, in their actions and words, displayed some degree of awareness of something unrevealed in their families that neither of them knew exactly.

Leila, on the other hand, had what appeared to be unconscious knowledge of what was unrevealed. Neither her actions nor her words suggested that she had knowledge pressing into consciousness of what her parents left unsaid about her origins. That is, though I believed she had an unconscious inkling, it was not in her preconscious—it was not pressing for clarification.

So as is true in our efforts as clinicians to aim our interpretations at just what is pressing into awareness but not quite known to our patients—for the purpose of maximizing the likelihood of their being able to hear and absorb our observations—I believe that we must be attuned to developmental and individual readiness of children to hear the unrevealed truths that surround them in their families. We have to try to listen to the actual questions of children and their preconscious derivatives and not read into these questions what we as adults may sense is more deeply motivating them unconsciously. This was the case in addressing Leila's preconscious preoccupations with comings and goings, as reflected in her play and words, which may well have had unconscious roots in more buried issues about her origins. We have to look at adolescents' behavior as sometimes an expression of preconscious fantasies put into actions rather than words. This is particularly the case when these actions show aspects of what has been left unsaid, as was true with Imelda.

There is another important issue introduced by these cases: How do we (or perhaps, do we) distinguish normative developmental fantasies, such as the family romance fantasy in David's case, the common adolescent girl's fantasy of being forced to have sex in Imelda's case, and the oedipal child's stories about her parents' union in Leila's case, from those that are being represented in these clinical cases? What made me hear these as anything other than the usual musings of children and adolescents (i.e., the musings that require no particular intervention, which distinguish them from these two adolescent cases in which I felt active intervention was needed?

I believe that what is left unsaid in families sometimes becomes an irritant in the psyches of the children. What is unsaid but sensed by children creates a vacuum that is filled in with fantasy. When that is the case, especially in adolescence, where there is already a proneness to action (Inhelder & Piaget, 1958; Levy-Warren, 1996), the children enact their fantasies about what is unsaid. This is particularly true when what is unsaid is about the children themselves. The fantasies fill in the gaps in the children's real knowledge, the developmental proclivity to know through action takes hold, and the adolescents show us through primary process activity what they are on the verge of knowing in their secondary process thinking.

Adolescents are also deeply involved in coming to terms with how they see themselves in the world. In early adolescence, they are in the throes of redefining their relationships with their families. In middle adolescence, there is a concern with defining a sense of gender and sexuality, particularly in the world of peers. In late adolescence, there is a focus on forming intimate relationships and defining a clear and personal sense of values and goals (Levy-Warren, 1996).

In the context of all that is happening developmentally with adolescents, it is a likely time for unconscious issues about their origins to be raised into consciousness (or closer to consciousness). This may be reflected in both actual questions and behavior. It is also a likely time for real information about origins to be more fully understood. I would just like to make clear that I believe there needs to be evidence from the adolescents themselves about their readiness to hear the stories of their origins. Both David and Imelda presented such evidence.

In the instance of the Desais, however, I felt such evidence was lacking. When they consulted me about Leila's repetitive play, I was aware of their ever-present concerns about Leila knowing her origins. These concerns had certainly diminished, but her parents were troubled about how and when to talk to Leila about these issues. As a result, they seemed always poised to see evidence of her wondering about her origins. It also was clear that they found it helpful to talk with me to resolve some of their personal issues about their relations with their families and the cultural asynchronies of their lives.

Over the years, I have felt that my usual role was to underscore both the adult Desais' normalcy as parents and Leila's normalcy as a young child. I was concerned that they would overread the degree of her preoccupation with the physical differences between them and impose information on her out of their own need to reveal rather than her need or readiness to know. I felt that it was most important to give Leila the psychic space to notice their differences on her own, frame them as she needed to, and eventually to ask about what she wanted to know.

In saying this, I am aware that children protect their parents (C.

Gilligan, personal communication, August 1999) and sense their discomforts; therefore, sometimes they may not ask about issues of concern to them. I had no evidence that Leila was doing this: She was an open, articulate, and curious child who seemed not to hesitate to ask her parents questions when she had them to ask.

David, on the other hand, who knew something was not quite right in his relationship with his father, had a fantasy of their not being of the same world but did not quite know what was awry. I believe, in his case, that he was not formulating questions to ask because he sensed his father's acute discomfort and wished to protect his father from possible pain. Instead, the tension between them continued to build, and discharge was achieved through open conflict.

In Imelda's case, it seemed to me that everyone was bursting with the wish to know and the wish to tell. The obvious tension in the family from the moment they first appeared in my office suggested it. There was a clear necessity to dissipate the friction through revealing the truth. The immediate sense *I* had of not quite knowing what was going on in the family—of being left out of the discussion when we first met—was my first evidence of the need for the gaps of knowledge to be filled in. What was then revealed in the consultation with the family and the subsequent individual consultations confirmed this early sense I had that something important was being left unsaid.

Knowing and telling are ever-present concerns in families and in the consulting room. How we know what we do, what we mean by "knowing," when we know in a conscious sense, and when what we know is buried more deeply and not accessible to us—all of these questions we must continue to consider and reconsider, most particularly in the context of the new ways that families are formed. I am also aware that there may be times when it may *not* make sense for parents to tell all that they know about their child's origins—that there is information that may be painful and/or unnecessary for the child to know. This chapter is not meant to exhaust the many questions that are raised in families about children's origins; I offer it simply as a contribution to what I know will be an ongoing conversation about telling and not telling about origins among those of us who work with individuals and families.

12

New Forms of Parentage

Summary and Implications for Practice, Training, and Research

Most families at one time or another need to address specific crises in the lives of their children. In this book we focussed on the problems that can occur in the special contexts of complex adoption and ART. As the number of these families increases, practitioners will gain more experience with the issues associated with new forms of parentage across the life cycle. However, we have begun to identify some of the special problems that may emerge in the development of secure parent–child relationships and in the processes of identity formation. Over time, clinicians and researchers will learn more about the ways in which children in families formed through complex adoption or the assistance of ART come to integrate this aspect of their life history into the narrative of their adult lives and experiences of self. Thus, practitioners in a range of settings and via many intervention modalities may see issues relating to complex adoption and ART as part of their ongoing contacts with children, families, and adult clients.

Many families formed through complex adoption or ART seek guidance and support to help them identify and address the special biological, psychological, and social issues that often exist for parents and children. As our knowledge of new forms of parentage continues to accumulate, practitioners will develop more understanding of the individual differences and the great variation that can exist within this special population. Woven into forms of complex adoption and ART are important factors that influence the life experience of *all* parents and children. These include the health and well-being of both parents and children, the degree of stress and social support in the family's environment, cultural beliefs, the effects of prejudice and discrimination, economic security, educational status, and access to a range of social and economic resources.

Because the new forms of parentage described in this volume represent an emerging field of practice, few definitive models of assessment and intervention exist. Clinicians can, however, utilize the existing knowledge base of work with children and families to inform their work in complex adoption and ART. In addition, it is equally important that practitioners remain open to the unique aspects of complex adoption and ART that may not be fully described by existing theoretical frameworks and practice models. By valuing the special, and often unrecognized, knowledge and experience of parents and children in new forms of parentage, clinicians can work toward the development of collaborative partnerships with parents who seek support for themselves and on behalf of their children.

The primary goal of this chapter is to consider the ways in which our current understanding of new forms of parentage can inform therapeutic work within this emerging field of practice. While we direct our discussion in this chapter to those clinicians working with parents and children in a therapeutic context, we encourage the reader to consider the ways in which this discussion can be extrapolated to a wide range of practitioners. Child welfare workers, social workers, psychologists, physicians, lawyers, and teachers may be involved with important concerns of both parents and children at various points in a family's history. It is our hope that an increased understanding of complex adoption and ART will raise the awareness of the many professionals working with this special population of parents and children.

In our discussion of new forms of parentage we have attempted to integrate aspects of developmental theory, ecological systems theory, and an ethnographic approach to understanding issues of difference. This work requires clinicians to be highly self-reflective with regard to their beliefs and values related to the defining characteristics of complex adoption and ART. Toward this end, we begin our chapter with a brief discussion of the relevance of an ethnographic approach to working across differences with children and families, and of the importance of a value orientation that supports a respect for individual differences and a strengths-oriented approach to work with families.

THE ETHNOGRAPHIC PERSPECTIVE: FAMILY NARRATIVES AND PROFESSIONAL VALUES

Family Narratives

Ethnographers and narrative theorists have written about the cultural and life experiences of individuals living in minority groups or "outside the mainstream" (Prell, 1989; Rosenwald & Ochberg, 1992). The knowledge of what it is like to live outside the cultural inheritance of the mainstream can be referred to as "subjugated knowledge." The primarily untold stories of parents and children in complex adoption and ART may represent an important body of subjugated knowledge that is central to the development and implementation of services designed to support their well-being. Thus, clinicians working in this field must develop models of practice that are guided by existing theory but are also open to the elicitation and understanding of these families' subjugated stories and knowledge.

We suggest that a narrative approach to work in complex adoption and ART may be helpful to the clinician in finding ways to elicit, and listen to, the experience of families whose stories may be subjugated to some degree. Such an approach can support the clinician's ability to recognize the uniqueness of families formed through complex adoption and ART, while avoiding errors in overgeneralization with regard to an individual family's structure and experience (Lamb, 1999).

As has been described throughout this book, the idea of *new forms of parentage* encompasses a wide range of pathways to parenthood and contexts for child development. Complex adoption and ART exist within a variety of family structures (heterosexual or gay and lesbian couples, or single parents by choice) and in equally diverse social, psychological, economic, and cultural circumstances. Thus, individual families will differ in the extent to which they perceive themselves to have unique, or subjugated, experiences relating to parenthood and child development.

An "informed not knowing" approach can help clinicians to *utilize* their existing knowledge base, while remaining open to the ways in which it may not adequately describe the experience of people whose life stories, or narratives, contain important subjugated knowledge. This approach, built on ethnographic and narrative techniques, recognizes the training of the practitioner *and* the role of clients as experts in their own lives (Shapiro, 1995). Clinicians must be open to new data that may challenge their preexisting views of human behavior and development.

As we meet and come to know parents and children, we bring with us a core knowledge base and a related set of theoretical assumptions. For example, theories of human development focus to some degree on the importance of the child's early life experience within the context of critical attachment relationships. The psychological development of the child is noted by many theorists to be related to the complex dynamics of family life. A similar emphasis is found in the literature on exploring the relative balance of the influence of "nature" and "nurture" on child growth and development. While each of these issues is germane to aspects of complex adoption and ART, it is important for practitioners to realize that the study of complex adoption and ART may also add to, or revise, our existing knowledge of such basic processes of development in childhood.

Professional Values as a Base for Practice

As practitioners, we bring a core set of theoretical assumptions to our work with children and families. We use this understanding to guide the processes of relationship building, assessment, and intervention. These assumptions guide critical decisions such as our definition of *who the client is,* our understanding of *what is the matter,* and our formulations regarding the *factors responsible for precipitating and sustaining the presenting concerns.* In conjunction with parameters set by the various contexts in which practitioners work, core sets of professional and personal values influence important aspects of relationship building with clients and decision making with regard to assessment and intervention.

Work with families who are forging new pathways to parenthood requires that practitioners be highly self-reflective with regard to their theoretical assumptions and their own value orientation (Borden, 1992). Beliefs and attitudes about family formation and family life, the meaning of children in family and society, and the factors that drive child development are both personal and strongly held. Given that complex adoption and ART raise important questions in this regard, practitioners must be prepared to heighten their awareness of their own attitudes, beliefs, and biases in relation to the defining characteristics of new forms of parentage. Moreover, because complex adoption and ART exist, at times, within a variety of nontraditional family structures, the practitioner's ability to work across issues of difference is especially important.

Working across issues of difference requires a respect for a wide range of individual differences, a belief in the worth and dignity of all individuals, a focus on promoting self-determination and the capacity for coping, and a belief in the capacity for change. Such an orientation supports the ability of practitioners to form collaborative partnerships with parents and children whose experience may be, to varying degrees, outside that of the practitioner and/or the cultural mainstream. Practitioners can begin by developing sensitivity to the experiences of marginalization that potentially may be associated with nontraditional family life and by viewing clients as "experts" in their own lives. Practitioners' ability to remain open to new data that challenges their existing view of development and/or beliefs regarding children and families is central to the formation of supportive partnerships with parents and children in new forms of parentage (Borden, 1992).

THEMES IN CLINICAL PRACTICE IN COMPLEX ADOPTION AND ASSISTED REPRODUCTIVE TECHNOLOGY

Family Differences and a Range of Unique Treatment Needs

Parents and children in complex adoption and ART are likely to vary with regard to the presenting problems they bring to clinicians and other professionals. Parents may seek out professional help at various points: along the pathway toward family formation, in the experience of parenthood itself, and/or on behalf of helping their children. Thus, parents may have a range of needs for education, guidance, support, and therapeutic intervention. The experiences of children entering families through complex adoption, for example, vary considerably. Furthermore, children in complex adoption may have had traumatic early experiences that are quite different from the more typical early family experiences of children born through the assistance of ART. The wide range of professionals with whom a child or family may come into contact can provide an important array of both direct and indirect services. In addition to therapeutic intervention, these children are strongly affected by the well-being of their families and the ecology of their wider social surround (Webb, 1996).

It is important that clinicians be prepared to address a wide range of biopsychosocial concerns and to make appropriate referrals when issues arise that are outside their range of expertise. For example, it may be necessary for child welfare workers and other clinicians to make decisions about when a child may need a neuropsychiatric or medical evaluation as they make differential diagnoses about a child's condition. Similarly, practitioners must be aware of the ways in which extended families, neighborhoods, communities, and institutions have an indirect influence on the well-being of children and families in complex adoption and ART. Prejudice, discrimination, and lack of acceptance of difference can present great stresses for children and families. In such cases, clinicians can help families to recognize the indirect influence of the social surround and support the family's active efforts in coping with its experience.

The case vignettes we have presented in this book reflect the wide-ranging needs of families in complex adoption and ART. For example, in Chapter 6 on skipped-generation caregiving, we described the experiences of grandparents who become full-time caregivers to their grandchildren through either formal or informal adoption. The extensive needs of these families required a broad-based assessment of the families' requirements for economic and social services, advocacy, and the grandparents' physical and mental health concerns, and the emotional and developmental needs of their grandchildren (Aranda & Knight, 1997; Burnette, 1999).

The Complexity of Family Narratives

As we have discussed throughout this book, there are many themes within the story of complex adoption and ART. Families formed through these pathways to parenthood share much in common with all families. The desire for connection, the need for differentiation, the symbolic meaning of children in family life, and the need for change in response to shifting developmental needs are important tasks for all parents and children. In addition, for all families, the creation of a "family story," or narrative, is important to the development of a coherent family identity.

The creation of a "family story" that serves to integrate past experiences with current life events and hopes for the future can be an important cornerstone of psychological well-being for individuals and families that have experienced major losses or biographical discontinuities (Saari, 1991; Webb, 1999). In new forms of parentage, one of the most difficult tasks is resolving questions regarding how to construct a story of family heritage that is helpful and understandable to the child. Often, the story includes aspects of broken attachments and loss that are difficult for parents to tell and difficult for children to understand. An important focus of therapeutic work in this regard is helping parents and children to find a language with which it is possible to construct a "talk story," or family narrative, that touches upon the complexity of the emotional life of the family while being attuned to the capacity of the child to understand. This task is made more complex by the need of the practitioner and parent(s) to adjust both language and thematic content to accommodate the child's developing capacity for complexity and the way in which the symbolic meaning *to the child* of the "family story" is likely to evolve over time.

In different ways, parents and children in complex adoption and ART may face challenges in the development of a coherent narrative that supports their individual and family well-being. For example, young children have a tendency to see themselves as responsible for the events that occur around them. Thus, their story regarding their removal from their family of origin may include feelings of guilt, shame, anxiety or depression, and a sense of responsibility about their role in the loss of their birth parents. From the parents' point of view, the losses that preceded the choices of complex adoption or ART for family formation may have involved significant biographical discontinuities that required them to adjust their sense of self, time, place, and purpose. An important focus of clinical work is to provide opportunities for parents and children to express, in their own way, their story of what has happened in their lives and the efforts they have made to bridge the experiences of loss.

Long-Term Reverberations: Attachment, Loss, and Identity Formation

Themes of attachment, loss, and identity formation reverberate across the lifespan of families formed through complex adoption and ART. While these developmental tasks are perhaps central for all families, *complex adoption and ART may present altered sequences of attachment and loss.* The traumatic impact of atypical experiences of attachment and loss can present challenges to both children and parents in complex adoption and ART. For some parents, the process of resolving social and medical barriers to parenthood has included experiences of loss related to their anticipated identity of biological parenthood. From the point of view of some children in complex adoption, loss of parental figures and multiple family disruptions occur prior to the availability of a secure family environment. Both parents and children, therefore, may have to bridge severe discontinuities in their lives that contribute to an element of fragmentation in their identity formation. The need to rebuild a sense of personal and family coherence is an important part of clinical work that can help repair the breach in the development of identity formation.

In the case of loss or other traumatic experiences, the child's capacity for understanding and adaptation may be overwhelmed because both important social contexts and primary attachment relationships may be unavailable as auxiliary supports to the child's emerging ego capacities. Moreover, young children may lack the verbal or cognitive ability to modify their emotional experience via the use of language, and thus face important obstacles in readjusting or bringing a sense of coherence to their internal and social worlds.

An awareness of the ways in which complex adoption and ART often involve themes of attachment, loss, and identity, is central to clinical work. Practitioners must make efforts to be aware of the both the children's and parents' history of attachment and loss. Specifically, it is important that clinicians consider the ways in which this history may influence the development of new attachment relationships, such as that between the child and the practitioner, or the child and the new parent(s). This is particularly salient in work highlighting the ways in which the therapeutic relationship can provide important opportunities for vulnerable children to experience being understood, or to revisit or rework traumatic aspects of their development (Hurry, 1998).

For example, for children adopted internationally, the sequence of family formation is altered and often begins with early institutional care. Initially, the child may not have had access to an attachment figure and may never have felt personally significant. When adopted, he/she is almost certain to have experienced a loss of connection to place and social surround and only later they may realize that family life includes emotionally available caregivers. Moreover, the child often has an urgent need for medical and developmental evaluations and treatment. When the immediate crisis of adjustment has subsided, the parents may seek out additional therapeutic help to better understand the developmental, social, and emotional needs of the child and related problems in the formation of a mutually satisfactory parent–child relationship.

As we have seen in Chapter 5, in the case of Tanya, the meaning of the loss of her birth mother reverberated across time and raised important questions about her sense of identity and loss in relation to her birth heritage. For Tanya, the construction of her narrative continued to change as her cognitive ability to understand and express her experience evolved over time. She eventually developed the ability to talk about both her birth family, whom she did not know, and her actual family. The process of identity formation for Tanya included the importance of resolving grief, loss, and survivor guilt, and as she mourned the loss of her "unknown parents," she came to accept the possibility of a more optimistic future.

Early Family Experiences and Child Well-Being

Over the past decades, research on the development of children has focused on the importance of the early interpersonal experience with a small circle of caregivers as central to many aspects of child well-being (Ainsworth et al., 1978; Freud, 1965; Stern, 1985; Winnicott, 1965a). From various theoretical perspectives, researchers and clinicians have explored the ways in which qualitative differences in parent–child interaction are associated with a range of developmental outcomes.

The children we have described in this book vary considerably. Some have experienced extreme hardships with regard to early caregiving and the quality of their earliest holding environments. They may have lacked an available caregiver who was able to recognize their affective states and contingently respond to their expressed needs. In addition, these children are unlikely to have had consistent experience with caregivers who were able to use language to show them that they were understood. Such holding environments limit opportunities for the development of secure attachment relationships and the many indices of developmental competence associated with secure attachment, such as the regulation of feeling states, the development of self, and the ability to differentiate self and other.

The concept of the holding environment can be used to understand the therapeutic relationship as a "new kind of relational experience" for the child (Winnicott, 1965a). If the therapist is able to recognize and tolerate children's expressions of fear, anxiety, apprehension, and disappointment, children may have the opportunity to establish a more hopeful return to the developmental pathway. By providing the reflective and mirroring function absent from the child's earliest experience, the therapist can create a holding environment that keeps the maturational needs of the child in mind. In conjunction with guidance, education, and collateral work with parents, such therapeutic intervention may be very helpful over time.

Winnicott (1965a) introduced the concept of the "holding environment" to describe the circle of care that surrounds the developing infant and young child. The "good enough" holding environment is characterized by caregiving that is stable, consistent, reflective of the infant's needs, and infused with an understanding of the infant's emotional life and development. The "holding" of the infant initially refers to the physical holding and caregiving in ways that support the infant's modulation of physiological states. As development continues, the concept of holding broadens to include the gradual emergence of the child's psychological self in the context of primary caregiving relationships. By recognizing and accepting the broad range of the child's feelings, including anxiety, the parent is able to help the developing infant to modulate overwhelming states of arousal in ways that facilitate the emerging ego and related capacities for self-soothing and homeostasis.

The Therapeutic Relationship as a Holding Environment for Children and Parents

In his exploration of this function of the holding environment, Winnicott (1965a) was able to apply this concept to the nature of the therapeutic relationship. He suggested that the therapist is "holding the patient, and this often takes the form of conveying in words at the appropriate moment something that shows that the analyst knows and understands the deepest anxiety that is being experienced or that is waiting to be experienced" (p. 240). More recently, other writers have conceptualized the ways in which the concept of the holding environment can be used by a broad range of clinicians in multiple therapeutic contexts (Applegate, 1993).

For children who have experienced multiple disruptions and trauma in early caregiving, the quality of the therapeutic holding environment is especially significant (Applegate, 1993). These children may initially present as having little confidence in the ongoing concern of adults and/or the possibility of hopes for the future. Children who have experienced multiple disruptions and losses in their early holding environment may develop a negative view of themselves and of others' interest in them that may influence their ability to form relationships within a range of contexts. In response to absent, disorganized, or chaotic and neglectful caregiving, children may develop defenses to avoid the pain that comes to be associated with interactions that are painful because of either under- or overstimulation (Fonagy & Target, 1998b). Behavioral patterns of withdrawal, freezing, physical aggression, and disorganization are characteristic adaptations to holding environments that lack both protective and reflective caregiving. The ability of clinicians and other professionals to understand these behavioral patterns as indicators of past trauma, and as adaptive from the child's perspective, may enable them to create a therapeutic holding environment that contains great curative potential (Applegate & Barol, 1989; Redl, 1966).

Working with Parents

Parents often seek help when their own ability to assuage their child's distress has become depleted. By this time, they may be experiencing a sense of vulnerability and concern about their capacity to "make things better." Thus, practitioners who work with children must be sensitive to the needs of parents for support and empathetic understanding. Moreover, it is important to assess the way in which parents understand their children's difficulties and the efforts they have made to respond to either emotional distress or behavioral problems.

For all parents, seeking help on behalf of their children can be a difficult experience. Feelings of ambivalence, anxiety, guilt, and exhaustion can create obstacles for parents in deciding when professional help may be needed and/or in forming collaborative partnerships with practitioners on behalf of their children. On the other hand, the great desire of parents to care for their children, to assuage their distress, and to help them along the developmental path can also result in the parental wish that the practitioner be able to provide immediate reassurance that the "problems will be solved." For the practitioner who is highly sensitive to the psychic pain being experienced by the child and family, it is important to be able to tolerate the anxiety associated with the "waiting and seeing" necessary to support the processes of in-depth assessment, problem formulation, and the formation of a trusting and effective therapeutic relationship.

Parents who seek help in cases of complex adoption and ART may contact practitioners with a wide range of presenting concerns at various points during the child's development. These concerns, described throughout this volume, can range from seeking support and guidance in anticipation of family situations to seeking help at times of acute crises. Practitioners must be prepared to help families differentiate acute problems from more ongoing concerns and be willing to start "where the family is," moving in a strengths-oriented manner to a broad-based assessment of the family's strengths and vulnerabilities. In this way, practitioners demonstrate from their first contacts that the child and family are to be considered "experts" in the experience of their own lives and that despite early experiences of loss and trauma, hope for recovery and growth does indeed exist.

From the point of view of the parents, the experiences of complex adoption and ART may be associated with a range of unvoiced issues. The practitioner must listen for information about the parents' history with regard to family formation, and feelings often hidden within their descriptions of other life events. In complex adoption and ART, parents usually have experienced a range of social and biological barriers to parenthood. Losses in relationship to fertility, to pregnancy, or to the idea and hope for a genetically related child can be acutely felt. In the case of skipped-generation care, grandparents may experience losses with regard to the "hoped for" relationship with their own children and the expectations they may have held for their own lives.

The desire for a child and the extraordinary efforts involved in complex adoption and ART may prematurely foreclose opportunities to resolve feelings of grief that may be associated with many of these losses. Practitioners working with parents on behalf of their children may need to focus on the dual tasks of responding to the parents' potential feelings of ambivalence, loss, and mourning related to the need for complex adoption or ART, while supporting their ability to provide empathic and attuned care for their children, often under difficult circumstances. In this regard, practitioners must develop skills in listening to parents' narratives with an ear for the symbolic meaning of their journey to parenthood and experiences with their child(ren).

Many of the parental concerns associated with complex adoption and

ART mirror issues that are present for all children and families. In all families, feelings of parental efficacy, entitlement, and agency are central to the ability of parents to make and carry out decisions in the best interests of their children. In addition, the ability of parents to accept differences between themselves and their child, and to allow for the transformation of the parent–child relationship as the child's development moves forward, are important indices of family well-being. In complex adoption and ART, issues of difference can range from the "overt" differences in transracial adoption to differences associated with partially heritable characteristics, such as temperament and individual personality. As clinicians work with families around issues of difference, it is vital that they work to heighten their self-awareness of both personal and professional value orientations that are relevant to work in this field of practice.

DEVELOPMENTALLY INFORMED PRACTICE IN THE CONTEXT OF COMPLEX ADOPTION AND ASSISTED REPRODUCTIVE TECHNOLOGIES

Developmentally informed therapy takes into consideration the importance for the child of the opportunity for a "new kind of relational experience" that a therapist can provide. The therapist can come to understand the child's fears, anxieties, and apprehensions that may interfere in relationships with others, as well as the capacity for spontaneous self-expression. Children who have had vulnerable early attachment relationship experiences may not have developed a positive model of themselves and may not feel a sense of personal agency and self-worth. Therapeutic treatment for the child, and guidance, education, and interpretive work with the parents, may be helpful in providing an opening for the child to develop and incorporate new capacities for the expression of feeling, understanding, trust, and positive expectations in personal relationships. Each of these areas is central to the child's more hopeful return to the developmental pathway.

In order to facilitate the kind of developmental growth described here, clinicians must establish a supportive holding environment and keep in mind the maturational needs of the child and especially the child's expressed views of self and his/her place in the world. The modalities of play and verbal and nonverbal communications are helpful to the clinician in getting to know the internal world of the child. Through these modalities, the child can find ways to represent important themes in his/her emotional life and sense of self in relation to the broader social surround.

The use of play is an important modality in child-focused work because it offers the child opportunities to communicate via displacement, in a manner that is less threatening. Children can construct stories of "other" children, of imaginary friends, or of fantasies and wishes. Over time, children may reveal their experiences at different levels of depth and with an increased ability to maintain communication about themes and experiences that are associated with anxiety or other painful affects.

A therapeutic relationship that supports children's ability to communicate through play can be extremely important. In work with children who have experienced major disruptions and/or crises, it is important that the clinician and child connect at a level that the child initiates and can sustain. In this way, the therapist becomes a new "figure" for the child, one who can listen and put the child's feelings into words, join in play and explorations, allow the child to reveal painful feelings, and provide containment for anxiety. The therapist provides the child with the sense that his/her feelings are important and have value and that he/she has a right to be protected and to grieve and mourn endured losses. At times children who have experienced abuse, neglect, or the absence of consistent caregiving try to engage the therapist in repeating dangers they have experienced. The therapist can set limits, which prevents the repetitions of dangerous actions (Downey, 2000; Hurry, 1998). As children get older, it may be possible to use more interpretations to increase their capacity for insight and to modulate their emotional experience.

Acute versus Chronic Problems

Differentiating between acute and chronic problems in childhood is a complex task that requires clinicians to take a detailed history. By understanding the ways in which children's current status either reflects or diverges from their past level of functioning, clinicians can work to identify important areas of child health and decrease the focus on the assessment of psychopathology. The nature of development in childhood can make it difficult to distinguish between acute problems and more chronic conditions. Because child development proceeds along multiple developmental lines and growth across lines of development may be uneven, it can be hard to form a complete picture of a child's overall developmental status. Moreover, experiences of crisis or trauma can precipitate regression in behavior that, if viewed outside the context of the child's history, could paint a misleading picture about the child's overall development and adaptive capacity. Through a combination of history taking and developmentally informed observation and assessment, the clinician may be able to identify past levels of competence and experiences of resiliency in both the child and his/her family. When possible, it is important for the practitioner to elicit information from multiple sources and to "listen" to the child's own story as it emerges through his/her unique pattern of expression.

Complex adoption poses a challenge to the process of assessment because the child's needs are likely to be multiple and interrelated, requiring a highly skilled process of differential diagnosis. When children are adopted following early experiences of disruption and/or deprivation, families may have a range of medical, social, and developmental concerns. They may need support in locating various professionals who can respond to concerns as they arise and are trained to recognize the special issues and circumstances associated with complex adoptions. For example, it may be difficult for some parents to obtain an adequate assessment of their child's health status. It is important that both medical professionals and others who work with children become familiar with the signs and symptoms of prenatal exposure to drugs, of malnutrition, and of a range of neurologically based conditions that can affect child behavior and development. If clinicians are aware of the ways in which the presenting symptoms and developmental status of children may be affected, or explained, by a range of biological and psychological factors, it is more likely that the children's treatment needs will be "understood." The increasing number of international adoptions has precipitated an increased awareness among medical doctors of the special health concerns of these children and this has become a new speciality in some medical centers.

As we have seen in Chapter 11, families formed through the assistance of ART may face particular problems in being able to communicate with their children about the special nature of their birth history. Often, as in adoption, there is a tendency for parents to overemphasize the impact of the special birth history on children's developmental problems, without fully considering other aspects of family dynamics. While a family may seek help at a moment of crisis, clinical help can assist parents to identify more accurately the particular family issues that may in fact be inhibiting children's emotional and developmental growth.

Developmental History

The developmental history of most children involves forward and backward movement along many developmental lines, or trajectories. Developmental shifts with regard to a child's dependence on attachment figures combine with changes in physical, cognitive, and emotional spheres to influence developmental well-being. Furthermore, the rapidity of development in childhood creates complexity for the practitioner, because development across spheres may be synchronous or dysynchronous. For example, a child may be at age level with regard to physical maturation but markedly delayed in terms of relational development. This understanding must also be placed in the context of awareness of important influences on development derived from the many familial, cultural, and societal contexts in which development occurs.

Communicating with Children: The Need for Action and the Role of Play in Clinical Work

Clinicians who work with children understand the struggle of facilitating children's ability to communicate about their internal or emotional lives (Chethik, 2000). The elicitation of a child's "story," or narrative, requires a developmentally informed approach to practice and both sensitivity and flexibility on the part of the practitioner (Chethik, 2000; Gardner, 1991; Hurry, 1998; Webb, 1996, 1999). Age-related maturational differences between children and adults require that practitioners be highly sensitive to the ways in which children experience and/or are able to articulate important life events and emotional states (Gardner, 1991; Siegel, 1999).

The context of child-focused work is strongly defined by developmental characteristics of children (Chethik, 2000). The relative inability of young children to identify and articulate feeling states, the importance of action and play as vehicles for communication, children's developing conception of time and perceptions of causality, and the primacy of young children's dependence on caregivers combine to create important parameters for practice. Thus, the elicitation of children's "stories" requires a range of intervention techniques infused with an understanding of children's developmental status. These may include the use of verbal interviews, developmental observation, play and storytelling, and collateral work with significant adults in children's lives (Webb, 1996, 1999).

Work with children requires a dual focus on the part of the clinician. In addition to assessing and responding to presenting concerns, the pace at which children develop requires that clinicians also focus on supporting the children's potential for future growth and maturation (Lieberman, 1990). Presenting concerns must be understood not only in terms of the way they affect current functioning and maturational status but also in terms of their implications for future growth and development.

While the development of language facilitates the ability to communicate, young children may be unable to identify and verbally articulate feeling states or other aspects of emotional experience. When young children have experienced either acute or chronic trauma and/or are experiencing states of anxiety and depression, their ability to communicate about their affective lives may be limited even further. The ability to modify their emotional lives through language may be limited not only by maturational status but also by disruptions in primary attachment relationships and/or the absence of emotionally available caregivers. When clinicians are assessing children who have experienced trauma, it is important to differentiate between long-standing developmental vulnerabilities and more acute reactions to current circumstances.

Indeed, the emotional life of young children is often experienced not in words but in behavior and the ways in which they relate to important people in their lives. Perhaps unable to identify and/or articulate feeling states, children may have bodily and affective memories of their experiences (Terr, 1991). Thus, their narrative, or description of important events, themes, and relationships, is often told through action and affective reactions rather than verbal reconstructions. The elicitation of a child's narrative requires that the practitioner bring developmental understanding, technical flexibility, and great sensitivity to the task.

The narratives of children's early experiences can sometimes be inferred from observation of their relationships with caregivers, and the quality and content of their play. Through a combination of verbal interviews, developmental observation, the use of play and storytelling, and collateral work with parents and other caregivers, practitioners can begin to develop an appreciation of the child's maturational status, as well as important themes in his/her emotional life. In addition to tracking important themes as they emerge in assessment and observation, it is important for practitioners to find ways to understand the child's emotional, or affective, reaction to particular content areas *and* the ways in which he/she attempts to modulate his/her affective life (Greenspan & Greenspan, 1991).

For children who experienced trauma in their early years, and for others who are experiencing distress related to unresolved family conflicts, play is an important therapeutic modality. Often children express their memories, feelings, and anxieties through constructed stories and other expressions representing their internal life. (Terr, 1991; Webb, 1999). If clinicians can avoid a too heavy or too early reliance on interpretations, and can accept the metaphors and hidden stories in the child's play, shared empathic understanding of the child's concerns can result.

IMPLICATIONS FOR PRACTICE

Direct Work with Parents—Education and Guidance over Time: A Case Example

Adoption at birth has the great benefit of the potential for the adoptive parents and their child to engage immediately in a relationship that can help lead to a secure parent–child attachment. Therapeutic experience with children who have been adopted at birth, however, reveals that the symbolic meaning of adoption takes on new hues and colors as the children reach new phases of development. The symbolic meaning of adoption presents a crisis for children as they begin to understand the issues of loss and abandonment associated with adoption (Brodzinsky & Schechter, 1990). In open adoption, the dynamics of adoption are different from those in traditional adoption, as children must deal in an early and concrete way with the reality of dual sets of known parental figures.

Sarah, whose case was discussed in Chapter 7, began her life with her adoptive parents and met her birth mother when she was 3 years old. At this time, Sarah was a happy, robust, comfortable child, who looked forward to meeting this special person she came to identify as Phoebe. Feeling secure within the circle of her adoptive parents and adopted younger sister, Sarah was happy to greet Phoebe, the important person who had given birth to her. Sarah's parents had continued to work with the counselors at the adoption agency to receive guidance related to building appropriate family relationships in the context of the open adoption. Sarah had been told that she had grown in Phoebe's tummy, but this concrete statement had little emotional meaning to her at this time. Being a happy and well-loved child, she felt that Phoebe was a welcome visitor in her parent's home, but Sarah's emotional ties and sense of connectivity were to her adoptive parents. At 3 years of age, Sarah's understanding of adoption was concrete, and she had developed a strong sense of family identity and a positive attachment relationship to her parents.

As Sarah matured, she grew to have a more conceptual understanding of how babies are born and the special genetic relationship she had with her birth mother. This awareness led to a series of new questions and a deeper search for understanding. For example, she began to wonder which characteristics she had inherited from her birth parents and which from her adoptive parents. She raised questions of loyalty regarding where she belonged and had concerns about permanence. Eventually, Sarah began to ask her adoptive mother questions such as, "Are you always going to be my Mom?" and "Could I ever live with Phoebe?" Her parents continued to respond to Sarah with empathy for the underlying concerns and worked to respond to Sarah's growing conceptual understanding of the meaning of the adoption. For example, Sarah's mother explained that she was and would always be her mom, but Phoebe also would be a special person in her life. She allowed Sarah to consider what values and traits she had inherited from each parent but reassured Sarah that she would develop her own pathway and would always be their child. Sarah, being secure within herself and knowing that she could rely on her adoptive parents, said, "I'm lucky to have two moms" (in Gritter, 1989, p. 14). Sarah, spent many years integrating this dual heritage in forming her own identity and made a successful transition to University and to creating an independent life.

Sarah's early relational experiences had been established on a bedrock of trust, understanding, and responsive care from her adoptive parents. She had internalized a view of family belonging that was secure, loving, and accepting, and this early care contributed to her strength and resilience. This early confidence in being loved enabled her to negotiate the complex relational patterns inherent in open adoption. She was able to cope with the potential threats to her identity posed by the symbolic loss in adoption and to integrate the dual family identity into a coherent narrative. This coherent family story was a useful foundation for her own pathway of identity development.

In this particular family, the parents sought guidance and education about the impact of open adoption from the family clinic that had helped arrange the adoption. Rather than seek therapeutic help for Sarah, they used the support and help of the adoption counselor to openly address the new questions they faced with Sarah. In this way, they used a developmental approach to recognize the changing meaning of adoption to Sarah and to respond according to her level of understanding.

Direct Work with Children in Post-Foster Placement, International Adoption, and Kinship Adoption

In clinical work with children in complex adoption, the therapist offers children a relationship and a safe space in which they can express the affective memories of their earlier life. In this context, the children can gain empathy, acceptance of their feelings, and find new avenues for expressing their needs and feelings. In some ways, the therapist can not only begin to acknowledge the child's feelings but also put words to the feelings, and offer new ways to think about life experiences.

For example, Naomi, a child from Romania, who had lived in an impoverished orphanage, was adopted at 2 years of age but she remembered her early experiences through reenactment of the caregiving she received. A dominant figure in her life had been a kitten that was frightened of anyone who approached, scurrying off to hide. Naomi often took the role of the kitten, curling up in a corner of a chair, shaking, or pretending to be dead. Her story took many tracks but all reflected themes of abandonment and being left in the presence of strangers.

She remembered her preverbal experience, describing in play and drawings the way people dressed and how children were treated. Her story was communicated to the therapist through reconstructions of her early life, but Naomi did not speak using the pronoun "I" for a very long time. Rather, she told her story through displacement in play. When the therapist commented on the story and the feelings of the little girl, Naomi felt some acknowledgment of her earlier experiences and began to form an attachment based on sharing some part of her life experiences and receiving empathy from the therapist.

At school, however, telling the story about her family was harder and contributed to Naomi's feelings of being left out. She could not put into words or even tell what she had endured. In general she observed others and hid her inner thoughts and feelings. As she got older, Naomi was given assignments at school that required her to reflect on, and share with others, her "family history." Although this was difficult for her, it presented an opportunity to begin to communicate about herself and her sense of family history to her peers. This experience was very complicated. While some of the children expressed empathy for her, others recoiled at the description of her early memories. For Naomi, this assignment contributed to her realization of the great differences that existed in her history, especially in relation to experiences of abandonment, as compared to the histories of her classmates.

Over time the story that Naomi told herself and others was shaped and altered as her increased understanding allowed her to make more sense of what had happened. She moved from the concrete repetition of actions to describing the feelings of the children in the dramas she was developing, putting into words some of these events had happened to her, and eventually was able to describe in a narrative her longing to know her birth mother and father.

Work with Families Formed through Assisted Reproductive Technology

In both complex adoption and collaborative parenthood, the life stories of children and parents have painful, poignant, and redemptive themes. Typically, the formation of the family is based on an unexpected disruption of certain biological ties, whether in adoption or ART. While both parents and children can and do come to form strong attachments for each other, the unusual beginnings are often of a very private nature because they include painful and intimate experiences. Telling the story may not match the "idealized" core of family stories, often represented in the drawing of the family tree. The traditional family tree is a linear model of family formation that connects traditional or classical genealogical ties across the generations. Even when there are breaks caused by divorce, death, and family cutoffs, we have the words to explain the connections between members of the family and what has happened to the relationships between the generations. The generally shared cultural story of family formation is often moralized and mythologized, resulting in the premise that each little girl or boy is "destined" to have a mommy and daddy who is biologically related and who loves them. Most children bring this traditional model of family history to school to comfortably explain his/her unique heritage. For those children with a unique family history, the painfulness of being different is often acute, and the heightened awareness of difference precipitated at school often raises emotional questions for the parents and their child.

In families being formed through the assistance of ART, the phases of conception, pregnancy, birth, and parenting are very different from the usual routes to parenthood. ART is used by infertile couples, by couples who have medical histories that create risks related to conception and childbearing, and by single parents by choice and gay and lesbian couples. Although the psychological issues are very different in each contextual situation of the family (see Chapters 8, 9, and 10), medical clinics are now recognizing the need for interdisciplinary treatment teams that can address the psychological as well as physiological needs of the parents (Burns & Covington, 1999; Leiblum, 1997).

For married couples, the decision to utilize ART may follow discovery of infertility or medical factors that alter decision making with regard to parenthood. The loss and grief that may be associated with this process may result in the parents' need for crisis intervention, support, guidance, and education about their choices and options. If the couple agrees to undertake fertility treatment, the strain on the family can be great. This road to parenthood may be filled with uncertainty, loss, and mourning. Couples may disagree on vital decisions, including the use of ova and/or sperm donor, the number of trials they feel they are able to undertake, the assistance of a surrogate birth mother, and questions relating to disclosure to the child and/or extended family about the child's birth heritage. Studies show that men and women can have different emotional reactions to all of these issues.

In the situations described here, therapeutic help can be important for many reasons. The physiological and psychological strain of ART can be overwhelming. Interventions focused on individual, couple, and/or group therapy can each be useful in providing support, education, and guidance. In addition to the resolution of feelings relating to infertility, it is important that parents reflect on the symbolic meaning, to them, of the kinds of collaborative parenthood made possible by ART. Feelings around the loss of a genetic tie to their child and decision making regarding disclosure are often important areas of work. Clinical experience reveals that the use of ART introduces difficult questions about the meaning of biological and psychological parenthood. If the parents have not explored their true feelings about the use of sperm and ova donors, and collaborative parenthood, psychological barriers may develop that interfere with the parent–child relationship. Therapists in this field suggest that an important part of their work is to help families deal with the initial losses and difficult choices they confront, and help them reach consensus on major decisions.

A primary decision for parents who utilize forms of ART is whether and how to disclose the use of ART to their children. A uniquely personal decision, it may be important for parents to seek therapeutic support in identifying the symbolic meaning to them of questions relating to disclosure decisions (Zoldbrod & Covington, 1999). As described in Chapter 11, even when children are not told about their birth heritage, it may be possible that they sense a "family secret," and this may have an adverse effect on their sense of trust within their family. Children who are told about their birth heritage will raise different questions at different phases of development, requiring their parents to develop an evolving family narrative that gains in complexity as the children mature. Many parents' history with regard to ART is a private story, often unshared with others. Thus, it may be extremely difficult for the parents to seek help, because of the many aspects of ART that relate to their most intimate lives. For both parents and children, sensitive therapeutic support can help to identify and increase understanding of the symbolic meaning of ART. In addition, clinicians can support families in their efforts at coping with issues of difference relating to family structure and ART, and with questions and concerns relating to child and family identity.

A DEVELOPMENTALLY INFORMED APPROACH TO WORK IN VARIOUS SETTINGS

Our discussion in this chapter has focused primarily on direct clinical work with children and families. However, complex adoption and ART represent a field of practice that often involves the efforts of many professionals in a variety of settings and organizations. A range of advocacy, research, and intervention efforts is also central to children and families in new forms of parentage. Child welfare professionals, medical social workers, adoption workers, physicians, lawyers, and teachers are among those who may come into contact, knowingly or not, with parents and children in complex adoption and ART. There are many ways in which increasing the awareness and sensitivity of these professionals to the issues associated with complex adoption and ART can inform their work with children and families.

Child Welfare and Adoption Practitioners

Child welfare and adoption professionals are all too familiar with the effects on young children of abuse, neglect, and disruptions in primary attachment relationships. It is vital that people who work in child welfare and adoption receive training on the nature of development in early life and the ways in which experiences of trauma, abuse, and neglect can influence children's ability to form relationships with others, such as workers, foster parents, or adoptive parents. For example, such training can help raise practitioners' awareness of the ways in which children's transition to an adoptive family may be influenced by their preadoptive history within their family of origin and within experiences of out-of-home care.

Important lessons that have been derived from direct practice and research in the field of child welfare are central to our discussion of post-foster placement adoption. Studies on family reunification and the importance of permanency planning have raised important questions for future research and service delivery. An important area in child welfare is the need for advocacy and treatment for families whose children initially enter the child welfare system, to give them a significant chance to recover sufficiently to care for their own children. For example, in our discussion of the debate regarding cross-racial adoption, it is clear that the social ecology of low-income families may be characterized by the lack of access to prevention services. The lack of sufficient family resources of all kinds is related to the rise in entries into the foster care system and difficulties in family reunification.

Medical Social Work

The field of medical social work practice is very important both to complex adoption and ART. In complex adoption, many children may have a primary need for medical attention. In addition to the initial adjustment to adoption, many families must immediately access specialized medical services. Medical social workers can help families traverse complex medical systems and identify what kinds of medical assessment and intervention may be needed. For example, children adopted in international adoptions may have a variety of needs that result from experiences of malnutrition and medical neglect. Medical social workers can play important advocacy roles in providing education and guidance to families in this regard. In ART, medical social workers can also play an important role as members of treatment teams involved in all aspects of decision making and care with regard to an individual's or couple's choice to pursue various ART options. In particular, the medical social worker can play a vital role in advocating for the individual or couple, providing referrals to appropriate resources when necessary, promoting the family's self-determination, and protecting dignity and confidentiality within a potentially depersonalizing situation.

Teachers and School Social Workers

Teachers and social workers within school settings will increasingly come into contact with both complex adoption and ART. An increased awareness of the many issues associated with complex adoption and ART can raise the sensitivity of teachers and school personnel to important aspects of the child's experience. For example, a common assignment in the elementary years is for children to "draw" or "create" a family tree that can be presented to the class. For many children, the complexities of modern family life make this assignment a potentially difficult one. As the notion of the traditional "nuclear family" describes family life for a decreasing proportion of children in the United States, it may be important to revise the language in such assignments and/or to consider the kinds of informed discussion that may increase the comfort level of all children in the classroom. As always, sensitivity to issues of difference is important in creating an atmosphere of respect that is welcoming to all children in a given classroom. In cases of complex adoption and ART, children may already be struggling with a range of issues of "difference." It is important that teachers and school personnel be aware of the ways in which such assignments might confront children, some for the first time, with the ways in which their experience may be vastly different from that of their classmates. This is true because, particularly in the elementary school years, children develop the cognitive capacities for social comparison and begin to focus on the importance of a sense of belonging to a peer group (Casper et al., 1992).

ISSUES FOR EDUCATION, TRAINING, AND RESEARCH

As we have described throughout this book, work in the fields of complex adoption and ART requires a multidisciplinary, integrated approach.

We believe that the study of complex adoption and ART cannot only inform the general knowledge base of work with children and families but may also add to our understanding of the basic processes of risk and resilience in child and family development in general. Thus, we conclude our discussion of new forms of parentage with an effort to identify important areas of education, training, and research in this emerging field of practice.

Education

Working in the fields of complex adoption and ART requires an extensive educational foundation that draws on the clinical and research literatures in many fields. In addition to a broad-based understanding of work with children and families, students need to address the unique issues associated with new forms of parentage. Because the new forms of parentage described in this volume represent an emerging field of practice, students require a framework for exploration of developmental issues and a perspective that remains open to critical analysis of new data as they emerge. Several areas are central to the knowledge base for practice in this area, including the following:

- The biopsychosocial theories of human behavior and development.
- The etiology of mental health and illness in childhood and adolescence.
- A multisystemic and multidimensional view of risk and resilience.
- The impact of poverty and discrimination on child and family well-being.
- The nature of crisis in childhood.
- Values in working with nontraditional families and issues of difference.

In addition, it is important that students become familiar with general modalities of child-focused work such as play therapy and storytelling, and with therapeutic processes central to working with children and parents in crisis.

Working with children and families in complex adoption and ART also is supported by raising students' awareness of the historical context of family formation, the changing structure and definition of the family, the biological and psychological dynamics of parenthood, and the role of children in families and society. Relatedly, educational efforts that encourage students to become aware of their own beliefs and values are an important aspect of professional development.

The ethnographic perspective highlights the importance of practitioners remaining open to the potentially subjugated experiences and stories of children and families in complex adoption and ART. In particular, it is important for students to receive clinical and supervisory experiences that help them to identify the ways in which themes of attachment, loss, and identity formation can reverberate throughout the life experience of children and families in new forms of parentage.

Training and Supervision

Students of child and family work may increasingly come into contact with the new forms of parentage described in this book. In a variety of settings, such as schools, clinics, hospitals, courts, agencies, and private practice, practitioners may require an understanding of the unique concerns associated with complex adoption and ART. Students who have increased awareness about complex adoption and ART, and who bring a sensitivity to working across differences, are in the best position to understand and offer support to these children and families.

The multiple systems and difficult experiences often involved in complex adoption and ART require that students receive attentive supervision as they take on new types of cases in this field of practice. The experiences of trauma and loss often associated with complex adoption and ART pose special challenges for student clinicians. The support of a supervisor can help these students to sustain professional contact with children and families under difficult and sometimes painful circumstances. In addition, supervision can help students to differentiate personal reactions from practice concerns. Supervisors can help students to heighten their awareness of personally held beliefs, biases, and values that can affect work with children and families negatively, if they are not well understood.

Research

Ongoing research on new forms of parentage can build on the literature on traditional adoption and the emerging literature on complex adoptions and ART. As has been true in the study of other special "populations," research efforts must consider the need to address diversity and unique individual differences in sample populations (Flaks, 1995; Lamb, 1999; Patterson & Chan, 1999). As we have discussed in our work, most of the research on complex adoption and ART focuses on the immediate process of family formation and on developmental outcomes in early childhood. More research is needed that explores the influence on development of these experiences over time. This is especially important because some of the core questions relating to complex adoption and ART, such as the symbolic meaning of these life experiences to parents and children, may not be overtly obvious. Understanding the nuances of these experiences may require long term, in-depth qualitative research. Long-term effects remain to be seen.

Research that provides a descriptive base of family dynamics and child development in complex adoption and ART is extremely important. As our experience with these new forms of parentage continues to increase, a broader understanding of their implications is developing. For example, the emerging field of "adoption medicine" provides important descriptive data about the immediate medical needs of children adopted internationally (Oleck, 2000). In addition to these kinds of data, it is important that research focus on the identification of individual differences among children and families in new forms of parentage. It is particularly important to focus on whether complex adoption and ART pose risks to child development and, if so, to identify the processes underlying both risk and resilience in these new forms of parentage. This kind of research may add to our understanding of important developmental processes in all children and families, and is central to the conceptualization of prevention and treatment services.

As our understanding of complex adoption and ART continues to accumulate, researchers and clinicians can begin to compare and contrast various approaches to prevention and intervention with this special population. For example, we currently have little empirical data on the kind of intervention best suited to particular circumstances in complex adoption and ART. Research can help us to understand more about the timing of services in complex adoption and ART. For example, *when* in the process of family formation and development are children and families best served by particular kinds of support and treatment services? It may be that in the case of ART, anticipatory guidance is very helpful. In some complex adoptions, it may be that parent education and guidance are needed, while more intensive therapeutic services may be required in other situations. Such attention to individual differences is central to a nuanced understanding of the children and families forging new paths through complex adoption and ART.

Parents and children in complex adoption and ART share much in common with all children and families. The desire for connection, the need for differentiation, and the importance of creating a coherent family narrative are central concerns for all parents and children. The altered sequences of attachment and loss that describe the lives of parents and children in new forms of parentage provide important opportunities to study anew the processes by which children grow and develop.

References

Abbey, A., Andrews, F. M., & Halman, L. J. (1991). Gender's role in response to infertility. *Psychology of Women Quarterly, 15,* 295–316.

Abma, J. C. (Ed.). (1997). Fertility, family planning and women's health: New data from the 1995 national survey of family growth. *Vital and Health Statistics, 23*(19), 1–14.

Achtenberg, R. (1990). *Preserving and protecting the families of lesbians and gay men.* San Francisco: National Center for Lesbian Rights.

Adoption and Foster Care Analysis and Reporting System (AFCARS). (2000). Washington, DC: U.S. Department of Health and Human Services, Administration for Children and Families.

Adoption and Safe Families Act of 1997. (Public Law 105-89).

Adoption Assistance and Child Welfare Act of 1980. (Public Law 96-272, 94 Stat. 500.

Ainsworth, M. D. S. (1979a). Attachment as related to mother–infant interaction. In J. B. Rosenblatt, R. H. Hinde, & M. Bushnell (Eds.), *Advances in the study of behavior* (pp. 1–51). New York: Academic Press.

Ainsworth, M. D. S. (1979b). Infant–mother attachment. *American Psychologist, 34,* 932–937.

Ainsworth, M. D. S., Blehar, M. C., Waters, E., & Wall, S. (1978). *Patterns of attachment.* Hillsdale, NJ: Erlbaum.

Alexander R., Jr., & Curtis, C. M. (1996). A review of empirical research involving the transracial adoption of African American children. *Journal of Black Psychology, 22,* 223–235.

Allen, K. R., & Demo, D. H. (1995). The families of lesbians and gay men: A new frontier in family research. *Journal of Marriage and the Family, 57,* 111–127.

Allen-Meares, P. (1995). *Social work with children and adolescents.* New York: Longman.

Amadio, C. M. (1991). Doing the right thing: Some ethical considerations in current adoption practice. *Social Thought, 17,* 25–33.

American Fertility Society Ethics Committee. (1994). Ethics and the new reproductive technologies. In T. Beauchamp & L. Walters (Eds.), *Contemporary issues in bioethics* (4th ed., pp. 201–206). Belmont CA: Wadsworth.

American Psychiatric Association. (1994). *Diagnostic and statistical manual of mental disorders* (4th ed.). Washington, DC: Author.

Andrews, L. B. (1999). *The clone age*. New York: Holt.

Anthony, E. J. (1981). The family and the psychoanalytic process. *Psychoanalytic Study of the Child, 36*, 3–34.

Anthony, E. J. (1983). Infancy in a crazy environment. In J. D. Call, E. Galenson, & R. L. Tyson (Eds.), *Frontiers of infant psychiatry* (pp. 95–109). New York: Basic Books.

Anthony, E. J., & Benedek, T. (Eds.). (1970). *Parenthood*. Boston: Little, Brown.

Anthony, E. J., & Chiland, C. (Eds.). (1998). *The child in his family: Vol. 8. Perilous development: Child raising and identity formation under stress*. New York: Wiley.

Applegarth, L. D. (1999). Individual counseling and psychotherapy (1994). In L. H. Burns & S. N. Covington (Eds.), *Infertility counseling: A comprehensive handbook for clinicians* (pp. 49–64). New York: Parthenon.

Applegate, J. S., & Barol, B. I. (1989). Repairing the nest: A psychodynamic developmental approach to clients with severe behavior disorders. *Clinical Social Work Journal, 17*(3), 197–207.

Applegate, J. S. (1993). Winnicott and clinical social work: A facilitating partnership. *Child and Adolescent Social Work Journal, 10*(1), 3–19.

Aranda, M. P., & Knight, B. G. (1997). The influence of ethnicity and culture on the caregiver stress and coping process: A sociocultural review and analysis. *Gerontologist, 37*, 342–354.

Aries, P. (1962). *Centuries of childhood*. New York: Knopf.

Assisted Reproductive Technology Success Rates 1997. (1999). In *National Summary and Fertility Clinics Report* (pp. 1–24). Atlanta, GA: Centers for Disease Control.

Bailey, J. M., Bobrow, D., Wolfe, M., & Mikach, S. (1995). Sexual orientation of adult sons of gay fathers. *Developmental Psychology, 31*, 124–129.

Bailey, J. M., & Dawood, K. (1998). Behavioral genetics, sexual orientation and the family. In C. J. Patterson & A. R. D'Augeli (Eds.), *Lesbian, gay, and bisexual identities in families* (pp. 3–18). New York: Oxford University Press.

Balint, M. (1968). *The basic fault*. London: Tavistock.

Baran, A., & Pannor, R. (1990). Open adoption. In D. M. Brodzinsky & M. D. Schechter (Eds.), *The psychology of adoption* (pp. 316–322). New York: Oxford University Press.

Barth, R. (1991). Educational implications of prenatally drug-exposed children. *Social Work in Education, 13*, 130–136.

Bartholet, E. (1993). *Family bonds: Adoption and the politics of parenting*. Boston: Houghton Mifflin.

Baumann, C. (1997). *Examining where we were and where we are: Clinical issues in adoption 1985–1995*. New York: Human Science Press.

Beauchamp, T., & Walters, L. (Eds.). (1994). *Contemporary issues in bioethics* (4th ed.). Belmont, CA: Wadsworth.

Beebe, B., Lachmann, F., & Jaffe, J. (1997). Mother–infant interaction structures and presymbolic self and object representations. *Psychoanalytic Dialogues, 7,* 133–182.

Beebe, B., & Sloate, P. (1982). Assessment and treatment of difficulties in mother–infant attunement in the first three years of life. *Psychoanalytic Inquiry, 1,* 601–623.

Bell, A. P., & Weinberg, M. S. (1978). *Homosexualities: A study of diversity among men and women.* New York: Simon & Schuster.

Belsky, J. (1984). The determinants of parenting: A process model. *Child Development, 55,* 83–96.

Belville, M., Indyk, D., Shapiro, V., Dewart, T., Mon, J., Gordon, G., & Sachapelli, S. (1991). The community as a strategic site for refining high prenatal risk assessment and interventions. *Social Work in Health Care, 16*(1), 5–19.

Benedek, T. (1952). Infertility as a psychosomatic defense. *Fertility and Sterility, 3,* 527–535.

Benedek, T. (1959). Parenthood as a developmental phase: A contribution to libido theory. *Journal of the American Psychoanalytic Association, 7,* 389–417.

Berry, M. (1993). Adoptive parents' perception of, and comfort with, open adoption. *Child Welfare, 72*(30), 231–253.

Bibring, G. (1959). Some consideration of the psychological processes in pregnancy. *Psychoanalytic Study of the Child, 14,* 113–121.

Blank, G., & Blank, R. (1974). *Ego psychology: Theory and practice* (pp. 19–26). New York: Columbia University Press.

Blanton, T., & Deschner, J. (1990). Biological mother's grief: The post-adoptive experience in closed and open adoption. *Child Welfare, 69*(6), 525–535.

Blos, P. (1967). The second individuation process of adolescence. *Psychoanalytic Study of the Child, 22,* 162–186.

Borden, W. (1992). Narrative perspectives in psychosocial intervention following adverse life events. *Social Work, 37*(2), 135–141.

Bos, C., & Cleghorn, R. A. (1958). Psychogenic sterility. *Fertility and Sterility, 9,* 84–95.

Bowlby, J. (1969). *Attachment and loss: Vol. 1. Attachment.* New York: Basic Books.

Bowlby, J. (1973). *Attachment and loss: Vol. 2. Separation: Anxiety and anger.* New York: Basic Books.

Bowlby, J. (1980). *Attachment and loss: Vol. 3. Loss: Sadness and depression.* New York: Basic Books.

Bowlby, J., Robertson, J., & Rosenbluth, D. (1952). A two-year-old goes to the hospital. *Psychoanalytic Study of the Child, 7,* 82–94.

Bozett, F. W. (1989). Gay fathers: A review of the literature. In F. W. Bozett (Ed.), *Homosexuality and the family* (pp. 137–162). New York: Harrington Press.

Braverman, A. M. (1997). When is enough enough? Abandoning medical treatment for infertility. In S. R. Lieblum (Ed.), *Infertility: Psychological issues and counseling strategies* (pp. 209–229). New York: Wiley.

Brinich, P. M. (1990). Adoption from the inside out: A psychoanalytic perspective. In D. Brodzinsky & M. Schechter (Eds.), *The psychology of adoption* (pp. 42–61). New York: Oxford University Press.

Brodzinsky, A. (1990). Surrendering an infant for adoption: The birth mother experience. In D. Brodzinsky & M. Schechter (Eds.), *The psychology of adoption* (pp. 295–315). New York: Oxford University Press.

Brodzinsky, D. (1993). Long-term outcomes in adoption. *Future of Children, 3*(1), 153–166.

Brodzinsky, D. (1997). Infertility and adoption adjustment: Consideration and clinical issues. In S. R. Leiblum (Ed.), *Infertility: Psychological issues and counseling strategies* (pp. 246–263). New York: Wiley.

Brodzinsky, D., & Schechter, M. (Eds.). (1990). *The psychology of adoption.* New York: Oxford University Press.

Brodzinsky, D., Smith, D., & Brodzinsky, A. (1998). *Children's adjustment to adoption: Developmental and clinical issues.* Thousand Oaks, CA: Sage.

Bronfenbrenner, U. (1977). Towards an experimental ecology of human development. *American Psychologist, 32*(7), 512–531.

Bronfenbrenner, U. (1979). *The ecology of human development.* Cambridge, MA: Harvard University Press.

Brooks, D., & Barth, R. (1999). Adult transracial and inracial adoptees: Effects of race, gender, adoptive family structure, and placement history on adjustment outcomes. *American Journal of Orthopsychiatry, 69*(1), 87–100.

Brown, P. (1990). Biracial identity and social marginality. *Child and Adolescent Social Work Journal, 7*(4), 319–337.

Bruni, F. (1998, June 25). A small-but-growing sorority is giving birth to children for gay men. *The New York Times*, p. A12.

Burnette, D. (1999). Custodial grandparents in Latino families: Patterns of service use and predictors of unmet needs. *Social Work, 44*(1), 22–34.

Burns, L. H. (1999). Parenting after infertility. In L. H. Burns & S. N. Covington (Eds.), *Infertility counseling: A comprehensive handbook for clinicians* (pp. 449–474). Pearl River, NY: Parthenon.

Burns, L. H., & Covington, S. N. (Eds.). (1999). *Infertility counseling: A comprehensive handbook for clinicians.* New York: Parthenon.

Burton, L. (1992). Black grandparents rearing children of drug-addicted parents: Stressors, outcomes, and social service needs. *The Gerontologist, 32*(6), 744–751.

Burton, L. (1999). Physical and emotional well-being of custodial grandparents in Latino families. *American Journal of Orthopsychiatry, 69*(3), 305–318.

Cadoret, R. J. (1990). Biologic perspectives of adoptee adjustment. In D. Brodzinsky & M. Schechter (Eds.), *The psychology of adoption* (pp. 25–419). New York: Oxford University Press.

Calkins C. A., & Millar, M. (1999). The effectiveness of court appointed special advocates to assist in permanency planning. *Child and Adolescent Social Work Journal, 16*(1), 37–47.

Caplan, A. L. (1994). The ethics of *in vitro* fertilization. In T. Beauchamp & L.

Walters (Eds.), *Contemporary issues in bioethics* (4th. ed., pp. 216–224). Belmont, CA: Wadsworth.

Capron, A. M., & Radin, M. (1994). Choosing family law over contract law as a paradigm for surrogate motherhood. In T. Beauchamp & L. Walters (Eds.), *Contemporary issues in bioethics* (4th ed., pp. 258–269). Belmont, CA: Wadsworth.

Carbone, L., & Decker, E. (1999). *A little pregnant: Our memoir of fertility, infertility, and a marriage.* New York: Atlantic Monthly Press.

Carter, L., & Larson, C. (1997). Drug-exposed infants. *Future of Children, 7*(2), 157–160.

Casper, L. M., & Bryson, K. R. (1998). Co-resident grandparents and their grandchildren: Grandparent maintained families. *Population Division Technical Working Paper 26.* Washington, DC: U.S. Bureau of the Census.

Casper, V., Schultz, S., & Wickens, E. (1992). Breaking the silences: Lesbian and gay parents and the schools. *Teachers College Record, 94*(1), 109–137.

Cassidy J., & Shaver, P. (Eds.). (1999). *Handbook of attachment: Theory, research, and clinical implications.* New York: Guilford Press.

Castle, J., Groothues, C., Brendencamp, D., Beckett, C., O'Conner, T., Rutter, M., & the ERA Study Team. (1999). Effects of qualities of early institutional care on cognitive attainment. *American Journal of Orthopsychiatry, 69*(4), 424–437.

Cath, S. H., Gurwitt, A., & Gunsburg, L. (Eds.). (1989). *Fathers and their families.* Hillsdale, NJ: Analytic Press.

Chase-Lansdale, P. L., & Brooks-Gunn, J. (Eds.). (1995). *Escape from poverty: What makes a difference for children?* New York: Cambridge University Press.

Chase-Lansdale, P. L., & Vinovskis, M. A. (1995). Whose responsibility? An historical change in roles of mothers, fathers, and society. In P. L. Chase-Lansdale & J. Brooks-Gunn (Eds.), *Escape from poverty: What makes a difference for children?* (pp. 11–37). New York: Cambridge University Press.

Chasnoff, I., Anson, A., Hatcher, R., Stenson, H., & Iaukea, K. (1998). Prenatal exposure to cocaine and other drugs: Outcome at four to six years. In J. Harvey & B. Kosofsky (Eds.), Cocaine: Effects on the developing brain. *Annals of the New York Academy of Sciences, 846,* 314–328.

Chess, S., & Thomas, A. (1991). Temperament and the concept of goodness of fit. In J. Strelau & A. Angleitner (Eds.), *Explorations in temperament: International perspectives on theory and measurement: Perspectives on individual differences* (pp. 15–28). New York: Plenum Press.

Chethik, M. (2000). *Techniques of child therapy: Psychodynamic strategies* (2nd ed.). New York: Guilford Press.

Chodorow, N. (1978). *The reproduction of mothering: Psychoanalysis and the sociology of gender.* Berkeley: University of California Press.

Cicchetti, D., & Cohen, D. J. (Eds.). (1995). *Perspectives on developmental psychopathology: Vol. 1. Theory and methods* (pp. 3–20). New York: Wiley.

Clunis, D. M., & Green, G. D. (1995). *The lesbian parenting book: A guide to creating families and raising children.* Seattle: Seal Press.

Cohen, S. (1996). Trauma and the developmental process: Excerpts from an analysis of an adopted child. *Psychoanalytic Study of the Child, 51,* 287–301.

Cole, E., & Donley, K. (1990). History, values and placement policy issues in adoption. In D. Brodzinsky & M. Schechter (Eds.), *The psychology of adoption* (pp. 273–294). New York: Oxford University Press.

Collins, L. (2000). Raising Kate. *In the Family, 5*(4), 12–13.

Congress, E. (1994). The use of culturagrams to assess and empower culturally diverse families. *Families in Society, 75*(9), 531–540.

Cooper, S. L., & Glazer, E. S. (1994). *Beyond infertility: The new paths to parenthood.* New York: Lexington Books.

Cote, J., & Levine, C. (1988). A critical examination of the ego identity status paradigm. *Developmental Review, 8*(2), 147–184.

Cox, C. (Ed.). (2000). *To grandmother's house we go and stay: Perspectives on custodial grandparents.* New York: Springer.

Crawford, S. (1987). Lesbian families: Psychosocial stress and the family building process. In *Boston Lesbian Psychologies Collective: Explorations and challenges* (pp. 195–214). Urbana: University of Illinois Press.

Daniluk, J. S. (1997). Gender and infertility. In S. R. Leiblum (Ed.), *Infertility: Psychological issues and counseling strategies* (pp. 103–128). New York: Wiley.

Davies, D. (1999). *Child development.* New York: Guilford Press.

De Parle, J. (1999, February 21). As welfare rolls shrink, load on relatives grows. *The New York Times,* B1.

Dewan, S. K. (2000, July 26). Growing up Asian and alone. *The New York Times,* p. B1.

Dickens, C. (1999). *David Copperfield.* New York: Oxford University Press.

Domar, A. D. (1997). Stress and infertility in women. In S. R. Leiblum (Ed.), *Infertility: Psychological issues and counseling strategies* (pp. 67–83). New York: Wiley.

Domar, A. D., Broome, A., Zuttermeister, P. C., Seibel, M., & Miedman, R. (1992). The prevalence and predictability of depression in infertile women. *Fertility and Sterility, 58,* 1158–1163.

Donovan, W., & Leavitt, L. (1992). Maternal self-efficacy: Illusory control and its effect on susceptibility to learned helplessness. *Child Development, 61*(5), 1638–1647.

Downey, W. (2000). Little orphan Anastasia: The opening phase of the analysis of a 5 year old encropetic adopted Russian girl. *Psychoanalytic Study of the Child, 55,* 154–179.

Elder, G. (1998). The life course as developmental theory. *Child Development, 69*(1), 1–12.

Emde, R. N., & Sorce, J. F. (1983). The rewards of infancy: Emotional availability and maternal referencing. In J. D. Call, E. Galenson, & R. L. Tyson (Eds.), *Frontiers of infant psychiatry* (pp. 17–31). New York: Basic Books.

Emery, J. L. (1993). Agency versus independent adoption: The case for agency adoption. *The Future of Children, 3,* 139–152.

Emond, M., & Scheib, J. (1998). Why not donate sperm? A study of potential donors. *Evolution and Human Behavior, 19,* 313–319.

Epstein, Y. M., & Rosenberg, H. S. (1997). He does, she doesn't; she does, he doesn't: Couple conflicts about infertility. In S. R. Leiblum (Ed.), *Infertility: Psychological issues and counseling strategies* (pp. 129–148). New York: Wiley.

Erikson, E. H. (1950). *Childhood and society*. New York: Norton.

Erikson, E. H. (1963). *Childhood and society* (2nd ed.). New York: Norton.

Eth, S., & Pynoos, R. S. (Eds.). (1985). *Post-traumatic stress disorder in children*. Washington, DC: American Psychiatric Press.

Evan B. Donaldson Adoption Institute. (2000a, March). *Adoption in the United States: A fact sheet update*. http://www.adoptioninstitute.org/tml.

Faderman, L. (1991). *Odd girls and twilight lovers: A history of lesbian life in twentieth-century America*. New York: Columbia University Press.

Falk, P. (1989). Lesbian mothers: Psychosocial assumptions in family law. *American Psychologist, 44*, 941–947.

Feigelman, W. (2000). Adjustments of transracially and inracially adopted young adults. *Child and Adolescent Social Work Journal, 17*(3), 165–183.

Fein, E. (1998, October 25). In search of a child: Secrecy and stigma no longer clouding adoptions. *The New York Times*, A1, A30.

Festinger, T. (1990). Adoption disruption: Rates and correlates. In D. Brodzinsky & M. Schechter (Eds.), *The psychology of adoption* (pp. 107–121). New York: Oxford University Press.

Flaks, D. K. (1995). Research issues. In A. Sullivan (Ed.), *Proceedings of the Fourth Annual Peirce–Warnick Adoption Symposium* (pp. 21–38). Washington, DC: Child Welfare League of America.

Fonagy, P., & Target, J. (1998a). Mentalization and the changing aims of child psychoanalysis. *Psychoanalytic Dialogues, 8*(1), 87–114.

Fonagy, P., & Target, M. (1998b). An interpersonal view of the infant. In A. Hurry (Ed.), *Psychoanalysis and developmental therapy* (pp. 3–32). London: Karnac Books.

Foster, H. H. (1973). Adoption and child custody: Best interests of the child. *Buffalo Law Review, 22*, 1–16.

Fraiberg, S. H. (1987a). The clinical dimensions of baby games. In *Selected writings of Selma Fraiberg* (pp. 362–387). Columbus: Ohio State University Press.

Fraiberg, S. H. (1987b). Pathological defenses in infancy. In *Selected writings of Selma Fraiberg* (pp. 182–202). Columbus: Ohio State University Press.

Fraiberg, S. H., Adelson, E., & Shapiro, V. B. (1975). Ghosts in the nursery: A psychoanalytic approach to the problem of impaired infant–mother relationships. *Journal of the American Academy of Child Psychiatry, 14*(3), 386–422.

Fraser, M. (1997). *Risk and resilience in childhood: An ecological perspective*. Washington, DC: National Association of Social Work Press.

Frazier, E. F. (1939). *The Negro family in the United States*. Chicago: University of Chicago Press.

Freud, A. (1965). *Normality and pathology in childhood*. New York: International Universities Press.

Freud, A. (1966). The ego and the mechanisms of defense. In *The writings of Anna Freud* (Vol. II). New York: International Universities Press.

Freud, A. (1981). The concept of developmental lines: Their diagnostic significance. *Psychoanalytic Study of the Child, 36,* 129–136.

Freud, A., & Burlingham, D. T. (1944). *Infants without families: The case for and against residential nurseries.* New York: International Universities Press.

Freud, S. (1957). Mourning and melancholia. In *The Standard Edition* (Vol. 14, pp. 243–258). London: Hogarth Press.

Furman, E. (1994). *A child's parent dies: Studies in childhood bereavement.* New Haven: Yale University Press.

Gadsden, V. L. (1999). Black families in intergenerational and cultural perspective. In M. E. Lamb (Ed.), *Parenting and child development in non-traditional families* (pp. 221–247). Mahwah, NJ: Erlbaum.

Gardner, R. (1991). *What children can tell us: communicating with children.* San Francisco: Jossey-Bass.

Garmezy, N., Masten, A. S., & Tellegen, A. (1984). The study of stress and competence in children: A building block for developmental psychopathology. *Child Development, 55*(1), 97–111.

Gibbs, J. T. (1987). Identity and marginality: Issues in the treatment of biracial adolescents. *American Journal of Orthopsychiatry, 57*(2), 265–278.

Gibbs, J. T. (1999). Biracial adolescents. In J. T. Gibbs & L. N. Huang (Eds.), *Children of color: Psychological interventions with culturally diverse youth* (pp. 305–332). San Francisco: Jossey-Bass.

Gibbs, J. T., & Huang, L. N. (Eds.). (1999). *Children of color: Psychological interventions with culturally diverse youth.* San Francisco: Jossey-Bass.

Gilligan, C. (1982). *In a different voice.* Cambridge, MA: Harvard University Press.

Glazer, E. (1993). Parenting after infertility. In M. Seibel, A. A. Kiessling, J. Bernstein, & S. Levin (Eds.), *Technology and infertility: Clinical, psychosocial, legal and ethical aspects* (pp. 399–402). New York: Springer-Verlag.

Goldberg, C. (2000, April 26). Vermont gives final approval to same- sex unions. *The New York Times,* p. A14 .

Goldberg, S., Gold, A., & Washington, J. (1997). Determinants of behavioral problems in Romanian children adopted in Ontario. *International Journal of Behavioral Development, 20*(1), 17–31.

Goldsmith, H. H., Buss, K. A., & Lemery, K. S. (1997). Toddler and childhood temperament: Expanded content, stronger genetic evidence, new evidence for the importance of environment. *Developmental Psychology, 33*(6), 891–905.

Goldstein, J., & Goldstein, S. (1996). Put yourself in the skin of the child, she said. *Psychoanalytic Study of the Child, 51,* 46–55.

Goldstein, J., Solnit, A. J., Goldstein, S., & Freud, A. (1996). *In the best interests of the child: The least detrimental alternative.* New York: Free Press.

Golombok, S. A., & Rutter, M. (1983). Children in lesbian and single-parent households: Psychosocial and psychiatric appraisal. *Journal of Child Psychology and Psychiatry, 24,* 551–572.

Golombok, S. A., & Tasker, F. L. (1996). Do parents influence the sexual orientation of their children? Findings from a longitudinal study of lesbian families. *Developmental Psychology, 32*(1), 3–11.

Gonsiorek, J. C., & Weinrich, J. D. (Eds.). (1991). *Homosexuality: Research implication for public policy* (pp. 197–214). Newbury Park, CA: Sage.

Gottman, J. S. (1990). Children of gay and lesbian parents. In F. W. Bozett & M. B. Sussman (Eds.), *Homosexuality and family relations* (pp. 177–196). New York: Harrington Park Press.

Green, G. D., & Bozett, F. W. (1991). Lesbian mothers and gay fathers. In J. D. Weinrich & J. C. Gonsiorek (Eds.), *Homosexuality, research implication for public policy* (pp. 197–214). Newbury Park, CA: Sage.

Green, R. (1978). Sexual identity of thirty-seven children raised by homosexual or transsexual parents. *American Journal of Psychiatry, 135,* 692–697.

Greenfeld, D. A. (1999). Recipient counseling for oocyte donation. In L. H. Burns & S. N. Covington (Eds.), *Infertility counseling: A comprehensive handbook for clinicians* (pp. 345–356). New York: Parthenon.

Greenfeld, D. A., Ort, S. I., Greenfeld, D. G., Jones, E. E., & Olive, D. L. (1996). Attitudes of IVF parents about the IVF experience and their children. *Journal of Assisted Reproduction and Genetics, 13,* 266–274.

Greenspan, S., & Greenspan, N. T. (1991). *The clinical interview of the child* (2nd ed.). Washington, DC: American Psychiatric Press.

Greenspan, S., & Porges, S. (1984). Psychopathology in infancy and early childhood: Clinical perspectives on the organization of sensory and affective–thematic experience. *Child Development, 55*(1), 49–71.

Greil, A. L. (1991). *Not yet pregnant: Infertile couples in contemporary America.* London: Rutgers University Press.

Griebenow, M. (2000). Chinese adoption. *In the Family, 5*(4), 7–9.

Gritter, J. L. (Ed.). (1989). *Adoption without fear.* San Antonio: Corona Publishing Co.

Gritter, J. L. (1997). *The spirit of open adoption.* Washington, DC: Child Welfare League of America Press.

Grotevant, H. D. (1997). Coming to terms with adoption: The construction of identity from adolescence into adulthood. *Adoption Quarterly, 1*(1), 3–27.

Grotevant, H. D., & Kohler, J. K. (1999). Adoptive families. In M. E. Lamb (Ed.), *Parenting and child development in non-traditional families* (pp. 161–191). Mahwah, NJ: Erlbaum.

Grotevant, H. D., McRoy, R. G., Elde, C. L., & Fravel, D. L. (1994). Adoptive family system dynamics: Variation by level of openness in the adoption. *Family Process, 33,* 125–146.

Hanafin, H. (1999). Surrogacy and gestational carrier participants. In L. H. Burns & S. N. Covington (Eds.), *Infertility counseling: A comprehensive handbook for clinicians* (pp. 375–390). New York: Parthenon.

Harden, A. W., Clark, R. L., & Maguire, K. (1997, June 20). *Formal and informal kinship care* (Vols. 1 and 2). Washington, DC: U.S. Department of Health and Human Services.

Harlow, H. (1958). The nature of love. *American Psychologist, 13,* 673–685.

Hartmann, H. (1939). *Ego psychology and the problem of adaptation.* New York: International Universities Press.

Hegar, R. L., & Scannapieco, M. (Eds.). (1999). *Kinship foster care: Policy, practice and research*. New York: Oxford University Press.

Hetherington, E. M., & Parke, R. D. (1999). *Child psychology: A contemporary viewpoint*. New York: McGraw-Hill.

Hodder, H. F. (1997, March 28). The new fertility. *Harvard Magazine*, pp. 54–64.

Hollingsworth, L. D. (1997, April). Promoting same-race adoption for children of color. *Social Work, 43*(2), 105–106.

Holt International Children's Services. (2000). *Update 3 - 2000*. Oregon.http.// www.hotintnl.org/ins1997.h.

Hoopes, J. L. (1990). Adoption and identity formation. In D. Brodzinsky & M. Schechter (Eds.), *The psychology of adoption* (pp. 144–167). New York: Oxford University Press.

Hoopes, J. L., Alexander, L. B., Silver, P., Ober, G., & Kirby, N. (1997). Formal adoption of the developmentally vulnerable African-American child: Ten-year outcomes. *Marriage and Family Review, 25*(3–4), 131–144.

Horowitz, R. M., & Maruyama, H. (1995). Legal issues. In A. Sullivan (Ed.), *Proceedings of the Fourth Annual Peirce–Warwick Adoption Symposium* (pp. 11–21). Washington, DC: Child Welfare League of America.

Howard, A., Royse, D., & Skerl, J. (1997). Transracial adoption: The black community perspective. *Social Work, 22*(3), 184–187.

Hurry, A. (Ed.). (1998). *Psychoanalysis and developmental therapy*. London: Karnac Books.

Indian Child Welfare Act of 1978, 1214, 95th Congress, Second Session. (1978).

Inhelder, B., & Piaget, J. (1958). *The growth of logical thinking from childhood to adolescence*. New York: Basic Books.

Institute for Science Law and Technology Working Group. (1998). Art into science: Regulation of fertility techniques. *Science, 281*, 651–652.

Jacob, M. C. (1997). Concerns of single women and lesbian couples considering conception through assisted reproduction. In S. Leiblum (Ed.), *Infertility: Psychological issues and counseling strategies* (pp. 189–209). New York: Wiley.

James, B. (1994). *Handbook for treatment of attachment trauma problems in children*. New York: Free Press.

Johnson, A. K., & Groze, V. (1993). The orphaned and institutionalized children of Romania. *Journal of Emotional and Behavioral Problems, 2*, 49–52.

Johnson, Y. (1999). Indirect work: Social work's uncelebrated strength. *Social Work, 44*(4), 323–334.

Joslin, D. (1999). Grandparents raising grandchildren orphaned and affected by HIV/ AIDS. In C. B. Cox (Ed.), *To grandmother's house we go and stay* (pp. 167–184). New York: Springer.

Josselson, R. (1987). *Finding herself: Pathways to identity development in women*. San Francisco: Jossey-Bass.

Kadushin, A. (1980). *Child welfare services*. New York: Macmillan.

Kagan, J., Arcus, D., & Snidman, N. (1994). The idea of temperament: Where do we go from here? In R. Plomin & G. McCleam (Eds). *Nature, nurture and psychology* (pp. 197–210). Washington, DC: American Psychological Association.

Kaler, S., & Freeman, B. J. (1994). Analysis of enviromnental deprivation: Cognitive and social development in Romanian orphanages. *Journal of Child Psychiatry and Allied Disciplines, 35*(4), 769–781.

Kamerman, S. B., & Kahn, A. J. (1988). *Mothers alone: Strategies for a time of change.* Dover, MA: Auburn House.

Kaufman, M. (1993). *Cracking the armour: Power and pain in the lives of men.* Toronto: Penguin Books.

Keye, W. R. (1999). Medical aspects of infertility for the counselor. In L. H. Burns & S. N. Covington (Eds.), *Infertility counseling: A comprehensive handbook for clinicians* (pp. 27–48). New York: Parthenon.

Kirk, H. D. (1964). *Shared fate: A theory of adoption and mental health.* New York: Free Press.

Kirk, H. D. (1981). *Adoptive kinship: A modern institution in need of reform.* Toronto: Butterworth.

Klempner, L. (1992). Infertility: Identification and disruption with the maternal object. *Clinical Social Work, 20,* 193–198.

Klock, S. C. (1997). To tell or not to tell: The issue of privacy and disclosure in infertility treatment. In S. R. Leiblum (Ed.), *Infertility: Psychological issues and counseling strategies* (pp. 167–188). New York: Wiley.

Kohut, H. (1972). Thoughts on narcissism and narcissistic rage. *Psychoanalytic Study of the Child, 27,* 36–40.

Kovacs, G. T., Mushin, D., Kane, H., & Baker, H. W. (1993). A controlled study of the psychosocial development of children conceived following insemination with donor semen. *Human Reproduction, 8,* 788–790.

Kroger, J. (2000). *Identity development: Adolescence through adulthood.* Thousand Oaks, CA: Sage.

Laird, J. (1993). Lesbians and lesbian families: Multiple reflections. In J. Laird (Ed.), Lesbians and lesbian families: Multiple reflections. *Smith College Studies in Social Work, 63*(3), 209–295.

Lamb, M. E. (Ed.). (1999). *Parenting and child development in nontraditional families.* Mahwah, NJ: Erlbaum.

Leiblum, S. R. (1994). The impact of infertility on marital and sexual satisfaction. *Annual Review of Sex Research, 4,* 99–120.

Leiblum, S. R. (Ed.). (1997). *Infertility: Psychological issues and counseling strategies.* New York: Wiley.

Leiblum, S. R., & Greenfeld, D. A. (1997). The course of infertility: Immediate and long-term reactions. In S. R. Leiblum (Ed.), *Infertility: Psychological issues and counseling strategies* (pp. 83–102). New York: Wiley.

Lemery, K., Goldsmith, H. H., Klinnert, M. D., & Mrazek, D. (1999). Developmental models of infant and childhood temperament. *Developmental Psychology, 35*(1), 189–204.

Levine, C. (1990). AIDS and changing concepts of family. *Millbank Quarterly, 68*(1), 35–36.

Levy-Warren, M. H. (1996). *The adolescent journey: Development, identity formation, and psychotherapy.* Northvale, NJ: Aronson.

Lieberman, A. (1990). Culturally sensitive intervention with children and families. *Child and Adolescent Social Work Journal,* 7(2), 101–120.

Lifton, B. J. (1976, January 25). The search. *The New York Times Magazine,* pp. 15–19.

Lifton, B. J. (1977). *Twice born: Memoirs of an adoptive daughter.* New York: Penguin Books.

Lifton, B. J. (1988). *Lost and found: The adoption experience.* New York: HarperCollins.

Lifton, B. J. (1994). *Journey of the adopted self: A quest for wholeness.* New York: Basic Books.

Lugaila, T. (1998). Marital status and living arrangements. *U.S. Bureau of the Census, Current Population Reports, Series P. 20–514.* Washington, DC: U.S. Government Printing Office.

Lyons-Ruth, K., Bronfman, E., & Parsons, E. (1999). Maternal frightened, frightening or atypical behavior and disorganized attachment patterns. *Monographs of the Society for Research in Child Development, 64*(3), 67–96.

Macklin, R. (1994a). *Surrogate mothers and other mothers.* Philadelphia: Temple University Press.

Macklin, R. (1994b). Artificial means of reproduction and our understanding of the family. In T. Beauchamp & L. Walters (Eds.), *Contemporary issues in bioethics* (4th ed., pp. 191–197). Belmont, CA: Wadsworth.

Mahlstedt, P. (1985). The psychological component of infertility. *Fertility and Sterility, 43,* 335–346.

Mai, F. M., Munday, R. N., & Rump, E. E. (1972). Psychiatric interview comparisons between infertile and fertile couples. *Psychosomatic Medicine, 12*(1), 46–59.

Marcia, J. E. (1994). The emprical study of ego identity. In H. Bosma & T. Graafsma (Eds.), *Identity and development: An interdisciplinary approach* (pp. 67–80). Thousand Oaks, CA: Sage.

Maslow, A. H. (1954). *Motivation and personality.* New York: Harper.

Masten, A. S., Best, K. M., & Garmezy, N. (1990). Resilience and development: Contributions from the study of children who overcome adversity. *Development and Psychopathology, 2*(4), 425–444.

Masten, A. S., Hubbard, J., Gest, S., Tellegen, A., & Garmezy, N. (1999). Competence in the context of adversity: Pathways to resilience and maladaptation from childhood to late adolescence. *Development and Psychopathology, 11l*(1), 143–169.

McCormick, R. A. (1981). *How brave a new world: Dilemmas in bioethics.* Garden City, NY: Doubleday.

McKenzie, J. K. (1993). Adoption of children with special needs. *The Future of Children, 3*(1), 62–76.

McLanahan, S., & Sandefur, G. (1994). *Growing up with a single parent: What helps, what hurts.* Cambridge, MA: Harvard University Press.

McLanahan, S., & Teitler, J. (1999). The consequences of father absence. In M. E.

Lamb (Ed.), *Parenting and child development in nontraditional families* (pp. 83–102.) Mahwah, NJ: Erlbaum.

McLoyd, V. C. (1990). The impact of economic hardship on black families and children: Psychologial distress, parenting and socioemotional development. *Child Development, 61*, 311–346.

McNamee, W. (1999, September 24). *The New York Times*, p. A1 (photograph).

Menning, B. E. (1980). The emotional needs of infertile couples. *Fertility and Sterility, 34*, 313–319.

Meyers, M., Diamond, R., Kezur, D., Scharf, C., Weinshel, M., & Rait, D. (1995a). An infertility primer for family therapists: I. Medical, social, and psychological dimensions. *Family Process, 34*, 219–229.

Meyers, M., Diamond, R., Kezur, D., Scharf, C., Weinshel, M., & Rait, D. (1995b). An infertility primer for family therapists: II. Working with couples who struggle with infertility. *Family Process, 34*, 231–240.

Miller v. Youakim, 440 U. S. 125 (1979).

Miller, B. (1979). Gay fathers and their children. *Family Coordinator, 28*, 544–552.

Miller, L. C. (1999). Caring for internationally adopted children. *New England Journal of Medicine, 341*(20), 1539–1540.

Miller, N. (1992). *Single parents by choice: A growing trend in family life.* New York: Plenum Press.

Minkler, M., & Roe, K. M. (1993). *Grandmothers as caregivers: Raising children of the crack cocaine epidemic.* Newbury Park, CA: Sage.

Minkler, M., Roe, K. M., & Price, M. (1992). The physical and emotional health of grandmothers raising grandchildren in the crack cocaine epidemic. *The Gerontologist, 32*(6), 752–761.

Mintz, S., & Kellogg, S. (1988). *Domestic revolutions: A social history of American family life.* New York: Free Press.

Multiethnic Placement Act of 1994, Public Law 103–382, 42: United States Congress.

Murray, T. H. (1996). *The worth of a child.* Berkeley: University of California Press.

Muzio, C. (1993). Lesbian co-parenting: On being with the invisible (m)other. In J. Laird (Ed.), Lesbians and lesbian families: Multiple reflections. *Smith College Studies in Social Work, 63*(3), 215–231.

Myerhoff, B. (1978). *Number our days.* New York: Touchstone Press/Simon & Schuster.

Nelson, C., & Bloom, F. (1997). Child development and neuroscience. *Child Development, 68*(5), 970–987.

New York State Task Force on Life and the Law. (1998). *Assisted reproductive technologies: Analysis and recommendations for public policy.* New York: Author.

Norris, M. (1991, July 8–14). The class of crack's innocent victims: The first wave of drug-disabled children jolts the ill-prepared schools. *Washington Post National Weekly Edition,* p. 11.

Notman, M. T., & Lester, E. P. (1988). Pregnancy: Theoretical consideration. *Psychoanalytic Inquiries, 8*, 139–145.

Noyes, R. W., & Chapnick, E. M. (1964). Literature on psychology and infertility. *Fertility and Sterility, 15*(5), 543–548.

Oates, J. C. (1998). The adoption: A play in one act. In J. C. Oates (Ed.), *New plays* (pp. 257–263). Princeton, NJ: Ontario Review Press.

Oleck, J. (2000, February 14). Science and technology: The kids are not all right. *Business Week,* pp. 74–76.

Painter, N. I. (1996). *Sojourner truth: A life, a symbol.* New York: Norton.

Pakizegi, B. (1990). Emerging family forms: Single mothers by choice—Demographic and psychosocial variables. *Maternal–Child Nursing Journal, 19*(1), 1–19.

Paret, I. (1982). Night waking and its relation to mother–infant interaction in nine-month-old infants. In J. Call, E. Galenson, & R. L. Tyson (Eds.), *Frontiers of infant psychiatry* (pp. 169–171). New York: Basic Books.

Paret, I., & Shapiro, V. (1998). The splintered holding environment and the vulnerable ego: A case study. *Psychoanalytic Study of the Child, 53,* 300–324.

Parks, C. A. (1999). Lesbian identity development: An examination of differences across generations. *American Journal of Orthopsychiatry, 69*(3), 347–362.

Pattatucci, A. M. L., & Hamer, D. H. (1995). Development and familiality of sexual orientation in females. *Behavior Genetics, 25,* 407–420.

Patterson, C. J. (1992). Children of lesbian and gay parents. *Child Development, 63,* 1025–1042.

Patterson, C. J., & Chan, R. W. (1996). Gay fathers. In M. E. Lamb (Ed.), *The role of the father in child development* (3rd ed., pp. 245–260). New York: Wiley.

Patterson, C. J., & Chan, R. W. (1999). Families headed by lesbian and gay parents. In M. E. Lamb (Ed.), *Parenting and child development in nontraditional families* (pp. 191–221). Mahwah, NJ: Erlbaum.

Pavao, J. M. (1998). *The family of adoption.* Boston: Beacon Press.

People. (1998, October 12). Miracle babies, pp. 64–69.

Perry, B. D. (1994). Neurobiological sequelae of childhood trauma: Post-traumatic stress disorders in children. In M. Murberg (Ed.), *Catecholamines in post-traumatic stress disorder: Emerging concepts* (pp. 253–276). Washington, DC: American Psychiatric Press.

Perry, B. D., Pollard, R. A., Blakely, T. L., Baker, W. I., & Vigilante, D. (1995). Childhood trauma, the neurobiology of adaptation, and use-dependent development of the brain: How states become traits. *Infant Mental Health Journal, 16*(4), 271–289.

Phinney, J. S., & Rosenthal, D. A. (1992). Ethnic identity in adolescence: Process, context and outcome. In G. R. Adams, T. P. Gullotta, & R. Montemayer (Eds.), *Adolescent identity formation* (pp. 145–172). Thousand Oaks, CA: Sage.

Pierce, W. (1990, November 28). Family secrets. *CBS News: 48 Hours. Cable News Network*, Transcript 132.

Pine, F. (1990). *Drive, ego, object, self.* New York: Basic Books.

Prell, R. E. (1989). The double frame of life history in the work of Barbara Myerhoff. In Personal Narratives Group (Ed.), *Interpreting women's lives*. Bloomington, IN: University Press.

Provence, S., & Lipton, R. C. (1962). *Infants in institutions.* New York: International Universities Press.

Pruett, K. D. (1992). Strange bedfellows: Reproductive technology and child development. *Journal of Infant Mental Health, 13*(4), 312–318.

Pruett, K. D. (2000). *Fatherneed: Why father care is as essential as mother care for your child.* New York: Free Press.

Pynoos, R., Steinberg, A., & Wraith, R. (1995). A developmental model of childhood traumatic stress. In D. Cicchetti & D. J. Cohen (Eds.), *Developmental psychopathology: Vol. 2. Risk, disorder and adaptation* (pp. 72–95). New York: Wiley.

Redl, F. (1966). *When we deal with children.* New York: Free Press.

Reitz, M. (1997). Groundswell change in adoption requires anchoring by research. *Child and Adolescent Social Work Journal, 16*(5), 327–354.

Reitz, M., & Watson, K. (1992). *Adoption and the family system: Strategies for treatment.* New York: Guilford Press.

Rich, A. (1976). *Of motherhood as experience and institution.* New York: Norton.

Richmond, M. E. (1922). *What is social case work?* New York: Russell Sage Foundation.

Rivera, R. (1991). Legal issues in gay and lesbian parenting. In F. Bozett (Ed.), *Gay and lesbian parents* (pp. 199–227). New York: Praeger.

Robertson, J. (1953). Some responses of young children to the loss of maternal care. *Nursing Times, 49*, 382–389.

Rohrbaugh, J. B. (1989). *Choosing children: Psychological issues in lesbian parenting.* New York: Haworth Press.

Rosenthal, J. A., Groze, V., Curiel, H., & Westcott, P. A. (1991). Transracial and inracial adoption of special needs children. *Journal of Multicultural Social Work,* (1), 13–31.

Rosenwald, G., & Ochberg, R. (Eds.). (1992). *Storied lives: The cultural politics of self-understanding.* New Haven, CT: Yale University.

Rushton, A., & Minnis, H. (1997). Annotation: Transracial family placements. *Journal of Child Psychology and Psychiatry and Allied Disciplines, 38*, 147–159.

Rutter, M. (1990). Psychosocial resilience and protective mechanisms. In J. Rolf (Ed.), *Risk and protective factors in the development of psychopathology* (pp. 181–214). New York: Cambridge University Press.

Rutter, M., & the English and Romanian Adoptees (ERA) Study Team. (1998). Developmental catchup, and deficit, following adoption after severe global early privation. *Journal of Child Psychology and Psychiatry, 39*, 465–476.

Ryburn, M. (1994). *Open adoption: Research, theory and practice.* Brookfield, VT: Aldershot.

Saari, C. (1991). *The creation of meaning in clinical social work.* New York: Guilford Press.

Saffian, S. (1998). *Ithaka: A daughter's memoir of being found.* New York: Basic Books.

Sameroff, A. J. (1989). Principles of development and psychopathology. In A. J. Sameroff & R. N. Emde (Eds.), *Relationship disturbances in early childhood* (pp. 17–32). New York: Basic Books.

Sanchirico, A., & Jablonka, K. (2000). Keeping foster children connected to their biological parents: The impact of foster parent training and support. *Child and Adolescent Social Work Journal, 17*(3), 185–205.

Sandler, J., & Sandler, A. M. (1978). On the development of object relationships and affects. *International Journal of Pschoanalysis, 59*, 285–296.

Savage, D. (1999). *The kid*. New York: Penguin.

Schecter, M., & Bertocci, D. (1990). The meaning of the search. In D. Brodzinsky & M. Schechter (Eds.), *The psychology of adoption* (pp. 62–93). New York: Oxford University Press.

Scheib, J. E., Kristiansen, A., & Wara, A. (1997). A Norwegian note on sperm donor selection and the psychology of female mate choice. *Evolution and Human Behavior, 18*, 143–149.

Schore, A. (1994). *Affect regulation and the origin of the self: The neurobiology of emotional development*. Hillsdale, NJ: Erlbaum.

Seelye, K. Q. (1998, March 24). Specialists report rise in adoptions that fail. *The New York Times*, pp. A14.

Seligman, S. (1994). Applying psychoanalysis in an unconventional context: Adapting infant–parent psychotherapy to a changing population. *Psychoanalyitic Study of the Child, 49*, 481–500.

Selye, H. (1978). *The stress of life*. New York: McGraw-Hill.

Sengupta, S. (2000, March 28). Youths leaving foster care system with few skills or resources. *The New York Times*, pp. 1, 12.

Severson, R. (1994). *Adoption: Philosophy and experience*. Weaverville, CA: House of Tomorrow Partnership.

Shapiro, J. R., & Applegate, J. S. (2000). Cognitive neurobiology and affect regulation: Implications for clinical social work. *Clinical Social Work, 28*(1), 9–21.

Shapiro, J., Mangelsdorf, S., & Marzolf, D. (1995). The determinants of parenting competence in adolescent mothers. *Journal of Youth and Adolescence, 23*(6), 621–641.

Shapiro, V. B. (1994). *Bridging the losses in biolgraphical discontinuities through narrative reconstructions*. Unpublished dissertation, Smith College School of Social Work, Northampton, MA.

Shapiro, V. B. (1995). Subjugated knowledge and the working alliance: The narratives of Russian Jewish immigrants. *In Session: Psychotherapy in Practice, 1*(4), 9–22.

Shapiro, V. B., & Gyzinsky, M. (1989). Ghosts in the nursery revisited. *Child and Adolescent Journal, 6*(1), 18–37.

Shapiro, V. B., Fraiberg, S., & Adelson, E. (1976). Infant–parent psychotherapy on behalf of a child in a critical nutritional state. *Psychoanalytic Study of the Child, 31*, 461–491.

Sharp, D. (1999, July 1). After a lifetime of work, a second family to raise. *USA Today*, p. 1.

Shireman, J., & Johnson, P. (1986). A longitudinal study of black adoptions: Single parent, transracial and traditional. *Social Work, 31*(93), 172–176.

Siegel, D. (1999). *The developing mind: Toward neurobiology of interpersonal experience.* New York: Guilford Press.

Silverman, A. R., & Feigelman, W. (1990). Adjustment in interracial adoptees: An overview. In D. Brodzinsky & M. Schechter (Eds.), *The psychology of adoption* (pp. 187–201). New York: Oxford University Press.

Simon, R., Alstein, H., & Melli, M. (1994). *The case for transracial adoption.* Washington, DC: American University Press.

Smothers, R. (1997, December, 18). Accord lets gay couples adopt jointly.*The New York Times*, p. B4.

Snowden, R. (1990). The family and artificial reproduction. In D. Bromham, N. Dalton, & J. Jackson (Eds.), *Philosophical ethics in reproductive medicine* (pp. 70–78). Manchester, UK: Manchester University Press.

Solomon, J., & George, C. (Eds.). (1999). *Attachment disorganization.* New York: Guilford Press.

Sororsky, A., Baran, A., & Pannor, R. (1989). *The adoption triangle.* San Antonio: Corona.

Spar, K. (1997). Foster Care and Adoption Statistics. *Congressional Research Service,* 97–11 EPW. Washington, DC: Library of Congress.

Spitz, R. A. (1945). Hospitalism: An inquiry into the genesis of psychiatric conditions in early childhood. *Proceedings, American Association of Mental Deficiency, 44*, 114–136.

Spitz, R. A., & Wolf, K. (1946). Anaclitic depression: An inquiry into the genesis of psychiatric conditions in early childhood: II. *Psychoanalytic Study of the Child,* 2, 313–342.

Sroufe, L. A., & Waters, E. (1977). Attachment as an organizational construct. *Child Development, 48,* 1184–1199.

Stack, C. (1974). *All our kin: Strategies for survival in a black community.* New York: Harper & Row.

Stanton, A. L., & Burns, L. H. (1999). Behavioral medicine approaches to infertility counseling. In L. H. Burns, & S. N. Covington (Eds.), *Infertility counseling: A comprehensive handbook for clinicians* (pp. 129–148). New York: Parthenon.

Steele, H., Steele, M., Croft, C., & Fonagy, P. (1999). Infant–mother attachment at one year predicts children's understanding of mixed emotions at six years. *Social Development, 8*(2), 161–178.

Stern, D. N. (1985). *The interpersonal world of the infant: A view from psychoanalysis and developmental psychology.* New York: Basic Books.

Stevens, J. W. (1997). African-American female adolescent identity development: A three dimensional perspective. *Child Welfare,* 2, 145–172.

Stolberg, S. G. (1998, January 18). Quandary on donor eggs: What to tell the children. *The New York Times,* pp. A1, A20.

Stone, F. H. (1972). Adoption and identity. *Child Psychaitry and Human Development,* 2, 120–128.

Stone, L. (1979). *The family, sex and marriage in England 1500–1800.* New York: Harper & Row.

Strong, C. (1997). *Ethics in reproductive and perinatal medicine.* New Haven, CT: Yale University Press.

Sullivan, A. (1995a). Policy issues. In A. Sullivan (Ed.), *Issues in gay and lesbian adoption: Proceedings of the 4th Peirce–Warwick Adoption Symposium* (pp. 1–9). Washington, DC: Child Welfare League of America.

Sullivan. A. (Ed.). (1995b). *Isues in gay and lesbian adoption: Proceedings of the 4th Peirce–Warwick Adoption Symposium.* Washington, DC: Child Welfare League of America.

Sussal, C. M. (1993). Object relations couples therapy with lesbians. In J. Laird (Ed.), Lesbians and lesbian families: Multiple reflections. *Smith College Studies in Social Work, 63*(3), 301–315.

Swerdloff, R. S., Overstreet, J. W., Sokol, R. Z., & Raifer, J. (1985). Infertility in the male. *Annals of Internal Medicine, 103*(6 pt. 1), 906–919.

Talbot, M. (1998, May 24). Attachment theory: The ultimate experiment. *The New York Times Magazine,* pp. 24–32.

Tasker, F. L., & Golombok, S. (1991). Children raised by lesbian mothers: The empirical evidence. *Family Law, 21,* 184–187.

Tasker, F. L., & Golombok, S. (1997). *Growing up in a lesbian family: Effects on child development.* New York: Guilford Press.

Taylor, R., & Thornton, M. C. (1996). Child welfare and transracial adoption. *Journal of Black Psychology, 22,* 282–291.

Terr, L. (1991). Childhood traumas: An outline and overview. *American Journal of Psychiatry, 148*(1), 10–20.

Thomson, E., Hanson, T., & McLanahan, S. (1994). Family structure and child well-being: Economic resources vs. parental behaviors. *Social Forces, 73*(1), 221–242.

Tizard, B., & Hodges, J. (1978). The effect of early institutional rearing on the development of eight-year-old children. *Journal of Child Psychology and Psychiatry, 19,* 99–118.

Tobin, P. O. Z. (1998). *Motherhood optional: A psychological journey.* New York: Jason Aronson.

Tonning, L. M. (1999). Persistent and chronic neglect in the context of poverty—when parents cannot parent: Case of Ricky, age 3. In N. B. Webb (Ed.), *Play therapy with children in crisis: Individual group, and family treatment* (2nd ed., pp. 203–224). New York: Guilford Press.

Triseliotis, J., & Hill, M. (1990). Contrasting adoption, foster care, and residential rearing. In D. Brodzinsky & M. Schechter (Eds.), *The psychology of adoption* (pp. 107–121). New York: Oxford University Press.

Turner, P. H., Scadden, L., & Harris, M. B. (1990). Parenting in gay and lesbian families. *Journal of Gay and Lesbian Psychotherapy, 1,* 55–66.

U.S. State Department. (1999). *Immigrant visas issued to orphans coming to the United States.* Washington, DC: U.S. Department of Health and Human Services.

Vaughan, B., Egeland, B., Sroufe, L. A., & Waters, E. (1979). Individual differences in

infant–mother attachment at twelve and eighteen months: Stability and change in families under stress. *Child Development, 50*(4), 971– 975.
Verdelle, A. J. (1996). *The good Negress*. New York: Harper Perennial.
Vondra, J., Hommerding, K., & Shaw, D. (1999). Stability and change in infant attachment style in a low-income sample. *Monographs of the Society for Research in Child Development, 64*(3), 119–144.
Vroegh, K. S. (1997). Transracial adoptees: Developmental status after 17 years. *American Journal of Orthopsychiatry, 67*(4), 568–575.
Wallerstein, J. S., & Kelly, J. B. (1979). *Surviving the break up: How children and parents cope with divorce*. New York: Basic Books.
Webb, N. B. (Ed.). (1993). *Helping bereaved children: A handbook for practitioners*. New York: Guilford Press.
Webb, N. B. (1996). *Social work practice with children*. New York: Guilford Press.
Webb, N. B. (Ed.). (1999). *Play therapy with children in crisis: Individual, group, and family treatment* (2nd ed.). New York: Guilford Press.
Webb, R., & Daniluk, J. C. (1999). The end of the line: Infertile men and the experience of biological childlessness. *Men and Masculinities, 1*(1), 6–25.
Wegar, K. (1996). *Adoption identity and kinship: The debate over sealed birth records*. New Haven: Yale University Press.
Weider, H. (1977). On being told of adoption. *Psychoanalytic Quarterly, 46*(1), 22.
Weider, H. (1978). On when and whether to disclose about adoption. *Journal of the American Psychoanalytic Association, 26,* 793–811.
Weil, W. B., Jr., & Walters, L. (1994). Reproductive technologies and surrogate parenting arrangements. In T. L. Beauchamp & L. Walters (Eds.), *Contemporary issues in bioethics* (4th ed., pp. 187–271). Belmont, CA: Wadsworth.
White, M., & Epston, D. (1990). *Narrative means to therapeutic ends*. New York: Norton.
Williams, C. B. (1999). Claiming a biracial identity: Resisting social constructions of race and culture. *Journal of Counseling and Development, 77*(1), 32–35.
Wind, L. H. (1999). Developmental identity crisis in nontraditional families: Cases of Emma, age 8, and Chad, age 13, children of lesbian parents. In N. B. Webb (Ed.), *Play therapy with children in crises: Individual, group and family treatment* (2nd ed., pp. 318–338). New York: Guilford Press.
Winnicott, D. W. (1965a). *The maturational processes and the facilitating environment: Studies in the theory of emotional development*. Madison, CT: International Universities Press.
Winnicott, D. W. (1965b). The theory of the parent–infant relationship. In *The maturational processes and the facilitating environment* (pp. 37–56). Madison, CT: International Universities Press. (Original work published 1960)
Winnicott, D. W. (1965c). Ego distortion in terms of true and false self. In *The maturational processes and the facilitating environment* (pp. 140–152). Madison, CT: International Universities Press. (Original work published 1962)
Wright, J., Allard, M., Lecours, A., & Sabourin, S. (1989). Psychosocial distress and infertility: A review of controlled research. *International Journal of Fertility, 4,* 126–142.

Wright, J., Duchesne, C., Sabourin, S., Bissonette, F., Genoirt, J., & Girard, Y. (1991). Psychosocial distress and infertility: Men and women respond differently. *Fertility and Sterility, 55,* 100–108.

Zelizer, V. A. (1994). *Pricing the priceless child: The changing social value of children.* Princeton, NJ: Princeton University Press.

Zigler, E., & Hall, N. (2000). *Child development and social policy: Theory and applications.* New York: McGraw-Hill.

Zoldbrod, A. P., & Covington, S. N. (1999). Recipient counseling for donor insemination. In L. H. Burns & S. N. Covington (Eds.), *Infertility counseling: A comprehensive handbook for clinicians* (pp. 325–344). New York: Parthenon.

Index

Adolescence
clinical illustrations, 251–252, 253–266
clinical issues, 252, 272–275
in open adoption, identity conflicts and, 161
See also Birth origin; Child development; Family narratives; Loss; Trauma
Adoption
in gay and lesbian families, 235–236, 239–240
minority families in, 127
international policies, social and political factors influencing, 100–101
legal and social transformations leading to open adoption, 150–155
nature/nurture dynamic of child development and, 31
psychological reactions of parents to, 155-156
right of access to genealogical history and, 170, 192
See also Traditional adoption; Complex adoption
Adoption agencies
full open adoption and, 167
in international adoption, 109
modified open adoption and, 166–167
Adoption and Safe Families Act, 60, 74, 128
Adoption and the Family System (Reitz and Watson), 170
Adoption Assistance and Child Welfare Act, 128
Adoption law, history of, 150–152
"Adoption medicine," 301
Adoption of Tammy (legal case), 236
Adoption triad, 149–150, 155–162
Adoptive parents
in clinical practice, 285–287, 291–293
traditional adoption and, 151–152
family narratives and, 16–17
insights from studies of traditional adoption, 15–16
in international adoption
attachment relationships and, 99, 106, 110, 122, 123
children's experiences of separation and, 107
children's responses to, 104
clinical vignettes, 111–121
typical experiences in, 107–109
issues of "entitlement," 15–16
in open adoption
acceptance of risks in, 158
attachment relationship and, 158–159
problems encountered in, 27–28
relationship with birth parents, 157, 158, 169–170

Adoptive parents, in open adoption (*continued*)
  in post-foster placement adoption
    attachment relationship and, 39, 68, 70–73, 74, 75
    preplacement history assessments and, 66
  self-reflection and, 16
  tasks of, 159
  transracial adoption and, 64–65
  understandings of the child's temperament, 43–44
Adultmorphism, 34
AID. *See* Artificial insemination by donor
AID-formed families
  development of paternal identity, 215–216
    case vignettes, 217–218
  disclosing birth origin, 189, 190, 216–217
    clinical issues and illustrations, 251, 252, 253–259, 266–272, 273, 274, 275
  family identity and, 216
AIDS (Acquired Immune Deficiency Syndrome)
  foster care and, 57
  skipped generation care and, 216
Aid to Families with Dependent Children (AFDC), 128
Anxiety
  in ART-formed families, 222–223
  disruptions in holding environment and, 77–78
  in women undergoing infertility treatment, 204, 205
  See also Separation anxiety
ART. *See* Assisted reproductive technology
ART-formed families
  adjustments to pregnancy, 221
  anxiety in, 222–223
  attachment relationships in, 198, 222–224
  birth narratives and, 190, 191, 199
  broadened notions of family and, 175, 176–178, 202
  clinical practice with, 175, 294–296
    See also Clinical practice
  conflicts in fertility decision making, 207–208
  development of parental identity and, 223–224
  difficulties and challenges to, 174–175
  disclosing birth origin, 189, 190, 195, 198–199, 212, 216–217, 227(table), 289, 296
    clinical issues and illustrations, 212–214, 251, 252, 253–259, 266–275
  emotional and empathetic acceptance of children, 224, 225–226
  family identity and, 176, 202–203
  family narratives and, 18–19, 294–296
  fertility counseling and, 208–211
  identity formation in the child, 224–225
  importance of having a birth child, 178–180, 197
  maternal depression following birth, 222
  new patterns of family formation and, 3, 4–5
  parentage roles, 175, 187, 195
  phases of achieving parenthood in, 203
  psychological experiences of, 185
  psychological recovery following infertility treatment, 222
  risk factors for parents and children, 221–223
  significance of studying, 4–5
  therapeutic assistance and, 197–198, 203
  See also Collaborative parenthood
Artificial insemination, 182
  number of births per year from, 173
  See also Legal and ethical issues

Artificial insemination by donor (AID), 206
  case vignette, 189–190
  fertility counseling and, 211
  gender differences in responses to, 207
  legal issues, 188–189
  procedures in, 187–188
  psychological issues, 188
  therapeutic assistance and, 190
  See also AID-formed families; Sperm and ova donors
Asian children, transracial adoption and, 121–122
  See also Complex adoption; Transracial adoption
Assessment
Assisted reproductive technology (ART), 202
  access to, 179–180
  artificial insemination by donor, 187–190
  broadened notions of family and, 175, 176–178
  clinical practice issues, 4
  demands on birth mother, 184
  emergence of, 13
  family experiences and difficulties with, 174–175
  genetic roots and procedures in, 200
  growth of, 173–174
  legal and ethical issues in, 174, 185–187
    disposition of unneeded embryos, 186
    frozen embryos, 187
    multiple births, 186, 221–222
  medical social workers and, 298
  new patterns of family formation and, 3, 4–5
  number of births from, 173, 174
  opposition from the Catholic Church, 179
  ova donations, 192–195
  procedures used in, 182–183
  psychological and physical experience of pregnancy through, 184–185
  psychological parents and, 14–15
  responses to, gender differences in, 207
  See also ART-formed families
Assisted reproductive technology clinics, 186
Attachment relationships
  ART-formed families and, 198, 222–224
  brain development and, 38
  child development and, 6, 7, 25, 37–39
  with children adopted from abroad, 99, 106, 110, 122, 123
    clinical vignettes, 111–121
  clinical practice issues, 6–7, 36, 37–39, 282–283
  collaborative parenthood and, 223
  complex adoption and, 7, 36, 37–39
  developmental research on, 25, 37–39
  difficulties from early trauma and loss, 18, 36, 38, 39, 68, 70–73, 75, 133, 135–136
  "disorganized" relationships, 38
  early caregiving environment and, 35–39, 283–284
  ego function and, 37–38
  experiences of trust and security in, 133
  family narratives and, 16–19
  international adoption and, 99, 106, 110, 122, 123
    clinical vignettes, 111–121
  open adoption and, 158–159
  post-foster placement adoption and, 39, 68, 70–73, 74, 75
  psychological parents and, 198, 216
  skipped-generation families and, 135–136, 145

Biopsychosocial issues in development. *See* Child development

Birth fathers, 153
psychological reactions to adoption, 155–156
Birth mothers
demands of infertility treatment on, 183, 184
depression following birth, 222
ova donations and, 195
psychological reactions to adoption, 155, 156
Birth narratives
the meaning of children to parents, 178-180
in ART-formed families, 190, 191, 199
See also Children's narratives; Family narratives ; Complex adoption
Birth origin
disclosing in ART-formed families, 189, 190, 195, 198–199, 212, 216–217, 227(table), 289, 296
clinical issues and illustrations, 212–214, 251, 252, 253–259, 266–275
disclosing in complex adoption, 251–252, 260–266, 273, 275
Birth parents
adoption counselors and, 156
in closed adoption, 151, 152
open adoption and, 13, 27, 156–157
contact with child and, 160–162, 169
introducing to the child, 159
relationship with adoptive parents, 157, 158, 169–170
post-foster placement adoption and, 61
psychological reactions to adoption, 155–156
Births, multiple, 186, 221–222
Brain development
affect regulation and, 27, 38
attachment relationships and, 38
early trauma and, 36, 77
teratogenic exposure and, 44–46
Brown, Louise, 173, 182–183
Caregivers. *See* Primary caregivers
Catholic Human Services, 167
Cesarean deliveries, 221
Child development
adultmorphism concept, 34
attachment relationships and, 6, 7, 25, 37–39
differentiating acute vs. chronic problems in, 288–289
early caregiving environment and, 35–37, 283–284
ecological perspectives, 7
family narratives and, 16–19
identity formation and, 18, 40
impact of early trauma and loss on, 18, 36, 68, 74–75, 77–78, 93–95, 134–135, 142
impact of transracial adoption on, 63–65
institutional care and, 98, 101–103, 109, 122
maturational differences with adults, 35
minority status and, 34, 41, 57, 61, 62
multidimensional view of, 32
nature/nurture dynamic in, 30–31
nontraditional families and, 5
parent–child relationship and, 105
poverty and, 25, 30
prenatal exposures to risk and, 44–46, 140–141
risk and resilience in, 73
role of fathers in, 214–215
sociocultural context and, 29, 31–32
Child-focused therapy, 46–49, 293–294
Child health
assessment of, 102
biopsychosocial view of, 29
cognitive development and, 102
institutional care and, 101–102
prenatal exposures to risk and, 44–46, 140–141
Children. *See* Child development and Child health
adaptations to stress and deprivation, 104, 123
closed adoption and, 160, 161

concepts of time, 72
disclosing birth origin to. *See* Birth origin
in gay and lesbian families
coping with bias and prejudice, 241
formed after heterosexual marriage, 232–234
outcome studies on, 228–231
psychological issues, 191–192
importance of having, 178–180
preplacement history assessments
benefits of, 65–66
case vignette, 66–68
guidelines for, 69–70 (table)
right of access to genealogical history, 170, 192
in single-parent families, 243–245
trauma and loss. *See* Loss; Trauma
See also Attachment relationships; Child development; Child health; Infants
Children at Risk Resources and Intervention Program (CARRI), 146
Children's Home Society, 166–167
Children's narratives
characteristics of, 16–19, 281–282
eliciting in clinical practice, 290–291
See also Birth narratives; Family narratives
Child welfare advocates, 61
Child Welfare League of America, 155
Child welfare professionals, 297
China, adoption policies and, 100
Civil rights movement, 152, 154
Clinical practice
with adoptive parents, 285–287, 291–293
with ART-formed families, 175, 294–296
attachment relationships and, 6–7, 36, 37–39, 282–283
with birth parents, 156, 157
children with early histories of trauma and loss, 65, 75, 78, 95–96, 284–285
case study, 79–93
with complex adoption
assessment spheres, 29
attachment research and, 37–39
child-focused therapy, 46–49, 293–294
child temperament, 42–44
developmental lines concept and, 46–47
developmental psychology and, 47–48
early caregiving environment, 35–37
focus on early experience and, 48–49
identity formation and, 40–42
infant health and challenges for caregiving, 44–46
multidimensional view of development, 32
nature/nurture dynamic, 30–31
problems of psychological adaptation for children and parents, 26–28
sociocultural context and, 31–35
cultural diversity and, 33–34
developing state of, 276–277
developmental perspectives, 6–7
communicating with children in, 290–291
differentiating acute vs. chronic problems, 288–289
understanding developmental history and, 289–290
use of play in, 287–288, 291
disclosing birth origin
clinical illustrations, 253–272
issues in, 252, 272–275, 289
ecological perspectives, 7
educational foundation for, 299–300
ethnographic perspectives, 7–9, 19, 278–280
family narratives and, 7–9, 19, 278–279, 281–282
holding environment as therapeutic relationship, 78, 284–285
case study, 77, 81–86, 88–93, 95–96, 97

Clinical practice (*continued*)
"informed not knowing" approach, 278
integrated approach, 5–9
with international adoption
clinical vignettes, 111–121
interdisciplinary approach, 123–124
long-term dimensions, 110, 124
transition crises, 109–110
understanding preadoptive histories, 109, 122
issues and challenges, 4–5
issues of attachment, loss, and identity formation in, 282–283
with open adoption
working alliance with birth parents, 157
working with adoptive parents, 291–293
working with children in, 162
perspectives for foster care, 54–55
professional values as base for, 279–280
research needs and trends, 300–302
responding to family differences in needs and problems, 280–281
with skipped-generation families
assessments, 128–131, 146
working alliance with grandparents, 129–130
traditional adoption studies and, 15–16
training and supervision in, 300
with transracial adoption, 65
using play in, 287–288, 291
Clinton, Bill, 60–61
Closed adoption. *See* Traditional adoption
Cocaine. *See* Teratogens
Cognitive development, 102–103
Cohort effects, 34
Collaborative parenthood
artificial insemination by donor, 187–190
attachment relationship and, 223
birth narratives and, 190, 191, 199
broadened notions of family and, 202
disclosing birth origin, 189, 190, 195, 198–199
family identity and, 202–203, 224
family narratives and, 224
formation of single, gay, and lesbian families, 190–192
gender differences in perceptions of, 208
identity formation in the child, 224–225
ova donations, 192–195, 211–214
parentage roles in, 175, 187, 195, 202
therapeutic counseling and, 210–211
See also Assisted reproductive technology; Gay families; Lesbian families; Single-parent families
Communication, in open adoption, 159, 169
Community adoption agencies, 166–167
Community resources, skipped-generation families and, 131
Complex adoption
assessing acute vs. chronic problems in children, 289
assessment spheres, 29
attachment relationships and, 7, 36, 37–39
child-focused therapy, 46–49, 293–294
child temperament and, 42–44
clinical practice with. *See* Clinical practice
defined, 3
disclosing birth origin, clinical issues and illustrations, 251–252, 260–266, 273, 275
early caregiving environment and, 35–37, 285
emergence of, 11–12
forms of, 3, 12–13, 26–28
gay families and, 239–240
identity formation and, 40–42

medical social workers and, 297–298
new notions of family and family formation, 3–5, 9–10
number of children available for, 12
prenatal exposures to risk and, 44–46
problems of psychological adaptation for children and parents, 26–28
significance of studying, 4–5
sociocultural context and, 32–35
See also International adoption; Open adoption; Post-foster placement adoption; Skipped-generation families; Transracial adoption
Courts
defining best interests of children, 78–79
placement process and, case study example, 96–97
Cocaine. *See* Teratogens.
Culturagrams, 34
Cultural diversity, clinical practice and, 33–34
See also Post foster-placement adoption, International adoption, Skipped-generation care, Gay and lesbian families, Transracial adoption, Ethnographic narrative and Working alliance.

Delayed adoption
case study, 76–77, 79–97
implications for children, 59–60, 78
Developmental lines, 46–47
Developmental psychopathology, 47–48
Developmental research
and clinical practice, 24, 25, 26, 28–29, 30–32, 287–291
on attachment relationships, 25, 37–39
perspectives on traditional adoption, 25–26
trends and insights, 24–25
value of, 24
Disclosure
disclosing birth origin of the child, 189, 190, 216–217
clinical issues and illustrations, 217, 251, 253–259, 272, 275
appendix, 227
Discrimination, impact on transracial adoptees, 64
Disorganized attachment, 38
Disruptions. *See* Trauma
Divorce
impact on children, 232
leading to gay and lesbian families, 232–234
Drug-addicted parents
burden of care for children, 141–143
case vignette, 143–144
prenatal exposure of children to drugs, 140–141
trauma experienced by children, 142
See also Post foster-placement adoption, Teratogenic exposure.

Early caregiving environment
foster care children and, 53–54
impact on child development and attachment relationships, 35–39, 283–284
See also Holding environment
Ecological systems theory
assessment of skipped-generation families, 129–131, 146
perspectives on child development and nontraditional families, 7
sociocultural context of development and, 31–32
Egg donors. *See* Ova donors/donations
Ego development
attachment relationships and, 37–38
holding environment disruptions and, 93–95
Embryos, 183, 186, 187

Emotional development. *See also* Child development, Clinical practice
in children adopted from abroad, 106
clinical vignettes, 111–121
impact of chronic trauma on, 134–135
Empathy, 8. *See also* Clinical practice, Child development
English and Romanian Adoptees Study Team, 102–103
Entitlement, parental issues with, 15–16
Ethnographic theory
case vignettes, 8–9
in clinical practice, 7–8, 19, 278–280
See also Family narratives, Child narratives, Clinical practice, Non-traditional families
Ethnoracial identity, transracial adoption and, 63–65

Family. *See also* Family formation, Family identity
barriers to providing care for children, 55–56, 57
broadened notions of, 9–10, 154–155, 175, 176–178, 197, 202
importance of having a birth child, 178–180, 197
insights from studies of traditional adoption, 15–16
as subjective entity, 178, 197
Family formation
new patterns in, 3–5, 175
See ART, Complex adoption
Family identity
in ART-formed families, 202–203
assisted reproductive technology and, 176
broadened notions of, 9–10, 154–155, 175, 176–178, 197, 202
in collaborative parenthood, 224
disclosing birth origin and
clinical illustrations, 251–252, 253–272
issues in, 252, 272–275
in skipped-generation families, 135
with surrogate/gestational parenthood, 197
transracial/transcultural adoption and, 121–122
See also Post foster-placement adoption, Open adoption
Family narratives, 4
ART-formed families and, 18–19, 294–296
clinical practice and, 7–9, 19, 278–279, 281–282
collaborative parenthood and, 224
significance of, 16–19
in skipped-generation families, 135
unvoiced, 17–18
See also Birth narratives; Children's narratives; Ethnographic theory
Family trees, making in school, 298
Fatherhood
artificial insemination by donor and, 187–190
development of paternal identity, 215
in gay families, 240
psychological meaning of, 214–215
Fathers. *See* Fatherhood; Psychological fathers
Fecundity, 180
Female infertility/sterility, 181–182
depression in infertile women, 204
psychological impact of, 192, 203–205
use of ova donations, 192–195
Feminist movement, 152
Fertility, 180
Fertility counseling, 208–211
issues of collaborative parenthood, 210–211
issues of continuing fertility treatments, 210
issues of openness and disclosure, 211
therapeutic objectives, 209–210
Fetal development, exposure to teratogens and, 44–46. *See also* Teratogens

Fight–flight responses, 123, 134
Foster care
barriers to family provision of care for children, 55–56, 57
clinical practice and, 54–55
defining best interests of children and, 58–61, 78–79
delayed adoption and
case study, 76–77, 79–97
implications for children, 59–60, 78
early caregiving experiences of children and, 53–54
holding environment disruptions and, 78
long-term, affective meaning of, 73
minority children in, 57, 62
number of children eligible for adoption, 57
number of children in, 54, 56
placement of children in, 56
state monitoring of, 56
trends in, 57–58
See also Post-foster placement adoption
Freedom of Information Acts, 154
Frozen embryos, 183, 187
Full open adoption, 167–169

Gamete intrafallopian transfer (GIFT), 183
Gay parenthood
effects of prejudice and bias on, 228, 239, 240–241
experiences of parenthood in, 240
forming of, 190–191, 246
adoption and, 235–236, 239–240
after heterosexual marriage, 231–234
collaborative parenthood, 235
increasing numbers of, 228
insights gained from, 246
legal status and difficulties, 177, 235
numbers of, 229, 239
outcome studies of children in, 228–231
psychological issues for children in, 191–192
social acceptance of, 235
surrogate/gestational mothers and, 240
therapeutic assistance and, 246–247
Gender, adjustment to adoption and, 64
Gender identity, parental sexual orientation and, 230. *See* Adolescence
Genealogical history, right of access to, 170, 192
Genetic parents, 175, 187, 202
Grandmother-headed families, 125–126, 128–129. *See also* Skipped-generation families
Grandparents
children of parents with AIDS and, 57, 216
forming attachment relationships, 135–136
for grandchildren with drug-addicted parents, 141–144
historical perspectives, 127
modern trends, 127–128
in complex adoption, 34
forming working alliance with, 129–130
lifecycle significance of, 127
physical and psychological impact of skipped-generation care, 128–129
relationship with lesbian families, 236–237
See also Skipped-generation families
Grief reactions, family disruptions and, 72

Health care, grandmother-headed families and, 126
Holding environment
developmental significance, 25–26, 35–37
therapeutic, 78, 284–285
case study, 77, 81–86, 88–93, 95–96, 97

Identity formation. *See* Adolescence
in child development, 18, 40
complex adoption and, 40–42
conflicts in open adoption, 161

Identity formation (*continued*)
family narratives and, 16–19
issues for clinical practice, 282–283
in skipped-generation families, 135
transracial adoption and, 63–65, 121–122
Impaired fecundity, 181
Independent open adoption, 162–163
case illustrations, 163–165
Indian Child Welfare Act, 62
Infant development, 35–37. *See also* Child development
Infants
adaptations to stress and deprivation, 104, 123
attachment relationships and, 39, 68
classifications of temperament, 42–43
declining numbers released for closed adoption, 11–12, 154
early caregiving environment and, 35–37
prenatal exposures to risk and, 44–46
preplacement history assessments
benefits of, 65–66
case vignette, 66–68
guidelines for, 69–70(table)
Infertility
anthropological perspectives, 201–202
overview of, 180–181
psychogenic model, 203–204
psychological impact, 184, 201
on men, 206–207
on women, 192, 203–205
psychological sequelae model, 204
therapeutic assistance and, 197–198, 208–211
treatments, 181–182, 202
Infertility treatments, 181–182, 202
anxiety experienced by women during, 204, 205
demands on birth mother, 184, 205
family conflicts around, 207–208
psychological recovery following, 222
therapeutic intervention and, 208–211
See also Assisted reproductive technology; In vitro fertilization
Inracial adoption, 64
Institutional care
cultural and political reasons for child abandonment, 100–101
developmental risks to children, 98, 109, 122
cognitive development, 102–103
physical health, 101–102
experiences of loss in leaving, 106–107
Intentional parents. *See* Psychological parents
Internal narratives, 17–18
International adoption
adoption agencies and, 109
adoption medicine and, 301
attachment relationships and
clinical vignettes, 111–121
problems establishing, 99, 106, 110, 122, 123
children's experiences of loss and separation in, 106–107
children's responses to adoptive parents, 104
clinical practice and
clinical vignettes, 111–121
interdisciplinary approach, 123–124
long-term dimensions, 110, 124
transition crises, 109–110
understanding preadoptive histories, 109, 122
costs of, 100
developmental risks to children in institutional care, 98, 101–103, 109, 122
disclosing birth origin, 251–252, 260–266, 273, 275
emergence of, 99–100
emotional adjustments of Romanian children, 103–104
family formation and, 98–99, 283
issues of cultural diversity and, 33

medical social workers and, 297–298
problems in personal and family identity, 121–122
problems of psychological adaptation for children, 26–27
social and cultural context of, 99–101
typical experiences of parents in, 107–109
In the Best Interests of the Child (Goldstein et al.), 58
Intracytoplasmic sperm injection (ICSI), 182, 206
In vitro fertilization, 173, 202
artificial insemination by donor, 187–190
demands on birth mother, 183
disposition of unneeded embryos, 186
emergence of, 13
impact on notions of family, 175
legal status of frozen embryos, 187
multiple pregnancies and, 186, 221–222
number of children created from, 182
Catholic Church and, 179
procedures in, 182–183
risk factors for parents and children, 221–222
success rates, 183, 184

Kinship adoption. *See* Skipped-generation families

Lesbian families
effects of prejudice and bias on, 228, 240–241
forming of, 190–191, 234–236, 246
after heterosexual marriage, 231–234
increasing numbers of, 228
insights gained from, 246
legal status and difficulties of, 177, 235
maternal identity and parental roles in, 236–239
numbers of children in, 229
outcome studies of children in, 228–231
psychological issues for children in, 191–192
right of access to genealogical history, 192
selection of sperm donor, 191, 236
social acceptance of, 235
therapeutic assistance and, 234, 238–239, 246–247
Life histories. *See* Family narratives
Loss
inherent in the adoption experience, 53
experienced by children leaving institutional care, 106–107
experienced by children in foster care, 54, 57, 59, 61
issues for clinical practice, 282–283
inherent in the ART experience, 204–207, 209
experienced by infertile couples, 204, 205, 206–207
See also Attachment, Family narratives, Children's narratives, Trauma

Male infertility, 180, 181, 182
artificial insemination by donor and, 187–190
psychological impact of, 184, 206–207
See also Fertility and infertility
Massachusetts Supreme Court, 236
Maternal identity, in lesbian families, 236–239
Maternal self-efficacy, 44
Maturation, differences between children and adults, 35
Medical centers, assessment of internationally adopted children, 102
Medical social workers, 297–298

Men
  psychological impact of infertility, 184, 206–207
  responses to sperm and ova donations, 207
  See also Birth fathers; Fatherhood; Psychological fathers
Miller v. Youakim, 128
Minority children
  in foster care, 57, 62
  poverty and, 62
  in skipped-generation families, 126
  in transracial adoption, 61
Modified open adoption, 166–167
Motherhood, in lesbian families, 236–239
Mothers. *See* Birth mothers; Motherhood; Psychological mothers; Surrogate/gestational mothers
Multiethnic Placement Act, 61–62
Multiple pregnancies/births, 186, 221–222

National Association of Black Social Workers (NABSW), 61
National Committee for Adoption, 155
Nature/nurture dynamic, in child development, 30–31
Nicotine, 44. *See* Teratogens.
Nontraditional families
  child development and, 5
  clinical practice with. *See* Clinical practice
  ecological perspectives on, 7
  effects of prejudice and bias on, 240–241
  legal difficulties with adoption and ART clinics, 177
  new models of, 10
  See also ART-formed families; Collaborative parenthood; Complex adoption; Ethnographic theory
Nuclear family, 10

Open adoption
  adoption triad in, 149–150, 155–162
  adoptive parents and
    acceptance of risks in, 158
    attachment relationship with the child, 158–159
    clinical work with, 291–293
    communication issues, 159, 169
    introduction of birth parents to the child, 159
    relationship with birth parents, 157, 158, 169–170
    significance of knowing child's biological background, 159–160
  background and emergence of, 12–13, 150–155
  benefits and difficulties of, 13, 169–170
  birth parents and, 13, 27, 156–157
    contact with child, 160–162, 169
    introducing to the child, 159
    relationship with adoptive parents, 157, 158, 169–170
  characteristics of, 149
  child identity formation and, 42
  children in
    clinical work with, 162
    contact with birth parents and, 160–162, 169
    identity conflicts and, 161
    introducing to their birth parents, 159
  communication in, 159, 169
  defined, 3, 148
  effects on international adoption, 99
  full open adoption, 167–169
  independent open adoption, 162–165
  modified open adoption, 166–167
  nature/nurture dynamic of child development and, 31
  problems of psychological adaptation for children, 27–28
  right of access to genealogical history and, 170
  state laws and, 155

Orphanages. *See* Institutional care
Outreach services, skipped-generation families and, 131, 146
Ova donors/donations
advertising for, 194
cesarean deliveries and, 221
disclosing birth origin, 195, 212, 227(table)
clinical issues and illustrations, 212–214, 252, 266–272
gender differences in response to, 207
guidelines for, 193–194
medical, ethical, and legal issues, 193
number of women using, 192
payment questions and, 194
procedures in, 193, 211–212
psychological meaning of, 212
reproduction problems used for, 192–193
role of birth mother in, 195
See also Secrets

Parentage, new models of, 10, 175, 187, 195, 202
Parent–child relationship
birth parent–child contacts in open adoption, 159, 160–162, 169
effects on child development, 105
in skipped-generation families, 136, 142
See also Clinical practice
Parenthood
desire for, 10
in gay families, 240
See also Collaborative parenthood; Fatherhood; Motherhood; Surrogate/gestational parenthood
Parents
in clinical practice, 285–287
drug-addiction and, 140–143
genetic, 175, 187, 202
social, 187
See also Adoptive parents; Birth parents; Psychological parents
Paternal identity
in AID-formed families, 215–216
case vignettes, 216–218
impact on child development, 214–215
Permanency planning
Adoption and Safe Families Act, 60, 74
child welfare advocates and, 61
defining best interests of children and, 58–61, 78–79
key principles of, 58
Play, using in clinical practice, 287–288, 291
Post-foster placement adoption
Adoption and Safe Families Act, 60, 74
attachment relationships and, 39, 68, 70–73, 74, 75
birth parents and, 61
children's experience of permanency and belonging in, 73
child welfare advocates and, 61
child welfare professionals and, 297
delayed
case study, 76–77, 79–97
implications for children, 59–60, 78
early caregiving experiences of children and, 12, 53–54
identity formation and, 41
implications of early trauma and loss for children, 68, 70–73, 74–75
number of children available for, 12
preplacement history assessments
benefits of, 65–66
case vignette, 66–68
guidelines for, 69–70(table)
problems of psychological adaptation for children, 12, 26–27
Poverty
grandmother-headed families and, 126
minority children and, 62
Pregnancies, multiple, 186, 221–222

Pregnancy
ART-formed families and, 184–185, 221
lesbian women and, 237
psychological fathers and, 215
psychological impact of pregnancy loss, 205
reasons for desiring, 215
Preplacement history assessments
benefits of, 65–66
case vignette, 66–68
guidelines for, 69–70(table)
Primary caregivers
attachment relationships and, 35–36
holding environment for children and, 35–37
Primary infertility, 181
Primary prevention, skipped-generation families and, 146
Psychogenic infertility model, 203–204
Psychological fathers
attachment relationships and, 216
development of paternal identity, 215–216
case vignettes, 217–218
disclosing birth origin of the child, 189, 190, 216–217
clinical issues and illustrations, 217, 251, 253–259, 272, 275
spouses' support of, 215–216
supportive role in pregnancy, 215
See also AID-formed families; Collaborative parenthood
Psychological mothers, 205
Psychological parents, 202
assisted reproductive technology and, 14–15
attachment relationships and, 198, 216
conflicts in fertility decision making, 207–208
emotional and empathetic acceptance of children, 224, 225–226
fertility counseling and, 208–211
working with in clinical practice, 285–287
See also AID-formed families; ART-formed families; Collaborative parenthood; Surrogate/gestational parenthood
Psychological sequelae infertility model, 204
Psychopathology, developmental, 47–48

Racial identity, transracial adoption and, 63–65
Racism, impact on transracial adoptees, 64
Romania
adoption policies and, 100
emotional adjustments of adoptees from, 103–104
institutional care for children in, 101
Russia, institutional care for children in, 101

School social workers, 298
Sealed records laws
arguments for and against, 150
challenges to, 152–154
history of, 148, 151–152
Secondary infertility, 181
Secrets. *See* Disclosure
Self-reflection, parents and, 16
Separation anxiety, 41
in children with histories of early trauma and loss, 72–73
in single-parent families, 245
support networks and resources, 245
Separations
experienced leaving institutional care, 106–107
multiple, consequences for children, 72
See also Trauma
Sexual intimacy, having birth children and, 178–179
Single Mothers by Choice (SMC), 245
Single-parent families, 10, 154
case vignettes, 242–245
emergence of, 241–242

formation of, 190–191, 242, 246
increasing numbers of, 228
insights gained from, 246
psychological issues for children in, 191–192
right of access to genealogical history, 192
separation anxiety and, 245
therapeutic assistance and, 245, 246–247
Skipped-generation families
advocacy for and value of, 146–147
assessment of needs, 128–131, 146
attachment relationships and, 135–136, 145
birth parent–child relationship and, 136, 142
caregiving burdens of, 126
case illustrations, 136–140
clinical services and, 126, 145
with drug-addicted birth parents
burden of care for grandparents, 141–143
case vignette, 143–144
implications for children, 140–141, 142
family identity and, 135
grandmother-headed, 125–126
economic and health care issues for, 126
factors in the growth of, 128
physical and psychological impact on grandmothers, 128–129
impact of early trauma and loss on children, 132–136, 142
increasing numbers of children in, 125, 126
increasing prevalence of, 126, 127–128
interventions and social services for, 131, 146
overview of conditions in, 145
Sleep disorders, 222–223
Smoking. *See* Teratogens
Social deprivation, children's adaptations to, 104, 123
Social parents, 187
Sociocultural contexts
child development and, 29, 31–32
complex adoption and, 32–35
Sperm donors/donations
gender differences in responses to, 207
selection by single and/or lesbian mothers, 191, 236
See also Artificial insemination by donor
Spirit of Open Adoption, The (Gritter), 167
State Regulations
monitoring of foster care system, 56
regulation of assisted reproductive technology clinics, 186
Stress, children's adaptations to, 104, 123
Subjugated knowledge, 7–8, 278
Surgical infertility, 181
Surrogate/gestational mothers, 175, 187, 195, 202
case vignette, 220–221
gay families and, 191, 240
key issues for agreement with intentional parents, 219
legal issues, 219–220
number of births per year, 173
satisfaction with role, 218–219
Surrogate/gestational parenthood
case vignette, 220–221
custody cases and, 196–197
family identity and, 197
key areas for agreement between parties, 219
legal and psychological issues in, 195–196, 219–220
number of births per year, 173
overview of, 218
parentage roles in, 195
recommendations for public policy on, 196
role of gestational mother, 218–219

Teachers, 298
Temperament
classifications for infants, 42–43
as heritable characteristic, 43
issues in complex adoption, 43–44

Teratogens, 44–46
cigarette smoking and prenatal development, 44
crack cocaine and prenatal development, 141
effects of exposure on development, 44–46
Test tube babies, 173. *See also* Assisted reproductive technology
Therapeutic donor insemination (TDI), 236
Therapeutic relationship, as holding environment, 78, 284–285
case study, 77, 81–86, 88–93, 95–96, 97
Traditional adoption.
adoption triad in, 149
basic premise of, 148
critical issues with, 170
declining number of infants released for adoption, 11–12, 154
developmental research and, 25–26
history of, 150–154
insights relevant to clinical practice, 15–16
psychological issues for children, 160, 161
state laws and, 155
studies of impact on children, 153
Transaction, with social environment, 31
Transcultural adoption, 12, 121–122
See also Post foster placement adoption; International adoption
Transition crises
in international adoption, 109–110
clinical vignettes, 111–112, 117–118
separation anxiety, 72–73
Transracial adoption
alternative strategies, 63
controversial nature of, 61
emergence of, 61
family identity and, 121–122
federal legislation and, 61–62
identity formation and, 41–42, 121–122
issues of cultural diversity and, 33
negative effects of bias and prejudice on, 32
preadoptive history of children, 62
psychological impact studies, 63–65
Trauma (from early loss and disruptions)
attachment relationship difficulties and, 18, 36, 38, 39, 68, 70–73, 75, 133, 135–136
behavioral responses and problems, 36, 39, 71, 72–73, 134–135, 142, 285
case study, 79–93
children's experiences of, 76–77, 78, 132–136
developmental effects, 36, 68, 74–75, 77–78, 93–95, 134–135, 142
therapeutic relationship and, 75, 78, 95–96, 284–285
See also Loss

Withdrawal, 71. *See* Teratogens.
Women
demands of infertility treatment on, 183, 184, 205
depression following birth, 222
maternal self-efficacy, 44
psychological impact of infertility, 184, 203–205
reasons for desiring pregnancy and childbirth, 179
responses to sperm and ova donations, 207
See also Birth mothers; Psychological mothers; Surrogate/gestational mothers

Zygote intrafallopian transfer (ZIFT), 183